Life Course Research and Social Policies

Volume 3

D1824292

Series editors
Laura Bernardi
Dario Spini
Michel Oris

Life course research has been developing quickly these last decades for good reasons. Life course approaches focus on essential questions about individuals' trajectories, longitudinal analyses, cross-fertilization across disciplines like life-span psychology, developmental social psychology, sociology of the life course, social demography, socio-economics, social history. Life course is also at the crossroads of several fields of specialization like family and social relationships, migration, education, professional training and employment, and health. This Series invites academic scholars to present theoretical, methodological, and empirical advances in the analysis of the life course, and to elaborate on possible implications for society and social policies applications.

More information about this series at http://www.springer.com/series/10158

Michel Oris • Caroline Roberts • Dominique Joye
Michèle Ernst Stähli

Editors

Surveying Human Vulnerabilities across the Life Course

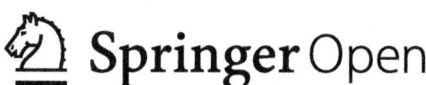

Editors
Michel Oris
CIGEV
University of Geneva
Geneva, Switzerland

Dominique Joye
Social Sciences Institute
University of Lausanne
Lausanne, Switzerland

Caroline Roberts
Social Sciences Institute
University of Lausanne
Lausanne, Switzerland

Michèle Ernst Stähli
FORS (Swiss Foundation for the
   Research in Social Sciences)
University of Lausanne
Lausanne, Switzerland

ISSN 2211-7776   ISSN 2211-7784   (electronic)
Life Course Research and Social Policies
ISBN 978-3-319-24155-5   ISBN 978-3-319-24157-9   (eBook)
DOI 10.1007/978-3-319-24157-9

Library of Congress Control Number: 2016931328

Printed on acid-free paper

This Springer imprint is published by Springer Nature
The registered company is Springer International Publishing AG Switzerland

Contents

Surveying Human Vulnerabilities Across the Life Course: Balancing Substantive and Methodological Challenges

Michel Oris, Caroline Roberts, Dominique Joye, and Michèle Ernst Stähli

1 Introduction

This book matches two concepts, one substantive, and the other methodological: 'vulnerability' and 'survey quality'. It concerns the challenges involved in conducting high quality social research using survey methods in non-standard contexts, to learn about vulnerable people and their experiences of vulnerability. The volume brings together nine contributions to a major Swiss research infrastructure named *'LIVES – Overcoming Vulnerability: Life Course Perspectives'*, each of which touches on the tension between the pursuit of elaborate, often delicate substantive research aims, and the demand for methodological rigour. The LIVES research programme has been funded by the Swiss Confederation through the National Science Foundation's National Centres of Competence in Research (NCCR) scheme, which

This chapter and this volume as a whole have been made possible by the support of the National Centre of Competences in Research "LIVES – Overcoming Vulnerability: Life course perspectives," financed by the Swiss Science Foundation (SNF). The authors express their gratitude to the SNF.

M. Oris (✉)
NCCR LIVES, IPs 213 & 214, Geneva, Switzerland

Centre for the Interdisciplinary Study of Gerontology and Vulnerability, University of Geneva, Geneva, Switzerland
e-mail: Michel.Oris@unige.ch

C. Roberts • D. Joye • M. Ernst Stähli
NCCR LIVES, IP 214, Lausanne, Switzerland

Social Sciences Institute, University of Lausanne, Lausanne, Switzerland

FORS (Swiss Foundation for the Research in Social Sciences), University of Lausanne, Lausanne, Switzerland

© The Author(s) 2016
M. Oris et al. (eds.), *Surveying Human Vulnerabilities across the Life Course*, Life Course Research and Social Policies 3, DOI 10.1007/978-3-319-24157-9_1

1

is designed to promote long-term research networks in areas of strategic importance for Swiss science, the Swiss economy and Swiss society. As the name 'LIVES' suggests, this multifaceted project aims to address human vulnerabilities across life trajectories, from the cradle to the grave. Yet while LIVES's defining feature and its raison d'être is its ambitious substantive focus, much of the research being carried out by the NCCR is equally driven and characterised by two specific epistemological features: the multidisciplinary nature of the work being undertaken, and a strong emphasis on quantitative methods and survey data collection. These features, along with the thematic focus of the research, present a double challenge to the researchers involved, the first of which is simply how best to obtain "meaningful" data about vulnerabilities and populations at risk, and the second of which is whether 'quality' is best achieved by applying standard, widely-accepted techniques for gathering new data, or by adapting these methods to the specific populations of interest, or research conditions.

The pertinence of this challenge – the methodological aspects of which have long troubled comparative researchers (Harkness et al. 2010; Davidov et al. 2010) – extends beyond LIVES and beyond Switzerland. In this sense the nine chapters of this volume contribute to crucial scientific debates in survey methodology, as well as in both psychological and social sciences. They provide detailed presentations of concrete experiences of conducting surveys and using other innovative approaches to study vulnerabilities and vulnerable individuals (belonging or not to populations considered to be vulnerable). Each one highlights the importance of a proper integration of theory, concepts, questionnaire content and design, procedures of data collection, analytical methods, and interpretations, to develop original perspectives in an area of research, which continues to gain in popularity. Indeed, the topic of 'vulnerability' has seen an explosion of interest in the scientific world over the course of the past 20 years, partly in response to demands from stakeholders and citizens, in spite of – or maybe because of – the fact that the concept of vulnerability is not clearly defined. Its many connotations and uses have both general and specific implications for the methods used to investigate the phenomena to which it pertains, and notably, for the various decisions involved in the design of quantitative surveys.

This book tackles the challenge of using survey research methodology – either on its own or in combination with other innovative approaches (such as social networks and observation) – to collect data from vulnerable population subgroups, to investigate their experiences of vulnerability and the resources available to them for surmounting 'vulnerabilising' contexts, events and life transitions. While at the same time aspiring to uphold the scientific standards of survey research methodology, researchers interested in vulnerability face a number of distinctive challenges. Many are extensions of existing problems affecting the quality with which any survey can be carried out.

Apart of being helpful for people working with data produced within the LIVES project, this book is mainly addressed to researchers specialized on topics around vulnerability, survey practitioners and survey methodologists who aim at questioning their routines, as well as to young researchers looking for examples of honest and innovating social science making.

After this introductory chapter, which discusses the contribution of the following chapters, the book is organized as follows: the first six chapters are grouped around the surveyed topics and populations: elder people for chapters "Representation of Vulnerability and the Elderly. A Total Survey Error Perspective on the VLV Survey" and "Adapting Quantitative Survey Procedures: The Price for Assessing Vulnerability? Lessons from a Large-Scale Survey on Aging and Migration in Switzerland", harsh events (such as widowing and cancer) during middle age for chapters "Vulnerability Following a Critical Life Event: Temporary Crisis or Chronic Distress? A Psychological Controversy, Methodological Considerations, and Empirical Evidence" and "A Survey of Couples Facing Breast Cancer in Women", working careers and disruptions for chapters "Career Pathways and Professional Transitions: Preliminary Results from the First Wave of a 7-Year Longitudinal Study and "How to Survey Displaced Workers in Switzerland: Ways of Addressing Sources of Bias". The last three chapters are more focused on a specific survey tool: life calendars for chapter "Using Life History Calendars to Survey Vulnerability", online social networks for chapter "Studying Youth Transitions Through a Social Network: First Impressions" and panels for chapter "Attrition in the Swiss Household Panel: Are Vulnerable Groups More Affected than Others?".

1.1 Background to This Volume

At the origin of this collection is an international workshop organized by LIVES called 'Methodological and Substantive Challenges in Measuring vulnerability across the Life Course', held at the University of Lausanne, Switzerland, in June, 2012. The aim of the workshop was to address some of the methodological challenges involved in measuring vulnerability and resilience using social surveys. The workshop brought together substantive specialists in researching these topics from within LIVES, and invited international experts in survey methodology to shed light on some of the shared methodological challenges being faced by the thematic research projects that make up LIVES. The challenges discussed at the workshop included (1) sampling and surveying 'hard-to-reach' populations; (2) the risk of low and differential rates of participation across important sub-groups, and attrition for surveys with a longitudinal design; (3) difficulties associated with using traditional data collection methods, including telephone under-coverage and the high cost of face-to-face interviewing, which have increased the demand for mixed mode data collection; and (4) measurement challenges including the collection of retrospective data (e.g. event histories and retrospective evaluations of personal wellbeing across different points of the life course), and the potential for interviewer effects on data quality. Understanding the nature of such challenges and the implications they have for the substantive aims of the LIVES project was one of the primary objectives of the workshop. A secondary, and relatively seldom pursued aim, was to forge a dialogue between substantive and methodological specialists, to try to seek solutions that could help to ensure the best possible synergy between the substantive goals of the LIVES research, and the methods used to gather new data. With this latter aim in mind, the program for the conference was based around three substantive areas of central interest to the LIVES project: (a) specific vulnerable populations – notably, national minorities, and younger and older people; (b) transitions in and out of employment, and (c) vulnerability in family life, with each session incorporating presentations from the methodological experts and the substantive specialists conducting research within the NCCR.

Though the specific focus of this volume is on the Swiss context (as for the workshop), the issues addressed have a broader significance in the social sciences, and provide lessons for quantitative researchers working in other European and North American contexts, as well as elsewhere. As in many countries, survey data in Switzerland play a central role in the social sciences, with more and more researchers carrying out secondary analysis of large-scale datasets available through national data archives, as well as conducting their own original data collection. In LIVES, major national studies of the general population (including notably, the Swiss Labour Force Survey (SLFS), and the Swiss Household Panel Survey (SHP)) have been supplemented by several purpose-designed quantitative surveys focused on different aspects of vulnerability and resilience among special subpopulations living in Switzerland. The chapters in this book have been contributed by the researchers responsible for designing and carrying out these new surveys and broadly reflect the three areas of focus addressed by in the workshop.

The LIVES surveys include (1) a study of a cohort sample of young adults, including an over-sample of second generation immigrants from Albanian-speaking countries in the former Yugoslavia being surveyed alongside the third sample of the SHP (Gomensoro and Bolzman 2015), and an associated pilot survey that was designed to field test a suitable sampling strategy (Elcheroth et al. 2011); (2) two studies investigating pathways out of unemployment, including a survey looking at the impact of mass redundancy among ex-employees of five firms that closed down between 2009 and 2010 (chapter "How to Survey Displaced Workers in Switzerland: Ways of Addressing Sources of Bias" in this volume), and a survey of the newly unemployed in the canton of Vaud (chapter "Studying Youth Transitions Through a Social Network: First Impressions"); (3) a seven-wave longitudinal survey of workers and the impact of individual characteristics and resources on professional trajectories (chapter "Career Pathways and Professional Transitions: Preliminary Results from the First Wave of a 7-Year Longitudinal Study"); (4) a two-wave extension of an existing panel survey of married and unmarried couples looking at changing family configurations in response to critical events (Widmer et al. 2013); (5) a two-wave panel study of the role of the couple relationship as a source of support for women facing breast cancer (chapter "A Survey of Couples Facing Breast Cancer in Women"); (6) a longitudinal survey of divorcees and widows investigating the effects of losing an intimate partner in the second half of life (chapter "Vulnerability Following a Critical Life Event: Temporary Crisis or Chronic Distress? A Psychological Controversy, Methodological Considerations, and Empirical Evidence"); (7) a survey of older adults aged 65 and over (called Vivre, Leben, Vivere, or VLV for short) investigating inequalities during old age (chapters "Representation of Vulnerability and the Elderly. A Total Survey Error Perspective on the VLV Survey" and "Adapting Quantitative Survey Procedures: The Price for Assessing Vulnerability? Lessons from a Large-Scale Survey on Aging and Migration in Switzerland"); and (8) a retrospective complement to the SHP (chapter "Attrition in the Swiss Household Panel: Are Vulnerable Groups More Affected than Others?") using a life history calendar (chapter "Using Life History Calendars to Survey Vulnerability").

In the next section, we discuss the concept of vulnerability, providing some definitions to help clarify the substantive ambitions of the authors of this volume. Then, we discuss issues related to survey quality, to provide a context for understanding the various methodological challenges related to surveying vulnerable individuals and populations, and measuring vulnerabilities in surveys. Along the way, we refer to the various contributions to the volume, touching on their substantive aims and their methodological concerns, in an effort to piece together the various pieces of the jigsaw. We conclude with a reflection on lessons learned, relating in particular to the need for close collaboration between substantive and methodological experts when producing new data, and the importance of transparency in interdisciplinary research.

2 Vulnerability

2.1 The Ambiguous Success of the Concept "vulnerability"

A simple search in English for the term "vulnerability" on Google Scholar shows its almost inexistence in the academic literature until the mid-1980s, its marginal presence in the 1990s and its sudden explosion from 2000, confirmed and amplified in more recent years. It seems that the original concept appeared in risk research when questions were raised about the naturalness of natural disasters. It was used at a macro and meso level to disentangle the physical hazard and the resulting disaster, and to take into account the various capabilities of structures and institutions to prevent or attenuate the consequences of a disaster, resulting in differential impact on and responses from different subpopulations (Henke 2015). The widespread appeal of the concept developed later, however, when vulnerability was adopted in many fields of research that have in common a micro – individual-level – approach to inequalities in human development, which has largely been promoted in recent decades by the life course/life span perspective (Mayer 2009; Oris et al. 2009). Hanappi and her colleagues (2015) have recently provided a statistical account of this association based on a content analysis of some 10,632 abstracts of articles published since 2000. They highlight the centrality of the concept of vulnerability across a variety of disciplines, from psychology to sociology and demography, and from youth studies to gerontology, covering more than 30 specific fields of study, including personality disorders and single motherhood, to take just two examples in a long list.

On the basis of this statistical assessment but also of a more qualitative literature review, Spini and colleagues (2013) conclude that the concept of vulnerability has a terrific advantage when you have interdisciplinary ambitions, which is its disciplinary neutrality.[1] However, at least a part of its success is related to the absence of an accepted definition, authorizing a range of uses of the term based on implicit disciplinary assumptions (see more in Perrig-Chiello et al. chapter "Vulnerability Following a Critical Life Event: Temporary Crisis or Chronic Distress? A Psychological Controversy, Methodological Considerations, and Empirical Evidence" of this volume). This field of research continues to grow tremendously but remains like the many pieces of still not unified puzzle. We do not have the arrogance to impose here the ultimate definition of vulnerability that could be recognized in the same way by all the many researchers concerned with the concept, but in the following we come up with one possible proposal and we make explicit how the contributors to this volume use the term, to then understand the questions they asked, to whom and how.

In LIVES, we see vulnerability "as a lack of resources, which in specific contexts, place individuals or groups at a major risk of experiencing (1) negative consequences related to sources of stress; (2) the inability to cope effectively with stressors; and (3) the inability to recover from the stressor or to take advantage of opportunities by a given deadline" (Spini et al. 2013, 19). Resources and stress are key elements in this definition that was inspired by the seminal works of Leonard Pearlin (1989) on stress, that consider the coping strategies and other resources individuals have to manage it. This definition of vulnerability, however, also reintegrates the notion of risk, and takes into account the context, the opportunities, as well as their temporality. Moreover, resources, stressors, and individual responses are all interrelated in a dynamic system that includes feedback, as well as spill-over effects across different life domains like family and work (Spini et al. 2013).

Generally speaking, vulnerability is considered as being particularly present in post-industrial societies, which can be characterized by growing uncertainty. According to this perspective, recent decades are contrasted with the Thirty Glorious Years (1945–1975) and the simultaneous apex of the welfare states after the Second World War. For Martin Kohli (2007), this period saw the peak of the life course institutionalisation with age-fixed related roles: being a child and studying, being a working adult and raising a family, and being retired. The life trajectories were highly standardized, the components of a transition like the one to adulthood were properly ordered and rapidly traversed. The whole resulted in a relatively normative but very transparent system, and provided a general sense of security about the life course. Then, with the globalization of the economy and increasing demands for

---

[1]This concept is not intrinsically linked to gerontology like frailty, or to sociology or socioeco-nomics like precariousness, etc.

flexibility in more competitive environments (Rudisill et al. 2010), with the myriad of changes affecting family and the multiplication and growing complexity of living arrangements (Fokkema and Liefbroer 2008), with the expansion of individualistic values (Giddens 1991; de Singly and Martucelli 2009), and the (albeit incomplete) gender revolution (Esping-Andersen 2009; Levy and Widmer 2013), life courses became de-standardized, desynchronized, more heterogeneous or disordered, more turbulent, less predictable, and increasingly insecure.

This double embedding of changes in history and in the individual life course makes up the dominant perspective in life course research. It is moreover completely coherent with the recent explosion of interest for the topic of 'vulnerability'. Although this vision is far from undisputed (see for example, Widmer and Ritschard 2009), its prevalence explains why two sets of theories are often contrasted with one another in the literature, the first one tending to be associated with the past, the second one with more recent dynamics: the social stratification versus biographization approaches. Given that our aim here is not to initiate a long theoretical discussion but to try to be concrete, we will mainly refer to the case studies that are discussed more in-depth in the remainder of this book.

2.2 The Social Stratification Perspective on Vulnerabilities

Social stratification is an old and prestigious area of research (Grusky 2001; Tillmann nd Voorpostel 2012) that found an echo in the early 1970s in the seminal works of Matilda Riley (see Dannefer et al. 2005) on the age stratification of society. In this perspective individuals are vulnerable if they are located in the inferior (dominated) classes or strata, as well as when they are unable to fulfil age-related duties. This is the case for young adults when they do not manage to cope with the education system and succeed in their transition to a stable job. This group is the focus of chapter "Studying Youth Transitions Through a Social Network: First Impressions" in this volume, by Eicher and her colleagues, who confirm what is well-known by life course specialists, i.e. that transitional phases of life are moments of increasing exposure to risks (Levy et al. 2005). At the opposite end of the age spectrum are the older adults aged 65 and over studied in chapter "Representation of Vulnerability and the Elderly. A Total Survey Error Perspective on the VLV Survey". Increasing longevity and the associated improvements in health and living conditions have been so great during the last few decades that we can no longer assume that the elderly are a vulnerable population just because of their age. However, rising life expectancies also implies that a growing proportion of people with limited resources, leading difficult lives, is now able to reach not only the age of retirement, but also very old age. In this sense, progress has resulted in growing inequality among the older population (Gabriel et al. 2015). A typical illustration are the old immigrants for whom vulnerabilities have been institutionally constructed through rules that have changed over time, and affected by other important determinants like their socioeconomic and family trajectories.

They are at the heart of Laure Kaeser's chapter "Adapting Quantitative Survey Procedures: The Price for Assessing Vulnerability? Lessons from a Large-Scale Survey on Aging and Migration in Switzerland".

More generally, social stratification is often associated with the theory of cumulative advantages and disadvantages (di Prete and Eirich 2006), which has gained great popularity in life course research and associated research designs (Elder et al. 2015). In this perspective, even modest initial differences in young age widen across life, little by little, leading to a maximal heterogeneity among the so-called "young old", until differential mortality reduces this diversity (Oris and Lerch 2009).

This heterogeneity entails related scientific challenges in terms of identifying the diversity of vulnerabilities (psychological or physical health, socioeconomic conditions, isolation, etc.) and their degree or intensity. Identifying vulnerable individuals within a given population or subgroup is an issue for the elderly in contemporary developed societies, but this is true for all potentially vulnerable groups since any a priori categorization has to be challenged. The classical dialectic of inter- versus intra-variance remains crucial for any empirical assessment of vulnerability. Chapter "Vulnerability Following a Critical Life Event: Temporary Crisis or Chronic Distress? A Psychological Controversy, Methodological Considerations, and Empirical Evidence" (by Perrig-Chiello, Hutchinson and Knöpfli) provides an excellent illustration of this difficulty since the authors not only compare people who experienced the breakup of a long marital relationship with people who are still married, but also, within the divorced group, the most vulnerable with the least, regarding, among others, the circumstances surrounding the divorce. This discussion is related to the fact that vulnerability can not only be viewed as a state, but also as a process. This has at least two methodological consequences. First, it entails a longitudinal perspective that considers how vulnerabilities are constructed across the life course, based either on a retrospective approach using life calendars, or on a prospective construction with panel data. Both pose specific methodological challenges but both are part of the analytical strategy (discussed in more detail in the next section). Second, this longitudinal approach puts more attention on transitions or events in one sense, or on sequences, on the order or disorder of life, on the structure of the life course (Ritschard and Oris 2005). These are also central concerns in the second most important body of literature related to vulnerability, discussed next.

2.3 The Biographization Approach to Vulnerabilities

The second main approach to inequality and vulnerability across the life course, biographization, can be seen as a by-product of the recent changes at the macro and micro levels that were briefly discussed above. In this perspective, lives nowadays are more turbulent, with more incidents. The norm of self-realization imposes on the individual a responsibility to face the trials of his or her plural life (professional, familial, etc.) and to be accountable for his/her successes, but consequently also for his/her failures. It is obviously a source of stress that can also result from uncertain or insecure social interactions in a "liquid" (Baumann 2006) and competitive world (Rudisill et al. 2010). Biographization is mainly concerned with event-based vulnerabilities associated with health problems, family discontinuities, and professional uncertainty. Typical examples addressed in this book are those who experienced the break-up of a long-term partnership (as mentioned, chapter "Vulnerability Following a Critical Life Event: Temporary Crisis or Chronic Distress? A Psychological Controversy, Methodological Considerations, and Empirical Evidence" by Pasqualina Perrig-Chiello and colleagues), couples where the woman has been diagnosed with breast cancer (chapter "A Survey of Couples Facing Breast Cancer in Women" by Linda Charvoz et al.), and displaced workers following the closure of an industrial enterprise (chapter "How to Survey Displaced Workers in Switzerland: Ways of Addressing Sources of Bias" of Isabel Baumann and colleagues).

In these kinds of contexts, the challenge for researchers is to capture the heterogeneity within the populations created by the event, not only associated with inequalities in personal and social resources, but also with the diversity resulting from the nature, intensity, and predictability of the stressor(s) (see here chapter "Using Life History Calendars to Survey Vulnerability" by Maggiori and his colleagues). Even more specifically, a crucial aim for these studies is to reveal the variety of responses to the event, which may include temporary crisis, chronic strain, adaptation, or even personal growth. The biographization theory tends to view more frequent life events as less harmful, provoking less permanent states and becoming part of more turbulent lives through a succession of limited failure and resilience phases (Vandecasteele 2010). However, some authors identify the long-term scarring effects of events like a dismissal (Antonini and Bühlmann 2015; Chauvel 2010). A similar debate contrasts psychological theories (see chapter "Vulnerability Following a Critical Life Event: Temporary Crisis or Chronic Distress? A Psychological Controversy, Methodological Considerations, and Empirical Evidence" by Pasqualina Perrig-Chiello and colleagues for an overview).

Of course, both from a social stratification and a biographization perspective, individuals are interconnected. Linked lives, significant others, social convoy and other forms of social support are not only significant resources, but they can also be a source of stress in case of inadaptive responses. Charvoz and her colleagues make this point very clearly in chapter "A Survey of Couples Facing Breast Cancer in Women" of this book, where they look at dyadic coping, at the reactions and interactions of couples where the woman is affected by breast cancer. Conversely Eicher and her co-authors (chapter "Studying Youth Transitions Through a Social Network: First Impressions") highlight the distinction between bridging and bonding social relations, their differential protective effects for individuals as well the potential importance of group identity for dealing with vulnerabilities. However, theories of post-modernity assume a decrease in formal, obliged, institutional ties, and an increase in elective relationships grouped in configurations that an individual has to animate using personal resources to manage this social capital (Widmer 2010).

Along the same lines, institutions other than family are also supposed to become less important, at least in their capacity to frame people's life courses and impose age- (and gender-) related norms. There is a consensus that formal recognition of vulnerability is a categorization process that often has negative drawbacks in terms of loss of self-esteem for the person or group being categorized, who become exposed to social stigmatization (Ruof 2004; Thomas 2008). There is also a general agreement that individualization implies an increasing role for the state and its various welfare components, which should be important in preventing vulnerability, and are particularly important in responses to so-called "social risks", old or new, and consequently in the public management of vulnerable situations and individuals (Leisering 2003; Ranci 2010). We can cite the education system, unemployment offices, hospitals, and institutions caring for the elderly as examples considered in this volume. They all tend to be affected by the "activation" paradigm which is coherent with the values of individualization, and it is now recognized that like family configurations, institutions can be a source of support but also of stress (Bonvin et al. 2014).

Stress is also present in the two main theoretical approaches discussed previously. Pearlin (1989) explicitly associated a lower position in the socioeconomic structure with greater exposure to stress. More recently, as we discussed briefly earlier, post-modern or post-industrial societies have also been seen as structural producers of stress through their demands for flexibility and competition (Rudisill et al. 2010) and, more generally, through the ambivalence of the ideal of self-realization (Giddens 1991), the burden of being the actor of his or her life (Ehrenberg 1998). Pressure, insecurity, chronic strain, daily hassles, incivilities are obvious sources of vulnerability when their effects accumulate over time. Their impact is maximized by contexts of discrimination, xenophobia, or other attitudes that challenge fairness. These negative associations are specifically discussed in chapter "Career Pathways and Professional Transitions: Preliminary Results from the First Wave of a 7-Year Longitudinal Study" by Christian Maggiori and colleagues in the context of professional life.

From a survey research perspective, the challenge for researchers interested in measuring vulnerability is to properly locate individuals in a web of social interactions that is more or less dense, with different actors that have to be identified. It is also to analyze those interactions from an individual's subjective point of view, in terms of *perceived* social support or discrimination (chapters "A Survey of Couples Facing Breast Cancer in Women" and "Career Pathways and Professional Transitions: Preliminary Results from the First Wave of a 7-Year Longitudinal Study"). It is finally to identify and measure chronic strain and daily hassles. Psychologists are of course the main contributors in relation to the latter (see chapters "A Survey of Couples Facing Breast Cancer in Women", "Career Pathways and Professional Transitions: Preliminary Results from the First Wave of a 7-Year Longitudinal Study, and "Studying Youth Transitions Through a Social Network: First Impressions") but all social scientists recognize the importance of subjective perception since another widely accepted definition of vulnerability is simply low levels of well-being (see chapter "Representation of Vulnerability and the Elderly. A Total Survey Error Perspective on the VLV Survey").

Finally, if social stratification and biographization are often contrasted, for example, in research on poverty, the preceding discussion has shown that they have a lot of associated concepts in common, although with different modulations. Indeed, these two theoretical bodies should not be seen as incompatible as their integration promises much. An illustration of this potential is provided by Isabel Baumann and her colleagues who, in chapter "How to Survey Displaced Workers in Switzerland: Ways of Addressing Sources of Bias", study a population defined by both its status and its experience of a vulnerabilising event: the workers of five factories which closed down, resulting in collective dismissals. They simultaneously lost their position and acquired an inferior one, as unemployed, because of an external shock that provoked a turning point in their professional lives and no doubt affected other domains, such as their family life.

3 Survey Quality

Survey research is at the center of the LIVES project, with over one hundred collaborators drawing on the new data sources described (as well as others) to develop new knowledge about the phenomenon of vulnerability and the resources people draw upon to overcome it, with a view to contributing to the development of innovative social policy measures informed by the findings of their research. The quality of the data collected is integral to the reliability and validity of these conclusions (Groves and Lyberg 2010), and the effectiveness of any recommendations derived from them. Yet the quality of all survey data is inevitably compromised by trade-offs made in the survey design process – trade-offs that even in general population surveys are becoming increasingly complex as a result of growing challenges associated with carrying out surveys using traditional tried-and-tested methods of data collection.

In particular, the LIVES studies face a unique set of challenges associated with sampling, and achieving an adequate representation of their chosen populations, many of which can be described as either 'hard-to-reach' or 'hard-to-survey', either because there are no suitable listings available for sampling purposes, or because they are notoriously hard to contact or reluctant to participate in surveys (see Riandey and Quaglia 2009; Tourangeau et al. 2014). Added to this, the substantive focus of the LIVES research poses quite particular, and often complex measurement challenges, such as how to ask about subjective phenomena likely to be perceived as sensitive by respondents, how best to capture life event histories (see chapter "Using Life History Calendars to Survey Vulnerability" by Davide Morselli and colleagues) or the configuration of social networks. To complicate matters, many of the LIVES surveys have a longitudinal design, incurring an additional threat to data quality due to the risk of selective sample attrition over the lifespan of the study (an issue addressed in chapter "Attrition in the Swiss Household Panel: Are Vulnerable Groups More Affected than Others?" by Rothenbühler and Voorpostel in relation to the SHP). Each of these challenges and the way in which they are managed in the survey design process has implications for the 'quality' (typically defined as accuracy) of the estimates derived from the data.

The accuracy of survey estimates is determined by the degree to which they are affected by different sources of error. In addition to sampling error, which can be controlled through the sampling design, these include a number of non-sampling errors: *coverage error* (associated with the failure to provide all eligible population members with a known and non-zero probability of being selected to participate in the survey); *nonresponse error* (resulting from nonparticipation among particular subgroups, and differences between the responding and nonresponding samples); and *measurement error* (resulting e.g. from problems with the design of the questionnaire, or the way in which respondents formulate their answers to the questions). Other sources of error may be present, such as data input errors, coding errors, processing errors (see Groves (1989) for a detailed discussion), but we focus on the principal sources here. The impact of survey errors on accuracy can be understood in terms of how each one affects the twin inferential processes of representation and measurement on which the accuracy of surveys depend (Groves et al. 2004). While the former concerns the process by which inferences to the population can be made on the basis of estimates derived from a sample (the success of which depends on the minimisation of coverage errors, sampling error, and nonresponse errors), the latter concerns estimate validity – the process by which inferences are drawn from survey statistics based on questions designed to tap the theoretical constructs of interest (for which it is essential to mitigate errors of measurement and processing errors and maximise reliability and validity).

This 'Total Survey Error' (Groves 1989) paradigm for thinking about survey quality continues to dominate the survey methodology literature and provides a helpful framework for thinking about the various challenges present in the LIVES empirical programme and comprehending the nature of the trade-offs that have been necessary in the survey designs. Nevertheless, it could be argued that surveying vulnerable populations presents such specific research challenges, that special rules in survey methodology should be applicable. Tourangeau et al. (2014), however, argues that the difficulties involved specifically in hard-to-survey populations can be classified in terms of the survey operations they affect – sampling, making contact, persuading people to participate, and measurement. In the following, we discuss how the different projects have negotiated these different features of the survey design in the context of surveying vulnerabilities and vulnerable populations.

3.1 *Sampling and Contacting Vulnerable Populations*

The populations studied in this volume are highly diverse, requiring diverse sampling strategies. For example, the entire Swiss population (resident in private households) is sampled by the SHP (chapter "Attrition in the Swiss Household Panel: Are Vulnerable Groups More Affected than Others?"); older adults, simply defined as all people aged 65 and over, are targeted by VLV, and those aged 40–89 by the study on the experience of divorce and widowhood (chapters "Representation of Vulnerability and the Elderly. A Total Survey Error Perspective on the VLV

Survey" and "Vulnerability Following a Critical Life Event: Temporary Crisis or Chronic Distress? A Psychological Controversy, Methodological Considerations, and Empirical Evidence"); while the working population of middle-aged adults (aged 25–55) is considered in chapter "Career Pathways and Professional Transitions: Preliminary Results from the First Wave of a 7-Year Longitudinal Study". For most of these studies, the sampling frame was the population register and random probability samples were drawn for the research teams, in most cases by the Swiss Federal Statistical Office (SFSO), but also sometimes by the cantonal administrations. Within each of these populations specific challenges appeared that were directly related to situations of vulnerability. For example, the unemployed form part of the active population but identifying them required the use of a different source, the national register of the unemployed held by the State Secretariat of Economy, as well as a screening procedure (chapter "Career Pathways and Professional Transitions: Preliminary Results from the First Wave of a 7-Year Longitudinal Study"). Elderly people with cognitive impairments also needed to be identified for VLV, but this was a post-identification by the interviewer.

Elderly people ageing in a country where they arrived as migrant workers illustrate another approach to sampling in vulnerability research: the selection of specific subpopulations assumed or at least suspected to be vulnerable. Older migrants or the unemployed are typically categorized in a social stratification perspective. Alternatively, event-based vulnerability is reflected in the choice of studying divorcees and widows or widowers or the couples where the woman faces breast cancer. To identify the former Perrig-Chiello and her colleagues used a large SFSO sample, which they decided to supplement with a convenience sample recruited through calls in the media (chapter "Vulnerability Following a Critical Life Event: Temporary Crisis or Chronic Distress? A Psychological Controversy, Methodological Considerations, and Empirical Evidence"). For the latter, Charvoz and her coauthors established a partnership with a university hospital (chapter "A Survey of Couples Facing Breast Cancer in Women"). Similarly, Eicher and her coauthors have obtained targeted samples of young adults from institutions. As noted above, chapter "How to Survey Displaced Workers in Switzerland: Ways of Addressing Sources of Bias" about the displaced workers uses both social stratification and event-based perspectives. In terms of defining the population to be studied, individually displaced workers are a selective group since the characteristics that provoked their layoff are highly likely to affect their probability of remaining unemployed. That is why Isabel Baumann and her colleagues provide a nice illustration of the "sociological imagination". Using data from plant closures where all workers were displaced they identify a group of job seekers, of some 1200 persons who worked in manufacturing plants, which closed their doors between January 2009 and August 2010.

Once a suitable sampling strategy has been implemented, finding and contacting the potential participants is the next step and an additional source of trouble for researchers. In the surveys considered in this volume, between 7.5 and 15 % of the postal addresses were no longer valid for the persons listed on the frame. Reasons include errors in the original registers, confusion between de jure and de facto populations (for fiscal or other reasons), death and mobility. The latter is especially important for some event-based vulnerabilities (divorce usually produces at least one change of residence) and for transitional life periods (like the transition to adulthood). This is one of the reasons why Véronique Eicher and her colleagues used an alternative approach involving an online social network. However, even there, from the 380 people initially sampled, some 23 % provided an invalid email address (see chapter "Studying Youth Transitions Through a Social Network: First Impressions"), radically reducing the size of the available sample with which further contact could be made.

3.2 Modes of Data Collection and Vulnerability

The potential participants who are successfully contacted may be confronted with various modes of data collection selected by the researchers. For example, the VLV survey of the elderly included two separate questionnaires deployed in a classical sequence with first a self-administered paper-pencil questionnaire, then a computer-assisted interview (CAPI) administered by a trained interviewer in a face-to-face interaction (chapters "Representation of Vulnerability and the Elderly. A Total Survey Error Perspective on the VLV Survey" and "Adapting Quantitative Survey Procedures: The Price for Assessing Vulnerability? Lessons from a Large-Scale Survey on Aging and Migration in Switzerland"). The study of marital break-up and that of displaced workers adopted an alternative, less expansive approach since the participants could choose between paper-pencil or online questionnaires (chapters "Vulnerability Following a Critical Life Event: Temporary Crisis or Chronic Distress? A Psychological Controversy, Methodological Considerations, and Empirical Evidence" and "Career Pathways and Professional Transitions: Preliminary Results from the First Wave of a 7-Year Longitudinal Study"). The research on the working population offered even more choices for their two-stage data collection design: a full online version, a phone interview (CATI) plus an online questionnaire, or a CATI plus a paper-pencil questionnaire. Estimations of the cost reduction associated with using the web-based instrument range from 15 to 20 % (chapter "Career Pathways and Professional Transitions: Preliminary Results from the First Wave of a 7-Year Longitudinal Study"). A shared rationale for the use of different modes is that sensitive questions are located in the self-administered questionnaires to give better comfort to the respondents who feel more reassured about their anonymity.

If mixed-mode approaches have obvious advantages, they can also have draw-backs. Measurement differences can appear when not all participants use the same response format since the stimulus of a question can vary across modes (de Leeuw 2005; Dillman and Messer 2010; and in-depth discussions in chapters "Career Pathways and Professional Transitions: Preliminary Results from the First Wave of a 7-Year Longitudinal Study" and "How to Survey Displaced Workers in Switzerland: Ways of Addressing Sources of Bias"). Linda Charvoz and her co-authors report different results relating to social support depending on whether self-administered questionnaires or interviews are used, the "leniency effect" varying according to the mode (chapter "A Survey of Couples Facing Breast Cancer in Women"). By contrast, in Maggiori and his colleagues' survey of the labour force, differences between the respondents answering in each mode exist but they are not very large (chapter "Career Pathways and Professional Transitions: Preliminary Results from the First Wave of a 7-Year Longitudinal Study"). The decision to mix modes is a question of searching for the best trade-offs (de Leeuw 2005), also because mixing survey modes is one of the available options for increasing the rate of participation to the surveys. This means that substantive researchers preoccupied by achieving a particular target response rate may be willing to accept a reduction in measurement quality.

3.3   Persuading Vulnerable Populations to Participate

Obtaining the cooperation of the potential participants is another crucial challenge and an increasing source of worry for survey researchers. In most developed countries, refusals to participate in surveys are growing, compounding increased difficulties associated with making contact. Nationwide, the field interviewers were confronted with refusals given without reasons, opposition to any form of survey, no interest in the topic, lack of time, language barriers, and frustration of people living a situation of vulnerability they do not want to speak about. The authors of chapter "Representation of Vulnerability and the Elderly. A Total Survey Error Perspective on the VLV Survey" emphasize the negative impact of aggressive phone calls for commercial purposes and the resulting importance of clearly communicating the scientific objectives of the research to the potential respondents. However, this may not be enough for some vulnerable populations since universities themselves are sometimes assimilated to the authorities. Martina Rothenbühler and Marieke Voorpostel (chapter "Attrition in the Swiss Household Panel: Are Vulnerable Groups More Affected than Others?") evoke the "cynicism against institutions" that even took an aggressive form among the older immigrants (chapter "Adapting Quantitative Survey Procedures: The Price for Assessing Vulnerability? Lessons from a Large-Scale Survey on Aging and Migration in Switzerland").

In the end, participation rates across the board were generally low, ranging from 32 to 40 % with however an exceptional 62 % in Baumann and colleagues survey of displaced workers. Different tactics were used to deal with this problem. In Maggiori et al.'s research on the working population, the private company hired by the researchers sent a first reminder by mail, then a second by phone. At the end of this process, a conversion-strategy was implemented and realized by specially-trained interviewers who tried to persuade those who initially refused to participate (see chapter "Career Pathways and Professional Transitions: Preliminary Results from the First Wave of a 7-Year Longitudinal Study", and a similar approach in chapter "How to Survey Displaced Workers in Switzerland: Ways of Addressing Sources of Bias"). Only the team working on the elderly (the VLV survey) took an ideological position and forewent conversion efforts, though they did invest considerable effort in making contact with the sample members and permitted the use of proxies to obtain a completed interview (chapters "Representation of Vulnerability and the Elderly. A Total Survey Error Perspective on the VLV Survey" and "Adapting Quantitative Survey Procedures: The Price for Assessing Vulnerability? Lessons from a Large-Scale Survey on Aging and Migration in Switzerland"). Another answer to low participation rates is the use of incentives, which is discussed in depth in chapters "Career Pathways and Professional Transitions: Preliminary Results from the First Wave of a 7-Year Longitudinal Study" (Maggiori et al.), "How to Survey Displaced Workers in Switzerland: Ways of Addressing Sources of Bias" (Baumann et al.) and "Attrition in the Swiss Household Panel: Are Vulnerable Groups More Affected than Others?" (Rothenbühler and Voorpostel). Additionally, a big frustration is when a participant starts, then renounces, a pattern which seems to be more common in the online mode of data collection where a simple click is all that is needed to drop out of the survey (see chapter "Career Pathways and Professional Transitions: Preliminary Results from the First Wave of a 7-Year Longitudinal Study").

The crucial issue is not so much the proportion of those sampled that participate but whether those that participate differ from those that do not on the key variables of interest. The principal concern is that those least likely to participate will also be those who are most vulnerable, resulting in bias in estimates based on the less vulnerable responding sample. People with lower levels of education, and especially those with literacy challenges are known to be less willing to participle in data collections that may be particularly cognitively demanding for them – particularly if the questionnaire is to be self-administered. A less nice way to say the same is that the survey could confront them with their ignorance and marginality (see chapter "Attrition in the Swiss Household Panel: Are Vulnerable Groups More Affected than Others?" by Rothenbühler and Voorpostel). This was found to be true among the older immigrants, who often cumulated limited or inexistent education opportunities in their native country together with a partial linguistic integration in their country of migration (see chapters "Adapting Quantitative Survey Procedures: The Price for Assessing Vulnerability? Lessons from a Large-Scale Survey on Aging and Migration in Switzerland" and "Attrition in the Swiss Household Panel: Are Vulnerable Groups More Affected than Others?"; and also Lipps et al. 2011, as well as many references in the survey literature).

Repeated contact attempts to improve response rates carry the risk of bringing more participants of the same type into the sample, while harder-to-reach "marginal" subpopulations that are more reluctant to contribute to surveys remain nonrespondents (Groves and Peytcheva 2008). Indeed, among displaced workers, Baumann and her colleagues found that repeated contact attempts increased the response rate but did not reduce nonresponse bias. Mode diversification, on the other hand, i.e. telephone interviews in addition to paper questionnaires, improved the participation of underrepresented subgroups. Remaining differences between respondents and non-respondents concerned age, education and occupational structures, but none were found on key variables such as the re-employment prospects of the respondents (see chapter "How to Survey Displaced Workers in Switzerland: Ways of Addressing Sources of Bias").

In chapter "Adapting Quantitative Survey Procedures: The Price for Assessing Vulnerability? Lessons from a Large-Scale Survey on Aging and Migration in Switzerland", Laure Kaeser discusses how the standard fieldwork procedures in use on the VLV survey had to be adapted to tackle the problem of nonparticipation among migrant elders. The survey included a number of oversamples of elderly migrants from Italy, Spain, and former Yugoslavia, but non-response due to both non-contact and refusal threatened to undermine the success of the project. Different strategies were employed by the fieldwork supervisors and interviewers to try to mitigate the problems, with varying degrees of success. Once again researchers cannot hope for a perfect solution but have to find the best trade-offs when they have to make a choice between adapting the procedures for a specific sub-population with the risk of impacting comparisons with other groups surveyed under different protocols, or strictly applying the same rules to not pre-construct differences associated with the risk of under-representing vulnerable persons.

3.4 Dealing with Time: Prospective and Retrospective Longitudinal Approaches

Of course, for panel surveys, which are so important when a the life-course perspective is adopted, these difficulties are even more important, as the challenge is not only to contact and obtain answers from sample members, but to keep them involved in the survey. The combination is complex between the first survey that has to be as complete as possible and the follow up, keeping as many sample members as possible in subsequent waves. Many of the LIVES surveys involve a longitudinal component, but at the time of writing most were still in their first wave of data collection. To retain participants and maintain their commitment to the survey goals, all the teams use tactics like a small gift, a yearly newsletter and access to the project website. In their research on the labour-market population Maggiori and his colleagues asked their respondents directly about their intention to participate in the next wave. Logistic regressions showed expected but also unexpected biases: young respondents, wealthier respondents, with a higher score on openness, a lower score on neuroticism, but also people with a high score on stress measures were more inclined to maintain their participation (chapter "Career Pathways and Professional Transitions: Preliminary Results from the First Wave of a 7-Year Longitudinal Study"). Of course, these authors were only looking at intention to participate in these analyses, while in chapter "Attrition in the Swiss Household Panel: Are Vulnerable Groups More Affected than Others?" Martina Rothenbühler and Marieke Voorpostel analyze the actual experiences of attrition from the SHP over a period of 14 years. They show a clear effect of education with a higher drop-out rate for people with lower levels. This is also the case for men and young single adults, the latter because of their increased mobility. Indeed, the authors are able to disentangle the reasons for drop-out between individuals who are not eligible anymore, people who left the household, the cases of missing contact information, the refusals, but also event-based vulnerabilities like having health and/or family-related problems. The authors ultimately show that in 80 % of 802 tested variables, the means and frequencies do not appear to be affected by attrition. The use of weights corrects the effect in 10.6 % of the cases but is unable to correct the biases in 8 % and even decreases the accuracy of the estimates in 1.1 %. The delicate issue of post-survey adjustments by means of weighting is also discussed in chapter "How to Survey Displaced Workers in Switzerland: Ways of Addressing Sources of Bias".

To deal with time and the interweaving of vulnerabilities into the life course – that is, to study vulnerability as a dynamic condition – researchers can be imaginative. Pasqualina Perrig-Chiello and her colleagues distinguish four marital disruption groups according to the time since the breakup or loss. Baumann and her co-authors surveyed displaced workers who lost their job 2 years ago to see whether and how they escaped from unemployment during this period. Basically, unlike the prospective approach that usually characterizes longitudinal research designs, these researchers use a retrospective perspective, which is discussed in-depth in chapter "Using Life History Calendars to Survey Vulnerability" by Davide Morselli and his co-authors. On the basis of a large literature review that crosses psychological and sociological perspectives on human memory, and using as an empirical basis three studies associated with the LIVES program, they discuss the advantages and limitations of these two approaches (among the latter being memory biases, omission or misreporting of life events). Research into solutions to minimize memory errors led to the development of event history calendars, a method that has been incorporated into the SHP, as well as in VLV. The calendar tool appears to be ideal for testing the theory of cumulative (dis)advantages, and the construction of vulnerabilities across the life course and across life domains. Moreover, the authors demonstrate its potential for confronting factual events with subjective interpretations. Adding to the literature results from cognitive interviews realized within LIVES, Morselli and his colleagues convincingly defend the provocative view that recall errors can, in fact, be a highly significant source of information.

Needless to say, research challenges are not restricted to those discussed above, which are only the most present in the contributions to this book. Issues like interviewer effects, respondent-interviewer social interactions, measurement errors, questionnaire design, unclear questions, misunderstandings, etc. are also touched on but only here and there. Furthermore, surveying vulnerable populations raises a number of important ethical challenges. Ethical considerations are already associated with identification (stigmatization) of vulnerable populations, with carrying out repeated contact attempts and handling refusals, with the effect our questions could have on the well-being of the respondents, and with the duty to include vulnerable people in data collections that are the foundations for scientific research likely to document political action. And this list is of course far from being exhaustive. Once again, this is a question about making trade-offs between upholding methodological ideals and negotiating the complex reality of pursuing substantive research aims in vulnerable contexts.

4 Surveying Vulnerabilities: Lessons Learned

In the preceding discussion, we have highlighted some of the challenges involved in conducting quantitative research into vulnerability across the life course. Drawing on theoretical perspectives from the literature on survey methodology that emphasize the need to mitigate potential sources of error, we discussed the various risks to quality present in the LIVES surveys, and the solutions and compromises to manage these risks reached by the researchers responsible for collecting new data. For each of the studies represented in the book, this involved finding a balance between the need to optimize measurement accuracy against the need to adapt to and respect the idiosyncrasies of particular subpopulations and research contexts. In this concluding section we reflect on the key lessons that have been learned as a result of these experiences, and the take-home conclusions of this book. The first concerns the significance of methodology and the collaboration between substantive researchers and methodologists. The second concerns the challenges of interdisciplinarity and its concomitant need for transparency in methodological matters.

4.1 Methodology Matters

The first take-home message concerns the central role of methodology in the pursuit of substantive research interests and the importance of dialogue between substantive researchers and methodologists when designing new research. Put simply, methodology matters. Firstly, data quality – meaning, in a conventional sense, the accuracy of estimates produced by a survey, or more generally, the reliability and validity of research findings – can be enhanced by seeking input from and acting on the empirically-based recommendations of methodologists. Given the popularity of research into vulnerability and its potential influence on policy development, quality is critical and fostering this collaboration should be a priority for future research. The beneficiaries of such collaboration are not only subject specialists, however, but also methodologists. Survey research methodology must be able to respond to the needs of life course researchers interested in vulnerability, which means methodologists involved in researching this field need to constantly interrogate common practices and dominant quality paradigms, to ensure they can adequately accommodate and adapt to the particular demands posed by studies of vulnerable people. As the preceding discussion testifies, conducting surveys of vulnerable sub-populations raises important questions about the extent to which conventional tools and procedures should be retained or adapted depending on the research context. This concerns all aspects of a research design from the methods used to ensure adequate representation of a particular target population, the tools developed for measuring pertinent theoretical constructs, to the procedures used to analyze the data.

Alongside the various challenges involved in data collection described earlier, vulnerability research presents numerous measurement and analytical challenges to which methodologists must be able to respond. Vulnerability is multidimensional, which means that we have to care about measurement quality and not rely on single indicators. Statistical methodology also has to take into account this multidimensionality, by using adequate analytical strategies. Equally, as we have seen, vulnerability can be seen as the result of tensions between stressors and resources. The evaluation of social resources can refer to different types of capitals: economic and cultural, but is also linked to a web of social relations. In this sense, research needs to take into account 'lives in context', that is how individuals fit within their social networks and the characteristics of the social and institutional contexts within which these are embedded. All these features of the research domain present unique challenges for future collaborations between substantive and methodological experts.

The rise in popularity of quantitative research into vulnerability has occurred at a time when survey methodologists are having to adapt the methods traditionally used to carry out surveys of the general population. This has been due to the deterioration of traditional sampling frames (particularly for telephone surveys), declining rates of participation, and rapid growth in information and communication technologies (Groves 2011). Survey research is changing. Paradoxically this revolution in how surveys are carried out comes at a time when survey methodology as a science has never been more knowledgeable or better equipped to both pre-empt and correct threats to data quality. Yet much of what has been learned so far has been derived from methodological research conducted alongside surveys of the general population. The empirical base is much more sparse for guidance about how best to survey those at the periphery of society, or how best to capture the dynamics of how individuals respond to major life transitions (whether they be normative or non-normative). In the context of turmoil surrounding mainstream survey methodology, building up specialized areas of expertise around specific substantive research objectives, topics and populations of interest will be of paramount importance. Longitudinal surveys, such as the household panel surveys, are playing a key role in the vulnerability domain – particularly where funding is explicitly made available for methodological research (e.g. in the case of the Dutch LISS Panel, the UK Household Longitudinal Survey). Via this book, the LIVES projects, along with the Swiss Household Panel Survey, are similarly making essential contributions to the methodology of vulnerability research.

A second argument for the essentialness of methodology concerns the use of the data themselves. The results of a survey are not simply "data" in the etymological sense of the word[2] but are also "produced" by the system that was used for observation and the context in which it operates (see Desrosières 2001; Héran 1984). This is not a limitation in the validity of surveys themselves, just an important point to keep in mind and to document before using data, and particularly when they have been collected in a complex, non-standard context. In other words, to take into account the characteristics of the data used and the way they were produced is a basic condition for their proper scientific use. It also means that it would be dangerous to separate the roles of methodologists and social scientists, as they are profoundly interdependent. This book as a whole demonstrates that the union of methodological and substantive issues is a prerequisite for a good scientific work.

4.2 Interdisciplinarity and the Need for Transparency

At the start of this chapter we noted two defining features of the LIVES research programme besides the shared substantive goal of investigating the experience of vulnerability at different stages and key transitions of the life course. These features were its interdisciplinarity – both within and across the various individual projects involved – and a predominant emphasis on quantitative methods. Yet while the overriding methodological approach of the LIVES projects relies on survey data collection, variations in implementation can be observed as a result of deeply entrenched, unique methodological traditions of the different disciplines involved. Each discipline has its own toolbox, which is not purely technical but also acts as a lens through which to look at social phenomena, and to produce, manipulate and interpret data. Such "traditions" are apparent when reading different journals,[3] but most of the time they manifest themselves as strong but implicit rules governing the conduct of research within a given scientific field. In this book, as in the LIVES project more generally, there has been no attempt to obviate this reality. As a result of varied disciplinary priorities, the various projects described have inevitably paid more or less attention to different sources of error in their data, or emphasised different notions of quality over others.

One example of this concerns measurement, where it is not just that the questions asked of respondents in different disciplines can differ, but also that the priorities, in terms of design, can vary: for example, psychologists tend to privilege "validated" scales, often long, while sociologists tend to favour shorter multi-item measures. Similarly, the way in which household income is considered will often be different in economic models where exact values are seen as important, while in other

---

[2]"The word data is the traditional plural form of the now-archaic datum, neuter past participle of the Latin dare, "to give", hence "something given"." From http://en.wikipedia.org/wiki/Data, accessed 29.03.2015.

[3]For example, discussion about representativeness and random sampling of subjects is not so common in psychology or social psychology, while it is rather crucial in sociology.

disciplines a more basic ranking (e.g. into deciles) will offer sufficient precision. A second example concerns what is considered as "ethical", which can similarly vary across disciplines: a practical exercise of walking in a room with elderly people is seen as routine by medical doctors, while a name generator network measure is seen as intrusive. For a sociologist, less at ease with the first case than the second one, the reverse is true.[4] In other words some crucial elements of design can vary between disciplines and one of the challenges is to initiate from the outset a space for multidisciplinary discussion, organised around the necessity of a common methodology.

This has implications not only at a practical level in terms of the day-to-day negotiations that must take place between the various stakeholders in multidisciplinary research, but also at a managerial level. Multidisciplinary work imposes more documentation requirements and a greater demand for transparency, particularly in relation to research methods. One reason for this is the need to make explicit the implicit methodological patterns at play, but it is also good research practice more generally. An interdisciplinary context should encourage the scientific use and exchange of data, but entails a need among participants to be prepared to accept and share the best practices of different disciplines, and to document the idiosyncrasies of different fields. One aim of this book, therefore, is to achieve this by recording not only the design decisions that have been made in executing the substantive research agenda of each project, but also reflections on the reasons behind decisions, for the sake of transparency and ultimately, to facilitate data sharing. This is of course important for every scientific program and is quite a general challenge.

5   Conclusion

In this introduction, we have emphasised the 'total survey error' framework as a theoretical basis for understanding the challenges involved in producing good quality data. However, we do so in recognition of the fact that central to this approach is a notion of quality, which may be at odds with the varied priorities of different disciplines. The ultimate goal in survey methodology is to find the optimal balance between errors and costs in survey design, while prioritising the accuracy of the estimates produced. But the goal of accuracy is often not the driving aim of researchers designing surveys, particularly where the survey concerns vulnerable populations, and the measurement of vulnerabilities. This raises the question of whether we should appeal to notions of quality other than statistical accuracy, given that in the real world, trade-offs and compromises are inevitable (even in studies of the general population). This question is especially pertinent at a time when survey research organisations worldwide are adapting the methods they have

---

[4]This is a real example, based on the remarks of the "Commission d'éthique du canton de Genève" when the VLV survey was planned.

conventionally relied upon, and with them, the quality framework that has governed best practices. Alternatives emphasise other standards besides estimator quality, such as the credibility, relevance and usability of a survey's results (their 'fitness for purpose'), as well as constraints such as ethical considerations and timeliness (Groves and Lyberg 2010; Weisberg 2005). Many of the chapters here underline the inherent tension involved in trying to apply standards of accuracy in hard-to-survey research contexts, and in many respects its publication is timely, providing an alternative perspective on the realities of implementing academically-led surveys in contemporary society.

Ultimately, the purpose is not to catalogue the difficulties, weaknesses, limits and sources of potential misinterpretation. On the contrary, the various contributions demonstrate that a reflexive attitude and a dialogue between methodological specialists and topic experts are the best means to develop intelligent research designs, avoid blind routines, make proper use of the data, and hopefully, also improve future survey research in this domain. It goes without saying that we cannot hope to completely eliminate all sources of error that affect the quality of the data we collect, but we can strive to make more transparent the various decisions involved in achieving the optimal trade-off between them.

References

Antonini, M., & Bühlmann, F. (2015). Towards a multi-dimensional theory of post-unemployment scarring: recurrence, instability and downgrading. *LIVES Working Papers, 2015*(37), 31 p.

Bauman, Z. (2006). *Liquid times: Living in an age of uncertainty*. Cambridge: Polity.

Bonvin, J. M., Otto, H. U., & Ziegler, H. (2014). Towards a more critical appraisal of social policies? The contribution of the capability approach. In H. U. Otto & H. Ziegler (Eds.), *Critical social policy and the capability approach* (pp. 231–248). Opladen/Farmington Hills: Barbara Budrich.

Chauvel, L. (2010). The long-term destabilization of youth, scarring effects and the future of the welfare regime in post-Trente Glorieuses France. *French Politics, Culture and Society, 23*, 74–96.

Dannefer, D., Uhlenberg, Fonner, A., & Abeles, R. P. (2005). On the shoulders of a giant: The legacy of Matilda White Riley for gerontology. *The Journals of Gerontology Series B: Psychological Sciences and Social Sciences, 60*, 296–304.

Davidov, E., Schmidt, P., & Billiet, J. (Eds.). (2010). *Cross-cultural analysis: Methods and applications*. New York: Taylor & Francis.

de Leeuw, E. D. (2005). To mix or not to mix data collection modes in survey. *Journal of Official Statistics, 21*(2), 233–255.

de Singly, F., & Martuccelli, D. (2009). *Les sociologies de l'individu*. Paris: A. Colin.

Desrosières, A. (2001). Entre réalisme métrologique et conventions d'équivalence : les ambiguïtés de la sociologie quantitative. *Genèse, 43*, 112–127.

Dillman, D. A., & Messer, B. L. (2010). Mixed-mode surveys. In P. V. Marsden & J. D. Wright (Eds.), *Handbook of survey research* (pp. 551–574). Bingley: Emerald.

DiPrete, T. A., & Eirich, G. M. (2006). Cumulative advantage as a mechanism for inequality: A review of theoretical and empirical developments. *Annual Review of Sociology, 32*, 271–297.

Ehrenberg, A. (1998). *La fatigue d'être soi. Dépression et société*. Paris: Odile Jacob.

Elcheroth, G., Fasel N., Gianettoni, L., Kleiner, B., Laganà, F., Lipps, F., Penic, S., & Pollien A. (2011, September). Minorities in general social surveys: What we can learn from the Swiss case and why the black box should be opened wider. *FORS Position Paper Series*.

Elder, G., Shanahan, M. J., & Jennings, J. A. (2015). Human development in time and place. In R. M. Lerhner (Ed.), *Handbook of child psychology and developmental science* (pp. 6–54). Hoboken: Wiley.

Esping-Andersen, G. (2009). *The incomplete revolution. Adapting to women's new roles*. Cambridge: Polity Press.

Fokkema, T., & Liefbroer, A. C. (2008). Trends in living arrangements in Europe: Convergence or divergence? *Demographic Research, 19*, 1351–1418.

Gabriel, R., Oris, M., Studer, M., & Baeriswyl, M. (2015). The persistence of social stratification? A life course perspective on old-age poverty in Switzerland. *Swiss Journal of Sociology, 41*(3), 465–487.

Giddens, A. (1991). *Modernity and self-identity. Self and society in the late modern age*. Cambridge: Polity.

Gomensoro, A., & Bolzman, C. (2015). The effect of socio-economic status of ethnic groups on educational inequalities in Switzerland: which 'hidden' mechanisms? *Italian Journal of Sociology of Education, 7*(2), 70–98.

Groves, R. M. (1989). *Survey errors and survey costs*. New York: Wiley.

Groves, R. M. (2011). Three eras of survey research. *Public Opinion Quarterly, 75*(5), 861–871.

Groves, R. M., & Lyberg, L. (2010). Total survey error, past, present, and future. *Public Opinion Quarterly, 74*(5), 849–879.

Groves, R. M., & Peytcheva, E. (2008). The impact of nonresponse rates on nonresponse bias: A meta-analysis. *Public Opinion Quarterly, 72*(2), 167–189.

Groves, R. M., Fowler, F. J., Jr., Couper, M. P., Lepkowski, J. M., Singer, E., & Tourangeau, R. (2004). *Survey methodology*. New York: Wiley.

Grusky, D. B. (2001). Social stratification. In N. J. Smelser & P. B. Baltes (Eds.), *International encyclopedia of the social & behavioral sciences* (pp. 14443–14452). Oxford: Pergamon.

Hanappi, D., Bernardi, L., & Spini, D. (2015). Vulnerability as a heuristic for interdisciplinary research: Assessing the thematic and methodological structure of empirical life-course studies. *Longitudinal Life Course Studies, 6*(1), 59–87.

Harkness, J., Braun, M., Edwards, B., Johnson, T. P., Lyberg, L., & Mohler, P. (Eds.). (2010). *Survey methods in multinational, multiregional, and multicultural contexts*. Hoboken: Wiley.

Henke, J. (2015). *Socioeconomic vulnerabilities among the Swiss elderly*. Doctoral thesis in Socioeconomics, University of Geneva.

Héran, F. (1984). L'assise statistique de la sociologie. *Economie et Statistique, 168*, 23–35.

Kohli, M. (2007). The institutionalization of the life course: Looking back to look ahead. *Research in Human Development, 4*, 53–271.

Leisering, L. (2003). Government and the life course. In J. T. Mortimer & M. J. Shanahan (Eds.), *Handbook of the life course* (pp. 205–225). New York: Springer.

Levy, R., & Widmer, E. (2013). *Gendered life courses between individualization and standardization. A European approach applied to Switzerland*. Wien: LIT Verlag.

Levy, R., Ghisletta, P., Le Goff, J. M., Spini, D., & Widmer, E. (Eds.). (2005). *Towards an interdisciplinary perspective on the life course*. Amsterdam: Elsevier.

Lipps, O., Laganà, F., Pollien, A., & Gianettoni, L. (2011). National minorities and their representation in Swiss Surveys (I): Providing evidence and analyzing causes for their underrepresentation. *FORS Working Paper*, (2), 20 p.

Mayer, K. U. (2009). New directions in life course research. *Annual Review of Sociology, 35*, 413–433.

Oris, M., & Lerch, M. (2009). La transition ultime. Longévité et mortalité aux grands âges dans le bassin lémanique. In M. Oris, E. Widmer, A. de Ribaupierre, D. Joye, D. Spini, & J.-M. Falter (Eds.), *Transitions dans les parcours de vie et constructions dans le grand âge* (pp. 407–432). Lausanne: Presses polytechniques et universitaires romandes.

Oris, M., Ludwig, C., de Ribaupierre, A., Joye, D., & Spini, D. (Eds.). (2009). *Linked lives and self-regulation. Life span – Life course: Is it really the same?*, special issue of *Advances in Life Course Research, 14*(1–2), 81 p. Elsevier.

Pearlin, L. (1989). The sociological study of stress. *Journal of Health Social Behaviour, 30*(3), 241–256.

Ranci, C. (2010). Social vulnerability in Europe. In C. Ranci (Ed.), *Social vulnerability in Europe: The new configuration of social risks* (pp. 3–24). Basingstoke: Palgrave Macmillan.

Riandey, B., & Quaglia, M. (2009). Surveying hard-to-reach groups. In P. Bonnel, M. Lee-Gosselin, J. Zmud, & J. L. Madre (Eds.), *Transport survey methods: Keeping up with a changing world* (pp. 127–144). Bingley: Emerald.

Ritschard, G., & Oris, M. (2005). Life course data in demography and social sciences: Statistical and data-mining approaches. In R. Levy, P. Ghisletta, J.-M. Le Goff, D. Spini, & E. Widmer (Eds.), *Towards an interdisciplinary perspective on the life course* (pp. 283–314). Amsterdam: Elsevier.

Rudisill, J. R., Edwards, J. M., Hershberger, P. J., Jadwin, J. E., & McKee, J. M. (2010). Coping with job transitions over the work life. In T. W. Miller (Ed.), *Handbook of stressful transitions across the lifespan* (pp. 111–131). New York: Springer.

Ruof, M. C. (2004). Vulnerability, vulnerable populations, and policy. *Kennedy Institute of Ethics Journal, 14*(4), 411–425.

Spini, D., Hanappi, D., Bernardi, L., Oris, M., & Bickel, J.-Fr. (2013). Vulnerability across the life course: A theoretical framework and research directions. *Working Paper LIVES*.

Thomas, H. (2008). Vulnérabilité, fragilité, précarité, résilience, etc. De l'usage et de la traduction de notions éponges en sciences de l'homme et de la vie. *Esquisses, 23*, 1–37.

Tillmann, R., & Voorpostel, M. (2012). Social stratification, social inequalities, and persistent social inequalities. *Swiss Journal of Sociology, 38*(2), 145–153.

Tourangeau, R., Edwards, B., Johnson, T. P., Wolters, K. M., & Bates, N. (Eds.). (2014). *Hard-to-survey populations*. Cambridge: Cambridge University Press.

Vandecasteele, L. (2010). Poverty trajectories after risky life course events in different European welfare regimes. *European Societies, 12*(2), 257–278.

Weisberg, H. (2005). *The total survey error approach*. Chicago: University of Chicago Press.

Widmer, E. (2010). *Family configurations: A structural approach to family diversity*. London: Ashgate.

Widmer, E. D., & Ritschard, G. (2009). The de-standardization of the life course: Are men and women equal? *Advances in Life Course Research, 14*(1–2), 28–39.

Widmer, E., Aeby, G., & Sapin, M. (2013). Collecting family network data. *International Review of Sociology, 23*(1), 27–46.

Representation of Vulnerability and the Elderly. A Total Survey Error Perspective on the VLV Survey

Michel Oris, Eduardo Guichard, Marthe Nicolet, Rainer Gabriel, Aude Tholomier, Christophe Monnot, Delphine Fagot, and Dominique Joye

1 Surveying the Elderly, Surveying Vulnerability

As its title suggests, this chapter takes inspiration from the literature on survey methodology, including the "total survey error" framework, and mainly deals with the different dimensions of its first component, which is the challenge of accurately representing a given population (Groves and Lyberg 2010, 856). The second component, minimizing the measurement errors, will only be touched briefly.

This paper has been made possible by the support of the Sinergia project, n° CRSII1_129922/1 and the IP 13 of the National Centre of Competences in Research "LIVES—Overcoming Vulnerability: Life course perspectives," both financed by the Swiss Science Foundation (SNF). The authors express their gratitude to the SNF. They are also happy to acknowledge the support of Pro Senectute Schweiz as well as the universities of Geneva and Bern.

M. Oris (✉) • E. Guichard • M. Nicolet • R. Gabriel • A. Tholomier • D. Fagot
NCCR LIVES, IP 213, Geneva, Switzerland

Centre for the Interdisciplinary Study of Gerontology and Vulnerability, University of Geneva, Geneva, Switzerland
e-mail: Michel.Oris@unige.ch

C. Monnot
NCCR LIVES, IP 213, Lausanne, Switzerland

Institute of Social Sciences of Contemporaneous Religions, University of Lausanne, Lausanne, Switzerland

D. Joye
NCCR LIVES, IP 214, Lausanne, Switzerland

Social Sciences Institute, University of Lausanne, Lausanne, Switzerland

FORS (Swiss Foundation for the Research in Social Sciences), University of Lausanne, Lausanne, Switzerland

M. Oris et al. (eds.), *Surveying Human Vulnerabilities across the Life Course*,
Life Course Research and Social Policies 3, DOI 10.1007/978-3-319-24157-9_2

Table 1 Participation and refusal in European surveys, 2004

Countries	Response rates	
	SHARE 2004	ESS 2004
Denmark	59 %	64 %
Germany	52 %	51 %
Italy	44 %	59 %
Netherlands	54 %	64 %
Spain	37 %	55 %
Sweden	41 %	65 %
Austria	45 %	62 %
France	69 %	44 %
Greece	55 %	79 %
Switzerland	**33** %	**49** %
Total	48 %	59 %

Sources: Börsch-Supan et al. (2008), Cheschire et al. (2011), De Luca and Peracchi (2005) and Scholes et al. (2009)

Consequently, this contribution is about issues like coverage error, unit and item non-responses, and influences of the questionnaire design, of contact procedures, of interviewers' and respondents' characteristics and their interactions on response. They are crucial to dealing with a real challenge: the impact of low and continuously declining rates of participation in large-scale surveys.

Major European comparative research has clearly established the special position of Switzerland, where the rates of refusals of inhabitants to participate in surveys are among the highest in Europe. By using the calculation standards of the American Association for Public Opinion Research, Table 1 shows that in the SHARE survey (Survey on Health, Ageing and Retirement in Europe), during the 2004 round, the acceptance rate varied from a maximum of 69 % in France to a minimum of 33 % in Switzerland (De Luca and Peracchi 2005, 90). The results for the European Social Survey the same year are similar although a bit better everywhere. Moreover, in most developed countries the trend in participation is declining (Rindfuss et al. 2015; Groves 2011). In Switzerland, more specifically in the cantons of Geneva and Valais, where surveys about living conditions among the elderly were done successively in 1979 and 1994 (see Betemps et al. 1997); then in 2011/2012, we observe a dramatic change: the refusal rate grew from 25 to 37 %, then to 47 %.

As we see from this evidence, participation has been decreasing in the long run and is especially low in studies about older adults as well as in Switzerland. It has already had a lot of effects on the costs of survey operations, an issue which is not trivial at all. Moreover, regardless of the studied population, the scientific implications are also of the utmost importance. Indeed, it is well known that standard procedures tend to over represent middle-class participants and to exclude people from the lower classes, who are more likely to not understand or not adhere to the survey project (Groves and Couper 1998). The problem is even bigger with the so-called "hard-to-reach," "hard-to-survey" groups (see Marpsat and Razafindratsima 2010; Tourangeau et al. 2014). So, all the individuals that could be labelled as vulnerable are disproportionately at risk of being missed. And low, decreasing rates of participation should increase those selective processes (Lessler and Kalsbeck 1992). Non-response is a particular challenge when surveying people affected by economic hardship, health problems, or life accidents.

The following sections of this chapter show how we have coped with this challenge in a survey named VLV (acronym of Vivre-Leben-Vivere, meaning "to live" in the three main languages of Switzerland) and devoted to the health and living conditions of the elderly in Switzerland. Our team conceived and managed this data collection in 2011 and 2012. First some design choices are discussed, including how the questionnaires were constructed and how some questions were designed to identify both latent and manifest states of vulnerability among the participants. We follow with the contact strategy before studying the reasons for refusal. Then we show that some procedures have been efficient in terms of including vulnerable persons in the sample of participants and have reduced the potential bias that would have been associated with a higher rate of refusal by the vulnerable. We also address this question through a comparison of the prevalence of poverty and health problems' in VLV and in the literature, and in other surveys. At this stage, from the response units we move to the response items; more precisely the non-response, the questions participants did not want to answer. The explanatory logic differs depending on the two modes of data collection that were used on the survey: the self-administered and the face-to-face questionnaires. For the former, we provide a full analysis to identify points of misunderstanding or reluctance to respond. For the latter, we consider two significant variables, household income and psychometric tests of cognitive abilities, in a model that takes into account interviewer and respondent characteristics as well as the context of the interview. A final discussion concludes.

2   Design Choices

2.1   VLV Objectives

The VLV research objective is to explore well-being among the elderly and the conditions for its maintenance throughout the ageing process. From a theoretical point of view, those conditions are constructed all along the life course, beginning early in life with a later accentuation of initial inequalities through processes of accumulation of advantages or disadvantages (Dannefer 2003) or under the impact of critical events (Bak and Larsen 2014). It is to capture those life course dynamics that life calendars have been implemented in VLV. This tool is discussed in this volume in the chapter of Davide Morselli and colleagues. Life trajectories result in a system of resources the aged person has at his or her disposal for ageing. The survey has to identify health, personality, cognition, social and human capital, lodging conditions, income, and wealth, which are some of those many resources. But to be effective, resources need to be used since it often happens that people do not make use of the assets they have. That is why we also surveyed the various practices of the elderly, especially social participation (Bickel 2014). In case of a deficit of crucial resources, in a society like Switzerland, the family and the welfare institutions are supposed to compensate, to take care. Their actions consequently need to be documented too, but from the point of view of the aged person who receives the care (Masotti and Oris 2015). Similarly, the final judgment can only come directly from the men and women themselves, who are the only ones who can tell us about their subjective well-being. Many of us define subjective well-being following Amartya Sen and his famous statement, "to lead the kind of lives they value—and have reason to value" (Sen 1999, 18). Psychologists of course have different references and make a distinction between cognitive (Diener et al. 1985) and affective (Girardin et al. 2008) components of well-being.

2.2   *Approaching Vulnerability*

Vulnerability, a central concept for the research pole LIVES and consequently for VLV too, could indeed be defined as low levels of well-being. However, in the following lines we emphasize another approach, very simple in its principle. We focus on a breakdown of the possible conditions, that is to say, a breakdown that goes beyond the "vulnerable versus invulnerable" dichotomy, which from the outset appeared unrealistic. The basic idea is simply to differentiate visible, evident, or realized situations of vulnerability from states of latent vulnerability, which are trickier to detect and assess but which are absolutely crucial for any policy, since it is there that useful measures of prevention can be applied. These latent conditions are linked to situations similar to those of realized conditions, but the evidence is no longer obvious, though the threat (or exposure to risk) is clearly present.

The above short development conceptualizes what has appeared, in fact, for two or three decades in several fields of study. Indeed, this idea applies to the distinction between poverty and precariousness that has become commonplace in sociology (Paugam 2000). Since we are here dealing with the aged, the field of gerontology sheds even more light. Between autonomy and dependency, the condition of facing "difficulties" is now the subject of a considerable number of studies. It has been developed and theorized through the concept of "frailty".[1] Up to a certain point, this is echoed in demography through the notion also named frailty, which describes more generically differential fragilities linked to phenomena of selection, in particular among the survivors, that is to say the aged, especially those of a very advanced age (Vaupel et al. 1979).

---

[1] With a touch of irony, Jean-Pierre Michel and his colleagues speak of fragility as an "unusual topic in the 1980s (less than 50 articles before 1990), an over-employed topic in the 1990s (1981 times between 1991 and 2000) and which had in 2001 and 2002 already been the subject of 724 publications in newspapers with an editorial policy" (Michel et al. 2005, 230).

To study vulnerability, we cannot remain with simple opposition between, for example, included and excluded persons, autonomous or dependent persons, etc. Adding more modalities, at least one, we must try to identify those who are at risk, we have to recognize that at the bottom of the scale but above obvious conditions, there is an ambiguous area that must be considered. As soon as it is accepted, the issue of choosing a "border", as with the definition of a threshold of poverty, becomes less important. Indeed, the border does not become entirely meaningless but much less crucial, since it is no longer a question of "isolating" a subpopulation (of poor people in this example) and comparing it with a global, undifferentiated "remainder." Concretely, in VLV, a bit <20 % of the participants have monthly incomes of <2400 SFr per individual, which is (almost) the official poverty threshold in Switzerland, but more than 30 % are located in the category just above (2400–3600). Those people are living above the poverty line but are very close and thus are vulnerable to economic stress, meaning they have an increased risk of falling below the threshold should they experience unfavorable circumstances (Gabriel 2015, 117). In his PhD, Rainer Gabriel (2015) considered various explanatory variables or factors associated with poverty, precariousness (the 2400–3600 income category), and the "secured" (3600 and above). Often, but not always, he identifies similar patterns for poor and precarious, such results being instructive for both science and policy.

In the questionnaires used in the VLV survey, tools were systematically selected, sometimes reconsidered, to support an approach that tends to spread the multiple dimensions to be taken into account in the identification and construction of human realities of vulnerabilities. The latter include material difficulties, as we have just seen above, but also health. For instance, Swiss researchers used the test of depression initially developed by Wang and his colleagues in 1975 and proposed a classification where the presence of four symptoms or more indicate a state of depression, while the presence of fewer than two symptoms is an indication of good mental health, and in between they also defined the ambiguous situation of people who are "worried" when two or three symptoms are observed (Lalive d'Epinay and Spini 2008, 90). This example shows that an "obvious" state of vulnerability is time- and context-dependent, since not everywhere is depression socially and institutionally recognized, but what is important here is that the proposed typology includes an intermediate latent state.

In this chapter, we will also illustrate our point by using another scale that is famous in gerontology and also well known to demographers of ageing (Robine and Jagger 2004), that of activities of daily living developed by Sydney Katz and his colleagues (1963). We have opted for the version with five assessments completed for three items on mobility. This tool very concretely indicates whether a given individual autonomously carries out elementary activities of his daily life (such as getting dressed, eating, etc.), whether the person can still do this but with difficulty, or whether, at this very basic level of daily life, he or she has become dependent on external assistance. These measurements, which are, after all, very human measurements of ageing, define in technical terms three statuses of functional health, the first reflecting an absence of vulnerability, the second a latent vulnerability, and the third an obvious one.

2.3   A Context-Dependent Survey

The development of the questionnaires for VLV raised another challenge related
to the issue of vulnerability. As it is implicitly said above and has to be made
explicit here, the aim was to consider the whole population aged 65 and over,
whatever their conditions or characteristics, and to identify the vulnerable persons
only in a second stage on the basis of the collected information. This approach
reflects changes in gerontological research that have been associated with objective
evolutions of life expectancy as well as health and living conditions. The above-
mentioned 1979 survey in Geneva and Valais was titled "Isolation and dependency
of older people." On one side, after several governmental reports for which only
experts were interrogated, a "knowledge from the bottom," was finally constructed
on the basis of the old persons' answers. On the other side, such a title expressed
the dominant view in the Western world after the Second World War that was still
prevalent at the end of the Seventies: a quite negative perception of ageing and of
the conditions of the elderly (see Bourdelais 1997). When this survey was repeated
in 1994, the title became "The autonomy of elderly persons in their socio-cultural
environment," and the comparison of the two waves revealed a "quiet revolution,"
i.e., significant socioeconomic and health improvements (Lalive d'Epinay et al.
2000). Both scientists and the public changed their vision of ageing, but only
partially; now there was a distinction between a "third age" of freedom and self-
realization versus a "fourth age" marked by senility and dependency, as well as
new age stratification like the young-old, old-old, or oldest-old (Dannefer 2001).
A research focus on the latter is reflected in the Swiss study of the oldest old that
longitudinally followed a sample of octogenarians among the participants of the
1994 survey, and demonstrated that frailty is now, by far, much more the fate of the
oldest old than dependency (Lalive d'Epinay and Spini 2008; Guilley and Lalive
d'Epinay 2008).

   In 2011, VLV considered first the other side of the coin, the young old. The
project was named "Old age democratization? Inequalities within progress in
Switzerland." This title expressed the ambition to assess (dis)continuation of the
improvements observed in 1979 (see more in Ludwig et al. 2014) and the idea that
in a country that has the second- or third-highest life expectancy in the world, even
people from the lower classes, with a low level of education, with an immigrant
background, etc., are now much more able to reach the age of retirement, and
even a very old age, than they were 15 or 30 years ago. This perspective implies
that progress indeed produces inequalities in the elderly population; more precisely,
we expect a maximal inter-individual variability from retirement until an advanced
age, where differential mortality reduces this diversity (Oris and Lerch 2009). This
is congruent with our objectives mentioned above and explains our motivation to
survey a large and highly heterogeneous population (aged 65–103), our rejection
of a vision of all old adults as a vulnerable population, and the need for tools
that can assess the variety of health and living conditions experienced within this
population. Concretely, it implied applying the same procedures and questionnaires

to as many people as possible, without which we would find differential rates of unit response and item response according, for example, to level of education or health status, which would create a biased sample of respondents. The only exception was a specific procedure for persons with cognitive impairments or serious physical problems who did not have the capacity to answer by themselves and had to be included through a proxy, to avoid skewing the results. Otherwise, the same questionnaires were applied to all the participants, regardless of their status or age.

2.4 Questionnaires

Constructing questionnaires is always about playing with constraints to create opportunities. The requirement to be able to study evolution over the last three decades imposed the obligation to keep enough questions from the 1979 to 1994 surveys (Ludwig et al. 2014), but offered the advantage that those old tools usually avoid academic jargon and are easy to understand. In addition, a holistic perspective on ageing implied the mobilization of several disciplinary competencies, which for VLV included geriatrics, psychiatry, psychology, sociology, social policy, and socioeconomics. All the disciplinary demands together imposed difficult challenges, requiring strict selection criteria. Selection criteria included coherence and comparability with other surveys worldwide like SHARE, internal coherence with the general and specific research objectives, interdisciplinary potential, and the desire to not make people feel uncomfortable. Questions on sexuality or tests of psychiatric troubles have been excluded for this reason, though of course those decisions were not undisputed. We reached a compromise between shortening the questionnaires and maintaining a minimal cohesion within the multidisciplinary research team.

The many questions that were left in the questionnaires have been regrouped in thematic chapters (for a description, see Ludwig et al. 2014, and Table 9 and Fig. 7). Following a general model (De Leeuw 2008) that has been applied for SHARE (Börtsch-Supan 2005) and the Berlin Aging Study (Baltes and Mayer 1999), the burden was distributed between a self-administered questionnaire and a standardized interview using the CAPI method. Intimate questions that were selected because of their importance were located in the former and some tests requiring vignettes, exercises and a trained interviewer were located in the latter. Within each questionnaire, the sequence was thought to deal with the old population heterogeneity; asking a question about incontinence to someone aged 67 could seem absurd, but if it is at the end of a series on medical problems the participant can understand the rationale and just answer "no." Also, some questions, especially some psychological tests where a positive formulation is systematically tested against a negative one, could appear heavy or boring and had to be alternated with more "funny" or attractive questions.

The self-administered questionnaire contained 150 questions and theoretically required one to one and a half hours to be properly filled out by the participant. The face-to-face questionnaire contained no <459 questions! Fortunately, they were never all asked, since several filters were used to identify widows or widowers, divorcés, foreigners, and other categories that called for specific sets of questions. Nevertheless, pre-test estimations of 90′–120′ for the interview duration were definitely too optimistic. Considering those lengths, researchers were concerned about the position of "their" questions to avoid loss of attention and non-answers. However, the following analyses will show us that those worries were not justified.

Finally, another problem was translation. We do not evoke here the immigrant oversamples, but the extension of the survey in two German-speaking areas (Bern and Basel) and an Italian-speaking one (Ticino). Running a survey in Switzerland implies a multicultural, multi-linguistic journey with the related challenges of translation validity and result comparability. As far as our central question here (capturing vulnerable persons) is concerned, we used the formal French, Italian, or German and not the dialects; although they are highly popular, especially in the German-speaking part of the country, but they are too diverse. This made the burden for the respondents even higher as standard German often makes the interaction very formal, administrative.

3   Fieldwork

VLV data have been harvested in five cantons representing the linguistic, political, and socioeconomic diversity of Switzerland. The objective was to question 3600 individuals aged 65 and over living in private households or in nursing homes (in Switzerland, "établissement médico-social," or EMS).

The individuals were randomly selected from the official lists of inhabitants, stratified by sex and according to six age groups[2] in each concerned canton in order to ensure the representativeness of our sample within each stratum, but also to have sufficient numbers for each sub-group. Table 2 shows the distributions of the completed interviews.

VLV has been a homemade product not only in its conception but also in its concrete realization. The research team recruited interviewers, organized their training, and supervised the fieldwork from the headquarters in Geneva, with two or three young researchers delegated to each of the five cantons to be in charge of the daily management of a little enterprise, attributing the sample units, controlling the quality of the work done by the employees, saving and transferring the various collected data, etc. This decision not to outsource to a private company was rooted in a tradition and justified with three reasons. Indeed, the 1979 and 1994 surveys were done the same way with approximately the same justifications: transparency, costs, and ideology. First, the idea was to keep complete control over the entire process of data collection from the first to the final stages. The statistics shown in this chapter are byproducts of this will. Second, it is likely that outsourcing would have been

---

[2]65–69 years, 70–74 years, 75–79 years, 80–84 years, 85–89 years, and 90 years and over.

Table 2 Complete interviews by stratum, VLV, five cantons, 2011

	Complete interviews							In percent of the persons solicited						
	Women													
	65–69	70–74	75–79	80–84	85–89	>90	Total	65–69	70–74	75–79	80–84	85–89	>90	Total
Geneva	59	58	61	57	55	61	351	37.3	32.2	33.9	31.8	30.7	34.3	33.3
Valais	58	61	58	59	60	61	357	32.0	31.4	27.6	31.6	36.4	38.6	32.6
Bern	63	65	64	62	62	61	377	37.5	34.0	29.6	24.5	29.0	24.5	29.2
Basel	68	59	59	60	58	60	364	35.1	24.5	24.3	22.5	22.4	17.8	23.6
Ticino	60	57	61	53	62	63	356	33.0	24.3	22.0	21.9	26.4	25.0	25.0
Total	308	299	303	291	297	306	1804	34.9	28.7	26.9	25.8	28.2	26.0	28.2
	Men													
Geneva	58	56	62	58	61	60	355	36.7	31.8	41.1	36.5	39.6	35.3	36.7
Valais	60	60	64	61	61	59	365	40.5	34.3	38.3	34.9	37.7	36.6	36.9
Bern	72	62	66	67	66	64	397	41.9	39.7	34.2	36.8	31.4	29.6	35.2
Basel	67	62	61	59	53	71	373	37.2	38.5	31.4	30.7	24.3	31.8	31.9
Ticino	58	72	56	59	59	61	365	36.9	39.8	27.1	27.6	28.5	26.4	30.5
Total	315	312	309	304	300	315	1855	38.7	36.7	33.9	33.0	31.5	31.5	34.0

more costly, as will be illustrated through the insistence strategy discussed below. Third, from 1979 until now it has always been the fundamental choice of the teams to refuse the distinction between the "noble" intellectual stages of research and the "lowest" ones, those stages concerning the hands-on technical and logistic aspects of carrying out a survey (see Bétemps et al. 1997; Nicolet and Oris (forthcoming). Simply said, managing an in-house survey is carried by the belief that researchers should not limit themselves to analyzing and theorizing about social science data; they should also go out and get their hands dirty while collecting it.

In the following, we discuss the survey procedures and contact strategy, the coverage errors, the refusals and their causes, and to what extent the procedures and their adaptations were efficient to "capture" vulnerable persons in the sample of participants, and we conclude with a comparison of the prevalence of socioeconomic and health vulnerability in VLV and in other data sources.

3.1 Procedures and Contact Strategy

To ensure data quality, a clear approach procedure that could be translated into the three languages was put together. The procedure took into consideration a number of situations that the interviewers would encounter:

- Ego[3] is apt (has the capacity to answer) and lives at home;
- Ego is apt and lives in a nursing home;
- Ego is unapt (at home or in a nursing home);
- Ego does not speak French, German, or Italian.

Before the procedure was launched, the sample members had to be allocated to the interviewers. For that purpose, the interviewers were given contact sheets that contained confidential information concerning ego (surname, forename, address, and phone number). The interviewers had to indicate each contact attempt, the date, whether there had been a visit or phone call, with whom the interviewer had spoken, the result, and in the case of a refusal, the reason(s) (Fig. 1).

The most concrete aspect of the approach procedure was making contact. The two first stages were common to all procedures, with small variations. First, ego received a leaflet presenting the study and a personalized contact letter announcing that an interviewer would phone. In the event that the respondent lived in a nursing home, the first letter was sent to the nursing home direction to inform that one of their residents had been selected to take part in the VLV survey and that an interviewer would contact the management before any other step was taken.

The question arose of which was the best solution for the first contact with ego: to phone or to make a visit at home? For the entire survey with its five regional fields, our team decided on an initial phone contact to ensure the best comparability with the 1994 survey and for other very pragmatic reasons. In some cantons, the

---

[3] "Ego" is the word used in the survey to refer to the interviewed person.

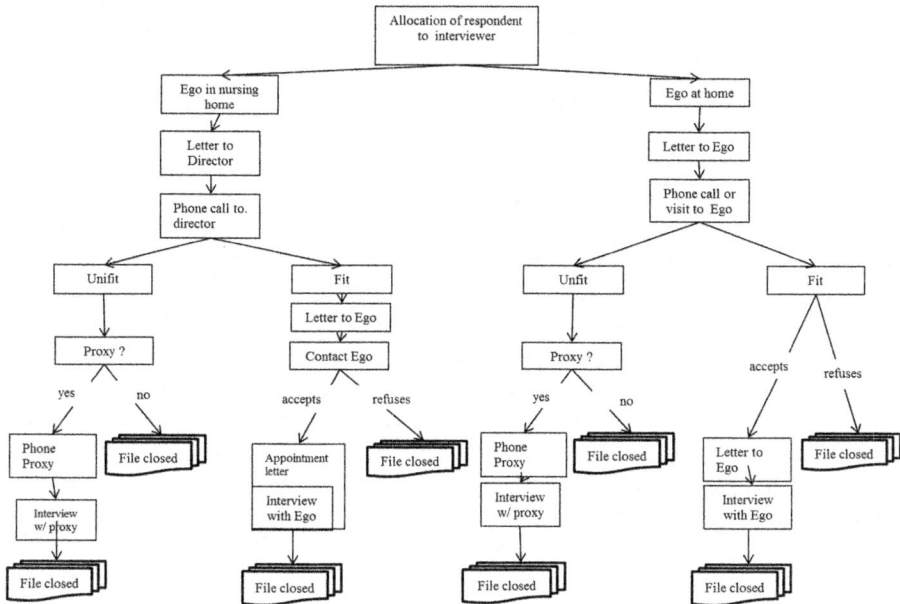

Fig. 1 Approach procedure

distances to be covered for each visit, especially if ego was living in a mountain village, could be long. This would have led to a substantial increase in the costs and would also have increased the time devoted to the survey by the interviewer who would have been reluctant to make such an effort with uncertain rewards.

A home visit was done in only two cases: firstly, when ego had no phone number and, secondly, when ego could not be contacted by phone for 2 weeks. It emerged that 5–26 % of elderly people do not have a phone number indicated in public phone directories, the proportion reaching its maximum in villages in the mountains of Valais, Ticino, and Bern Oberland. In Switzerland, for a population of eight million inhabitants, some four million phone solicitations are made each year for surveys, very often for marketing purposes. Combined with aggressive selling and the increased use of mobile phones, this creates an increasingly difficult environment for scientific surveys (Joye et al. 2012). In this respect, the initial letter was crucial in allaying certain fears.

When contact was made with ego, the interviewer could have been confronted with two situations: the person was apt, i.e. able to answer, and could therefore decide whether he or she agreed or refused to participate in the study, or ego was non-apt. During the phone call, the interviewer could already be able to detect whether ego had cognitive problems by asking simple spatial orientation or temporal questions:

– "Could you suggest a date for the appointment?"
– "Is there an entry code for where you live?"

– "Could you explain how to get to where you live?"
– "Could you remind me of your address?"

If ego appeared not to have the capacity to answer, the interviewer had to activate the so-called proxy procedure, asking the assistance of a close friend, relative, or caregiver to answer a short questionnaire of some 60 questions. Similarly, if ego was living in a nursing home, when the interviewer contacted the management, he or she would obtain information on ego's health, that is to say his or her ability to participate in the survey. If the reply was affirmative, a first contact letter was sent to ego to provide the person, just as the other sample members, with information on VLV and to allow him or her to express informed acceptance or refusal to take part. Otherwise, the proxy procedure was applied.

If ego was no able to answer, it was rare that the person could be directly contacted, but contact was made with a spouse, family member, guardian, or the nursing home. In such a case, the interviewer would suggest to one of the aforesaid to participate in the survey by replying to a limited number of questions on ego. This "proxy" procedure, as indicated above, was initially the only procedure to diverge from the standard one. It was essential to avoid the trap, still too frequent in gerontology surveys, of not gathering data on individuals who are in very bad physical health and/or suffering from cognitive problems. It was all the more crucial to ensure correct comparability with the 1994 survey, since the weight of diseases such as Parkinson's or Alzheimer's has constantly increased in the causes of death of the very old (80 years and more), in Switzerland as elsewhere (Berrut and Junker 2008). This procedure allowed us to interview 555 close friends, relatives, or caregivers, which represents somewhat more than 15 % of all the interviews collected (Table 3). Without this special procedure and its adapted questionnaire, an entire segment of the population would have been excluded and the sample of respondents seriously biased.

In the framework of the standard procedure, once contact had been made with ego or a proxy, several situations could arise:

1. Ego had died. The file was then closed for reason of death;
2. Ego was no longer living in the same place, with three possible situations:

Table 3 Number of proxy interviews by age and gender of ego, VLV, five cantons, 2011

Age	Women	Men	Total
65–69	4	3	7
70–74	8	9	17
75–79	17	15	32
80–84	45	45	90
85–89	75	63	138
90+	158	113	271
Total	307	248	555

- Ego had moved outside the territory concerned by the survey; his or her file was closed under the category "no reply" (NR),
- Ego had moved but had remained in the area of the survey; the first letter was forwarded to the new address,
- Ego had moved into a nursing home; the contact letter was sent to the director of the nursing home,

3. Ego had not received the first letter, so it therefore had to be sent again and ego had to be called a few days later;
4. Ego had received the letter.

When the interviewer was finally in situation 4, he/she was faced by one of three situations:

(a) Ego refused. The file was closed due to refusal;
(b) Ego hesitated and wished to see the questionnaire before deciding;
(c) Ego accepted and an appointment was made with the interviewer.

In cases b and c, a second letter was sent to ego. It contained:

- the self-administered questionnaire (SAQ)
- the personalized life history calendar (LHC)
- the information leaflet explaining in greater detail the survey and the confidentiality of personal data
- If an appointment was made, a letter of confirmation was sent.

Following the second letter, ego may:

- refuse by calling the interviewer or the cantonal office;
- in situation b, accept and set up an appointment with the interviewer.

3.2 Coverage Errors and Mistakes in the Samples

Figure 2 shows the concrete results of the procedures described above. We will discuss the refusals in the next section. Here, we deal with the coverage errors that affected no <13 % of the original sample.

People who cannot be found at the address provided by the cantonal and federal population or statistical offices reflect discrepancies between the target population and the sampling frame. These problems can be explained by the length of the VLV field and consequently a growing temporal duration between the samples extracted from the lists of inhabitants, but also because the latter are theoretically updated every 3 months, and obviously less often in some municipalities. Other discrepancies are due to the very nature of ageing, such as risks of dying or moving to an institution between the date of the population enumeration and the date of a contact attempt by a VLV collaborator.

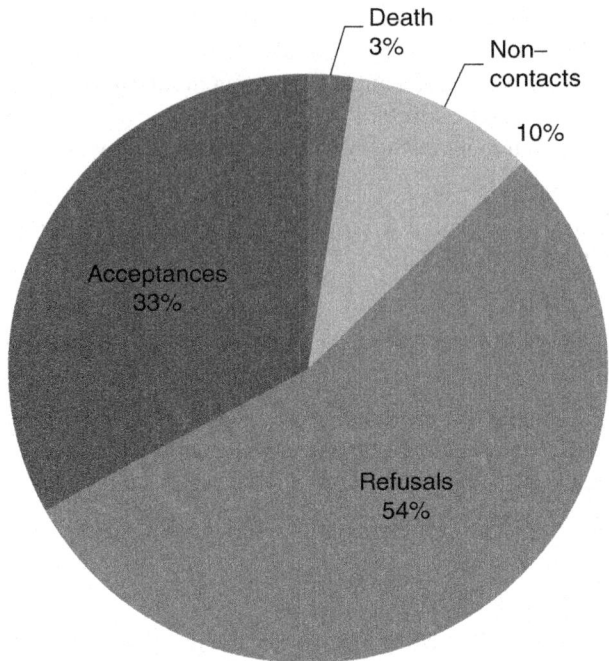

Fig. 2 Distribution of the four types of individual outcomes, VLV, five cantons, 2011

On the ground, it was decided that a home visit would be a last resort when unable to contact ego by telephone. Therefore, if there was no phone number and no reply after 2 weeks, the interviewer contacted the relevant commune (municipality) to find out whether ego was still living in the same place, had moved or had died. The communes and post offices (sometimes the priests also, and neighbors) proved to be very helpful throughout the data collection stage. Another source of coverage error appeared during the fieldwork. In Geneva, it happens that people have a postal box in the canton but in reality live in France, the former being their formal address, explaining why they were on the lists of inhabitants and were included in our sample. This comes from a law regarding civil servants that was abrogated some years ago, but the practice survived. In Valais, several persons have their formal residence in a chalet in the mountains while it is in fact a secondary residence. Usually this is for fiscal purposes. At the end, in 14.1 % of the 4105 files opened in Geneva and Valais, it was impossible to make contact with the person. For the five cantons altogether, 10 % of the files were in this situation, which is a bit less than the average proportion observed in European countries in the 2004 round of the Survey on Health, Ageing and Retirement (De Luca and Peracchi 2005, 94).

Those cases were costly in terms of management time. From the attribution of the contact sheet to the interviewer to the transfer of the complete interview to the headquarters, it took on average some 40 days for a full participation in the survey;

the length was 60 days in cases of non-contact (NR in Fig. 2), to harvest nothing at the end. It was consequently also very negative for the motivation of the interviewers who had to deal with those cases.

3.3   Many Refusals

Figure 2 shows that we ended with 54 % refusals against 33 % acceptances. For Groves and Couper (1998), individuals who refuse to take part in a survey are more likely to be uninterested in the topics of the survey; not have the time; or find it difficult to understand the language of the questionnaire, which would indicate a low level of education, or different origins and partial learning of the host society's language, or both. Analysis of the reasons for refusals bears out their first judgments (see Fig. 3, which reports the percentage of men and women citing each reason). For Geneva and Valais in 2011, the refusals "without reason" dominated, but among those who gave some justification, a lack of interest was top of the list, which justified more than one refusal in five. This was followed by health problems, being "too tired," or being "too old," with around 14 %; and inversely, being too busy with 8/9 %. Personal and family reasons, which often expressed a desire to protect one's intimacy, varied between 6 and 8 %; and a clear rejection of surveys ("I don't want to be a guinea pig") was manifested by 7/8 %. Men were somewhat more likely to refuse without explanation, while women more frequently indicated their absence of interest or desire. Globally, however, an obvious gender pattern does not emerge.

As we can see in Table 4, the two main causes are not particularly affected by age, but among the oldest old, 31 % of the nonagenarians refused without explanation. As we could expect, health problems or feeling tired or too old is a reason that

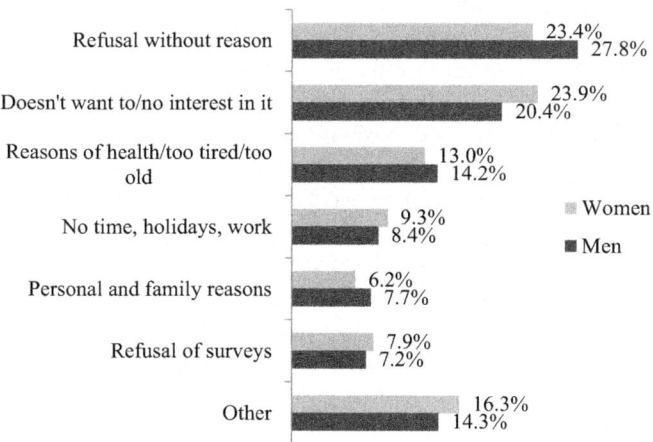

Fig. 3 Reasons for refusal to participate in the VLV survey, by sex, Geneva–Valais, 2011

Table 4 Reasons for refusal to participate in the VLV survey, by age, Geneva-Valais, 2011 (in %)

Age groups	65–69	70–74	75–79	80–84	85–89	90+	Total
Reasons							
Refusal without reason	25	26	24	24	24	31	25
Doesn't want to/no interest in it	24	26	25	22	18	17	22
Reasons of health/too tired/too old	8	7	10	16	22	23	14
No time, holidays, work	18	12	9	5	4	2	9
Refusal of surveys	11	9	7	7	7	4	8
Personal and family reasons	2	7	6	8	8	10	7
Other	12	14	18	17	16	13	15
Total	100	100	100	100	100	100	100

increases with age. Personal and family reasons show the same pattern, being a marginal factor among those aged 65–69, then growing in importance. Protecting intimacy is more of a concern for the oldest old. Interestingly, the rejection of the survey appears as more "modern"; it is more of a reason in the recent cohorts that in the older ones. Refusing "to be a guinea pig" and similar expressions reached 11 % among the 65–69 cohort and then continuously fall to 4 % among those aged 90 and more. As we could expect, being busy with work, holidays, or other activities was also important among those who had just retired and strongly decreased, becoming marginal from the age of 80.

This issue is crucial, since the credibility—and consequently, the survival—of surveys as a tool for the social sciences seems to be engaged when so many potential participants refuse to contribute. However, it is difficult to go deeper into this issue right now, because we know very little about these persons, aside from the little data provided by the administrative files when the samples were delivered. Some logistic regressions on refusals and acceptances, respectively, are not shown because they only brought limited additional information: higher participation of men and people living in urban areas, and those aged 80–84 showing the lowest propensity to contribute. In terms of interactions, the sex of the interviewer (whatever the sex of the sample member) and his or her age had no impact. While an initial recruitment condition to work for VLV was to have a bachelor's degree in social sciences (in a broad sense), it appears that the interviewer's level of education had no effect. Only the interviewer's accumulated experience increased the probability of obtaining an acceptance from the sample members, but this is a tautological result, since those with few successes were discouraged and gave up.

3.4 Adaptations and the Inclusion of Vulnerable Populations

Faced with so many refusals, the VLV team decided against using standard 'refusal conversion' efforts (see Groves and Lyberg 2010, 872) for ethical (ideological) reasons. A "no" has to be respected. However, to reduce the number of negative

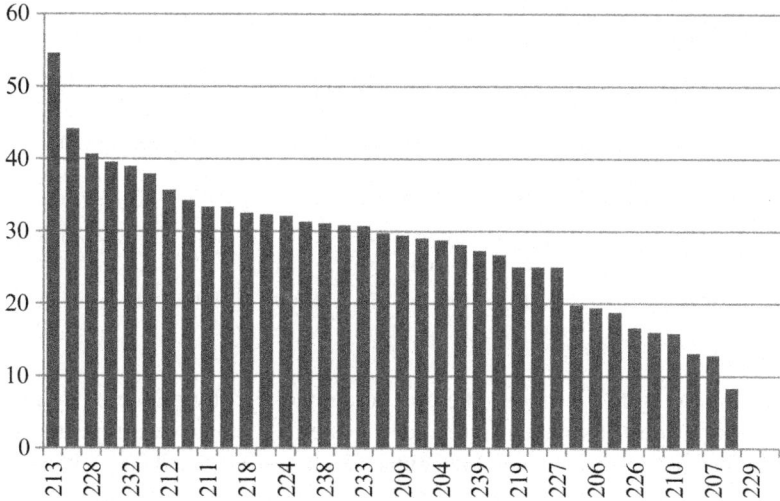

Fig. 4 Rates of acceptance per interviewer, VLV, Valais, 2011

answers as much as possible, we chose to have some interviewers specialize; they were requested to make the first phone contact, not only for themselves but for the entire team. The crucial nature of this first interaction has been studied for some 15 years (see Snijkers et al. 1999; Durrant et al. 2010) and now appears to be an explanation for national variations, as well as being likely to affect the comparability of results (Blom et al. 2011). In our case, certain interviewers clearly proved to be more effective than others in obtaining the cooperation of potential participants. Figure 4 shows the success rates per interviewer in Valais. A similar distribution was observed in the other four cantons. With a large majority of collaborators showing an average level of efficiency, with approximately one in every four being clearly less efficient, several champions emerge. In each field, they became famous as heroes of the survey journey. By distributing the appointments obtained by the more persuasive collaborators throughout the entire team, we managed to prevent any increase in interviewer effect. This is a typical illustration of our initial compromise: combining maximum flexibility to obtain as many acceptances to participate as possible, but applying the same questionnaires and interview mode to all of the participants, apart from those unable to answer, as rigorously as possible.

A second strategy was to show endurance and accept large extensions in the duration of the fieldwork. It was our wish to never force an individual to take part in the survey, but also to insist as much as possible until having a clear reply directly from ego. This obstinacy was costly, both in time and money. When the fieldwork was launched, it was estimated that we would need around 3 months per canton to gather the data—in the end, it took us 8 months per canton. Table 5 explains why. In Geneva and Valais, 4105 people were contacted to obtain 1428 acceptances (including both proxies and "normal" interviews). Roughly 25 % of the latter were

Table 5 Types of contact by final outcome type, Geneva and Valais, 2011

	Completed interviews		Found dead		Non-contacts		Refusals		All files	
	N	%	N	%	N	%	N	%	N	%
0–2 calls	749	52.45	67	66.34	118	20.38	1039	54.54	2001	48.75
3–4 calls	325	22.76	12	11.88	67	11.57	384	20.16	809	19.71
5+ calls	239	16.74	16	15.84	126	21.76	332	17.43	730	17.78
Visit	113	7.91	5	4.95	240	41.45	148	7.77	508	12.38
Not noted	2	0.14	1	0.99	28	4.84	2	0.1	57	1.39
Total	1428	100	101	100	579	100	1905	100	4105	100

obtained following five or more attempts to contact ego by phone or by a visit to the home to request his or her agreement. Generally, in surveys repeated calls is a well-known strategy to reduce noncontacts, while home visits are barely part of the procedures. Indeed, Groves and Lyberg (2010, 872) rightly insist on the costs of obstinacy. Take the example of a car drive through a mountain village with uncertain results. However, without those home visits and knocking directly on the door of ego, we would have lost almost 8 % of the final participants, and without calling five times and more (until 23), we would have missed 17 %. The potential related biases are assessed below.

This question of bias is important and less obvious that it seems at first glance. Indeed, if certain sub-populations reply less than others and efforts to increase the general response rate are made without taking this into account, such efforts would potentially result in an increase in the selective bias (Peytchev et al. 2009, 786; Roberts et al. 2014). However, when walking the tightrope between ethical evidence of respect for refusals and the wish to obtain a reply directly from ego, whatever this reply may be, could we consider that our procedures worked? Can we conclude that insistence and recourse to proxies allowed more vulnerable individuals to be included in the survey? Of course, we assume that the risk of capturing too many vulnerable people is illusionary.

To provide initial replies to this question, Figs. 5 and 6 represent the distribution of interviews obtained by age group, for men and for women. By differentiating the different procedures according to age and gender, we are able to conduct a more detailed analysis on the impact of our perseverance. We also take into account the proxies and individuals who were contacted by the standard procedure. We therefore have five categories: 1 or 2 calls to obtain participation, 3 or 4 calls, 5 calls and more, a visit (to ego's home), and proxy. In addition, Table 6 shows the statuses of functional health and each of the respective depression categories, which in both cases are distributed according to the type of procedure that allowed information to be obtained.

Among the participants, women aged 75–79 and men aged 75–84 were the most difficult to contact by phone. The 75–84 cohort required the heaviest procedure of a home visit most often. An initial explanation is linked to the availability of a phone

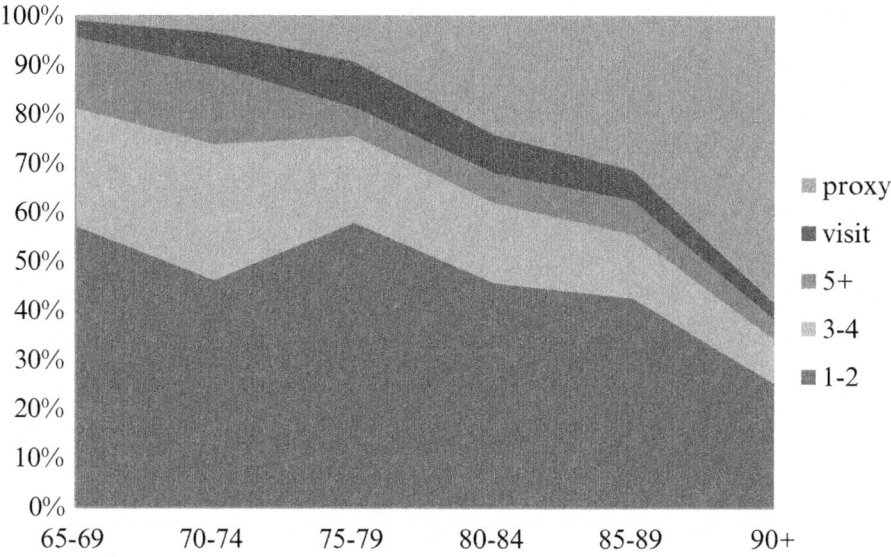

Fig. 5 Distribution of respondents by approach procedure and age group, Geneva–Valais, women, 2011

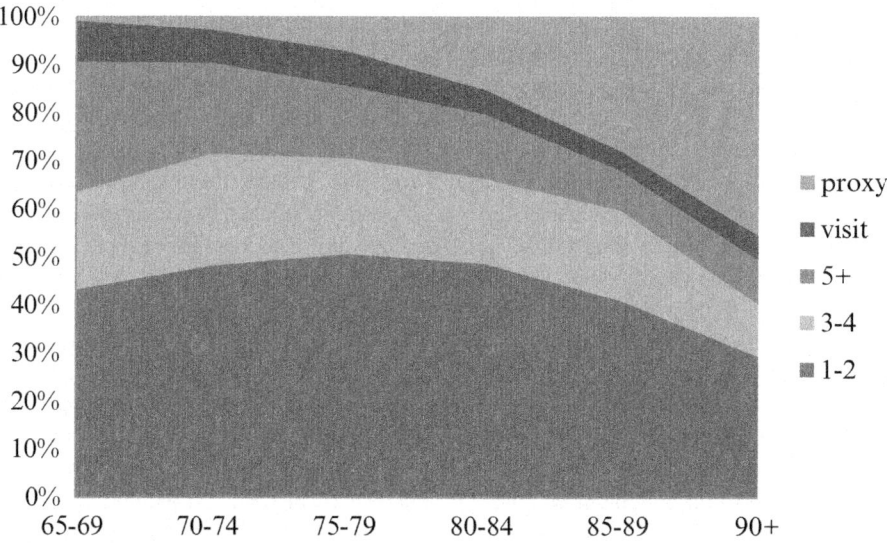

Fig. 6 Distribution of respondents by approach procedure and age group, Geneva–Valais, men, 2011

number. In Valais, we had no phone numbers to contact roughly 22 % of the women in this stratum. Both men and women aged 75–84 were also the groups in which the rates of refusal to participate in the survey were the highest, with reasons that mixed

Table 6 Statuses of functional health or depression by type of procedure, weighted data. VLV, five cantons

Procedure type/status	Call(s) 1–4		Calls 5+		Visit		Proxy	
	N	%	N	%	N	%	N	%
Functional health statuses								
Independent	786	80.5	164	81.4	72	76.6	20	12.9
In difficulty	123	12.6	24	12.2	14	15.1	24	15.1
Dependent	53	5.4	7	3.6	5	5.8	110	70.0
Unknown	14	1.4	6	2.9	2	2.5	3	2
Total	976	100	201	100	93	100	157	100
Depression categories								
Good health	582	59.6	124	61.2	47	50.5	19	12.1
Worried	237	24.3	46	22.9	34	36.6	23	14.6
Depressed	143	14.7	31	15.4	12	12.9	66	42.0
Unknown	14	1.4	1	0.5	0	0.0	49	31.2
Total	976	100	201	100	93	100	157	100

those of the oldest old and the young old (Table 4). Taking into account the evidence collected in another study (Duvoisin et al. 2012), we put forward the hypothesis that a fair proportion of individuals aged 75–84 tend to live their experience of ageing negatively. They are affected by biological changes, realize that their losses exceed their gains, and suffer from this evolution, which leads them to refuse useful offers from associations working for the elderly; similarly, they are also more likely to refuse to participate in a survey "on the old" (Duvoisin et al. 2012). This interpretation requires more research, of course, but all elements at this stage point in this direction. In any event, the complicated and costly procedure of home visits allowed the survey to include relatively isolated individuals in borderline age groups between what is widely referred to as the 3rd and 4th ages, that is to say, between 75 and 84.

In the same order of ideas, repeated phone calls—from 5 to as many as 23—mainly appeared useful for contacting and convincing the "young old," exactly those whose refusals were largely explained by a lack of time, holidays, or work. This is all coherent, and we must also give credit to obstinacy. Whilst this observation is valid for both sexes, the greatest effort had to be made to reach the men. Participation was obtained after five or more phone calls in around 15 % of the cases, versus a little <9 % among women for this type of recruitment. This originates from two phenomena. One is mechanical, since the number of proxies is lower on the male side (16.5 %, against 21.3 % for women). This confirms the well-known health–gender paradox, according to which women live longer than men but age with worse health (see Van Oyen et al. 2013). Another explanation has more of a psychosocial nature, since experience in the field showed that wives often blocked phone calls, feeling the need to protect their husband (who were generally older than they were) from aggressive phone canvassing or suspected risks of invasion of privacy. This does not emerge very clearly on Fig. 3, for which we wished to avoid overly subjective coding.

The proxy procedure obviously centers on the oldest individuals. Initially, it may appear less heavy than a standard procedure (shorter questionnaire, fewer letters to be sent), but the Valais figure for the time spent on each case shows that this approach required great perseverance to obtain the desired result, since it required just as much time, if not more, depending on the strata. An average of 43 days was needed to close a proxy file for the men, whereas 38 days were needed for a normal procedure. It could take time to discover that ego was non-apt (and/or moved into a nursing home), and contacting a close friend, relative, or caregiver of ego and making an appointment was more complicated than with the retired sample members, since at least 50 % of the proxies had a job.

With Table 6, we touch even more directly the central question: the inclusion of vulnerable people. Whilst we could have hoped that our insistence on contacting the sampled individuals by repeated phone calls would allow us to capture more vulnerable individuals, the results on functional health, in fact, point in the other direction: when we repeatedly insisted on participation by calling repeatedly, there were more independent individuals than those among the files obtained easily (after 1–4 calls), as many people in difficulty, and fewer dependents. This can be explained by what Figs. 5 and 6 showed—that is to say, the relative youth of the respondents recruited in this way. In their case, by seeking out dynamic seniors in this way, we tended to avoid a negative bias that would have underestimated their global good health and numerous activities.

Home visits, on the other hand, allowed significantly more people to be recruited whose functional status was described as "in difficulty," which can be considered a latent state of vulnerability. But the proxy procedure—although requiring great insistence—turned out to be even more important in accounting for the vulnerable aged than we expected. As a reminder, somewhat less than one file out of six was obtained in this way, but no <70 % of the individuals included in this way were in a situation of dependency.

When we look at the second panel of Table 6, which describes categories of mental health, we find confirmation that repeated calls did not help to capture more vulnerable people, when compared with those whose participation was obtained easily, which already included some 15 % of persons who were depressed but participated anyway. Home visits were once again—and in fact, much more clearly than for functional health—useful for obtaining the contributions of those in a latent state of vulnerability—the "worried"—to the survey. Additionally, the proxy procedure confirmed its usefulness for including people who were obviously vulnerable, with 4 or more symptoms of depression. However, Table 6 also shows a trade-off: in 32 % of the cases, we were not able to establish the category of mental health because of item non-response. Indeed, the questions that constitute the Wang test of psychic health were the only ones about ego's feelings in the proxy questionnaire, due to the importance of this dimension in any assessment of well-being among the elderly. But we can understand that approximately one in three proxies refused or were unable to guess ego's pleasure, sadness, etc.

At this stage, it is fair to note that the inclusive approach based on recourse to a proxy was recently criticized. In this critical perspective, an individual whose cognitive capacities have deteriorated should be excluded from the process; indeed, such an individual cannot really give his or her informed consent and someone who ego has not necessarily designated replies to questions concerning ego. Depending on how close this person is to ego, the social situation, socioeconomic status, and, a fortiori, past life of ego will be documented with some degree of uncertainty. It is this "silence by proxy" (Fillit et al. 2010) that is thus being denounced. An answer could be that the absence of impaired elderly in the survey, the scientific results, and ultimately the citizen debates about the social and political management of ageing would be another form of highly negative silence. At the same time, the ethical question, i.e. the point at which the individual's consent was informed, cannot just be rejected.[4] We face here a real tension.

3.5   Prevalence of Vulnerabilities in VLV and Other Data Sources

To the instructive but indirect evidence discussed above, this section adds the results of a benchmark approach, comparing the prevalence of forms of vulnerability in the VLV's final sample of respondents with the numbers that can be found in other data sources.

Being poor is an obvious state of vulnerability, since the poverty line is fixed by a confederation of Swiss institutions of social help and applied all across the country. This threshold is set at a monthly income of 2450 SFr. per person. In VLV, we used 2400 to simplify, and the poverty rate in the sample reached 17.9 % for men and 23.3 % for women. Table 7 offers a comparison with four other studies. Variations can generally be explained with the use of different sources, definitions, and temporal differences. However, between the SILC use of the 60 % median income level and the SKOS/CSIAS (2013) threshold, the difference is marginal (2450 versus 2500 SFr. in 2012). It can also be pointed out that there is no significant

Table 7 Estimates of poverty among the elderly in twenty-first century Switzerland

Rate(s) of poverty	Year	Source	Reference
17.9–23.3 %	2011–2012	VLV	Gabriel et al. (2015)
18–21.6 %	2008	OECD	Pilgram and Seifert (2009)
16.2 %	2008–2010	SILC[a]	Guggisberg et al. (2012)
13.3 %	2000	LIS[b]	Nolan and Marx (2009)
9.9–15.4 %	2003	Fiscal data	Wanner et al. (2008)

[a]Statistics on income and living conditions
[b]Luxembourg income study

---

[4]Dealing with the other point, the validity of the answers given by ego or a proxy, respectively, is part of the ongoing doctoral thesis of Aude Tholomier on octogenarians and nonagenarians.

evidence that the "Great Recession" from 2008 has affected the economic well-being of the Swiss elderly, as it did in many other European countries (Cavasso and Weber 2014). Globally, we can conclude that VLV faced the challenge of fair inclusion of the poor in the survey with success.

For functional health, the VLV estimates can be compared with two recent reports from the Swiss Federal Statistical Office on the elderly living in private households (Bundesamt für Statistik [OFS/BFS] 2014) and in institutions (Bundesamt für Statistik 2012). According to the findings of the VLV survey, 86.9 % of people aged 65 and more were found to be independent, as opposed to the 91 % claimed by the first OFS/BFS study. Moreover, VLV estimates that 6.9 % of elderly people are in a situation of difficulty, meaning that they are generally able to accomplish all activities of daily living themselves but uneasily for at least one of them. Additionally, an estimated 6.1 % are no longer capable of performing their daily activities independently, meaning that they require external help with at least one activity. Contrasting these results, the BFS/OFS report found 7 % of elderly people in Switzerland with difficulties[5] and 2 % being completely dependent. Based on the comparison with this first report, VLV seems to have slightly over-reported the prevalence of dependence in the population. The differences between the VLV data and the aforementioned report, however, are most likely due to differences in their samples: whereas VLV also included people living in nursing-homes, the OFS/BFS study exclusively considered those living in private households.

In the second report that focused exclusively on elderly people living in care institutions (Bundesamt für Statistik 2012) the numbers change drastically: 96 % of individuals were found to have trouble accomplishing at least 1 activity of daily living; thus, only 4 % of individuals were completely independent. The analysis was restricted to a population that was no longer living in their own households due to the importance of their restrictions in managing their daily lives, which explains these very high percentages. Given these two selective and therefore biased sources, however, it seems plausible that VLV generally captured a relatively representative sample of the general population, in terms of functional health, especially thanks to the proxy procedure.

Finally, comparing the mental health findings in VLV with those from other sources was not a straightforward task, since there are many indicators to measure depressive symptoms, different classifications to determine the actual categories and statuses of psychic health or to measure the intensity of depressive disturbances, and generally very little research on the topic of elderly people with depression. A relatively exhaustive report on depression among the Swiss population by the Swiss Health Observatory (OBSAM) estimated the prevalence of depressive symptoms among the elderly population (Baer et al. 2013). The results are summarized and contrasted with VLV figures in Table 8.

---

[5]The report distinguishes between "minor" and "major" difficulties, whereas these categories are collapsed in VLV. Thus, the percentages for minor difficulties (6 %) and major difficulties (1 %) are were merged to compare them to the VLV data.

Table 8 Comparison of two estimates of depression prevalence among the Swiss elderly (in %)

Depression categories	Baer et al.	VLV	Baer et al.	VLV
Age groups	65–74		75+	
No symptoms	74.8	74.4	65.7	58.9
Minor symptoms	23.0	18.1	31.2	26.4
Intermediary to strong symptoms	2.2	7.6	3.2	14.7

Despite the cautiousness needed when comparing these findings, it can be seen that depression was reported more often in the VLV data. Both studies found that roughly 75 % of the population was free from any symptoms of depression in the 65–74 age group. VLV, however, lowered the estimation of persons with minor signs of depression and suggested that there were more than three times as many people suffering from intermediary to strong depressive symptoms in this age group, compared to the OBSAN report. Among those aged 75 or higher, individuals who are not vulnerable or in a latent state of vulnerability were proportionally less represented in the VLV data, where we once again find much higher estimates for people who were obviously vulnerable, from a mental health point of view.

The challenge was to avoid or at least limit the risk of differential rates of answers between vulnerable and secure sample members leading to the exclusion of the former. Although the rate of participation for VLV was low and although it is not really possible to provide a strict, definite answer with the comparisons discussed above, all of the evidence is clearly positive and suggests a fair inclusion of the vulnerable elderly in the survey.

4 Responses and Non-response in the Questionnaires

The last part of this chapter considers item non-response, revealing questions that participants were unable to understand or that made them uncomfortable, if not reluctant to answer. In this perspective, we assume that non-answers are not equally distributed among the participants and could reflect vulnerabilities. Since we are not intrinsically vulnerable but vulnerable to something, through an analysis of non-response, we have a chance to identify some perturbing factors that have affected VLV respondents and could ultimately affect the validity of the measures based on this material (Groves and Lyberg 2010, 856).

Concretely, in the VLV leaflets as well as at the beginning of the interview, the participants were instructed that they could refuse to answer at any time, without justification, and move to the next question, or interrupt the process and renounce their participation.[6] Of course, the use of this freedom does not adhere to the same

---

[6]The cases of break-off were quite dramatic for the interviewer and took a large role in the team discussions, but they were ultimately statistically rare.

Table 9 Distribution of non-responses in the VLV self-administered questionnaire, by thematic chapter

Chapter	Non-response	Chapter	Non-response
B. Parents	4 %	J. Formal care	17 %
C. Children and grand-children	2 %	K. Lifestyles (health)	2 %
D. Pension	7 %	L. Relational life	5 %
E. Lodging	6 %	M. Religion	5 %
F. Media	14 %	N. Changes in life	13 %
G. Social life	27 %	O. Opinions	11 %
H. Transportation	13 %	P. Health and medical problems	6 %
I. Health	6 %	Total	11 %

logic when the old person is confronted with the self-administered questionnaire, what it means with him- or herself, compared with the face-to-face interaction with the interviewer. This is why we made a distinction between the two tools in the following, starting with a section on item non-responses in the first questionnaire, based on a systematic analysis. Then, we follow with a second section on two non-representative but especially eloquent cases of delicate information collected during the interview: household monthly incomes and the results of the cognition tests.

4.1 Non-responses in the Self-Administered Questionnaire

Table 9 shows the various thematic chapters in their order of appearance in the questionnaire. For the 3080 participants (proxy questionnaires excluded), non-responses represented an average of 11 %, but with a large variability, from 2 %, for the questions on children, to 27 %, when social life is concerned. Coming back to points that have been discussed at the beginning of this chapter, we did not observe a direct effect of the length of the questionnaire. We made the bet that locating the "health and medical problems" topic at the very end would provoke renewed attention, since it is an important concern for the elderly, and it seemed to have worked. Otherwise, the vision offered by Table 9 is too vague. It is clear that the probability of non-response is associated with some thematic chapters, but it does not suggest obvious explanations. To take further steps, we need to look at Fig. 7, which shows the distribution the item nonresponse rate across the 150 questions.

Generally, the average is artificially increased, since peaks of non-response are observed for the item "other(s)" all along the questionnaire, concluding long lists of possible answers. While it is easy to understand why the survey designers systematically included this option, many participants obviously did not understand the rationale of choosing this modality. Similarly but also differently, long, repetitive series of items produced misunderstandings. This happened in the "social life" chapter, in which the participants were asked if they were currently members of

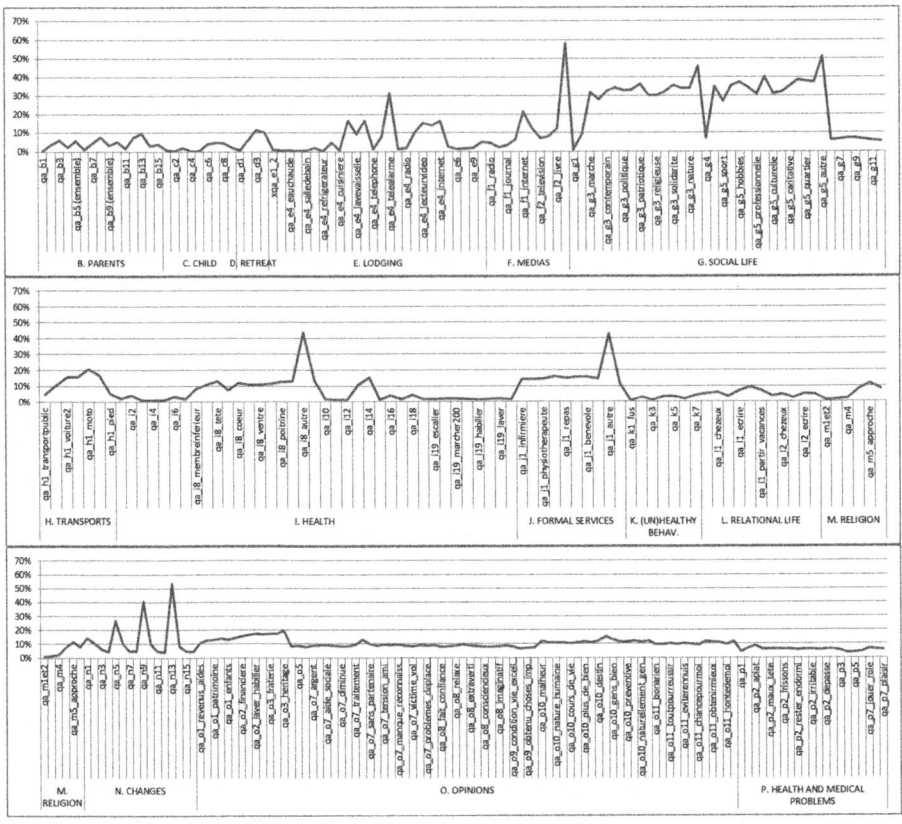

Fig. 7 Distribution of non-response in the VLV self-administered questionnaire

an association or not and were confronted with a list of 14 items.[7] Moreover, for obvious reasons of memory mobilization, the same list was asked just afterwards but concerning membership at the age of 45. Several checks showed that older participants ticked off the types of associations that they were or had been members of, but not the others, with an absence of responses meaning "no." Such behavior explains the high values in the "social life" chapter but also appears all across the self-administered questionnaire from time to time. Significantly, this behavior is not associated with the sex or age of the respondent.

Another logic emerges in chapters E and F on lodging and media, respectively. Indeed, non-responses are concentrated on specific technologies like microwaves, remote alarm, computers, and the Internet. Not surprisingly, this is associated with

---

[7]Walking clubs; sports associations; political, professional, patriotic, and religious, groups; charities; etc.

a strong age effect. It reflects a dis-adjustment process to recent technologies among the oldest old, who do not answer questions they do not understand.

The non-answers in the chapter on "care" call upon all the explanations discussed above. There are relatively moderate (12–16 %), but the value for the "other" item explodes to 43 %. This is a more frequent pattern among the oldest old, who are the more frequent users of care, by far, but who are confronted with a list of various caregivers and another list of various types of help and tick off only positive answers, leaving the unused responses blank.

Finally, people generally answered when asked to express their opinions, although some questions provoked a significant rate of non-response (10–15 %) and a few were rejected by 16–20 % of the participants. A more careful look shows that the second and third categories contain questions formulated in an impersonal way. Instead of engaging the surveyed person directly, they are of a general nature. For example, "Do you agree with the following sentences? 'Hard blows hurt people by chance.' 'Human nature is fundamentally good,'" etc. A fair proportion of the respondents felt unable to take a position and/or did not understand the rationale of such questions. Significantly, those questions were the only ones with significant percentages of non-valid answers (in most of the cases because two modalities of answers were ticked off, instead of only one). When financial issues are concerned,[8] the rates of non-response grew further still and women were more likely to refuse.

4.2 Non-response in the Face-to-Face Interview

We find a similar pattern when we move to questionnaire 2, which was administered during a face-to-face interview, and more specifically for the question on household monthly income. The delicate aspect of interrogating people on their revenues is well-known. In the 1970 survey in Geneva and Valais, this information was missing in 13.9 % of the cases; this proportion grew to 23.9 % in 1994. However, this trend was interrupted, since the figure for 2011/2012 is 14 % for the two same cantons, and 15 % when we consider the five cantons of the full VLV survey (Gabriel 2015). The participants were not asked to provide a number but just to make a choice between nine categories.[9] This approach was explicitly chosen to make the respondents' job easier and increase the answer rate. Generally, people do not answer such questions because they do not want to, but also because they do not know. To go deeper, Table 10 provides the results of a logistic regression on non-response to monthly household income.

---

[8]Question O2 offers a good illustration. Its formulation is "Generally, who—the family or the State—has to be responsible for:—financial help?" The modalities of the answers are only the family, mainly the family, both equally, mainly the State, and only the State.

[9]Less than 1200, 1200–2400, 2400–3600, 3600–4800, 4800–6000, 6000–7200, 7200–10,000, 10,000–15,000, 15,000 and more.

Table 10 Logistic regression on non-response, monthly household income, VLV, 2011

Variables	Exp(B)
Women	1.51***
Canton Valais (ref. Geneva)	0.92
Bern	0.57***
Basel	0.94
Ticino	1.61
Age group 70–74 (ref. 65–69)	1.24
75–79	1.04
80–84	1.52**
85–89	1.82***
90+	2.29***
Low education (ref. Apprenticeship)	1.03
Higher education	1.59***
Constant	0.09***
Observations	3038
Log likelihood	−1316.30
Akaike inf. crit.	2658.59

Note: *p < 0.10; **p < 0.05; ***p < 0.01

First, women had a 51 % higher probability of not answering the question on household monthly income, compared to men, and the oldest old were also much more prone to missing this information. The odd ratios were significantly higher from the age of 80 and continuously increased until reaching 2.29 among the nonagenarians, with 65–69 being the reference category. As far as those demographic groups are concerned, VLV is not different from other surveys in Europe and North America (Groves and Couper 1998; Malter 2013). More specific but difficult to interpret, the participants were more likely to give this information in the canton of Bern, where the poverty rate is low, and were much less likely to do so in the canton of Ticino, where the poverty rate is the highest. More conclusive are the results about education, which proved to be a robust indicator of social class (Gabriel 2015), largely predicting poverty in old age (Gabriel et al. 2015). Compared to those with apprenticeships, which is the reference group and also the largest group, people with low education had a similar probability of giving information on the revenues on their revenues. However, persons with superior diplomas were almost 60 % more likely to refuse to give an indication, even though they quite probably knew their incomes well. While the evidence discussed in the preceding part consistently suggests that poor elderly have been properly included in the VLV survey, we see here that the distribution of non-response cannot result in a measurement error, i.e., in an under-estimation of the socioeconomically vulnerable.

In a second analysis, we consider another crucial dimension that was quite delicate to ask questions about: cognition. It is a key variable when aiming to identify and explain the mechanisms that generate or avoid vulnerability and permit resilience in old age. Cognitive abilities are important resources when coping with developmental tasks and age-related challenges, and have been shown to be a powerful factor that affects successful regulation in the interplay between age, personal, motivational, and social resources, and well-being and functional health (e.g., Baltes and Lang 1993; Köhler et al. 2011). Well-preserved cognitive resources represent a core dimension of well-being and mental health in old age. On the other hand, Lawton et al. (1999) showed that over 60 % of the participants aged 70 and older in a US survey would not wish to live any longer under any condition of cognitive impairment. Cognitive decline was more threatening to older adults' quality of life than functional impairment or pain. Such fears are both expressed and nourished by the mediatization of the so-called "epidemics" of cognitive impairments, even though Alzheimer's disease and other diseases sharing the same etiology are not contagious at all. This context makes assessing cognition in large-scale surveys like VLV quite important and delicate at the same time.

To understand the reasons of non-response in the cognition items, we developed a more complete model than that for household incomes. This model indeed takes also the interviewer effect and the context into account.[10] The premise is that interviews are a complex process of information exchange, in which different elements that could introduce bias into the responses may interfere (Groves et al. 2004). In the existing literature about the interviewer effect, a set of variables is identified that can explain the phenomenon in an operational way and can be categorized into four fields that interfere in the "interviewing act": (a) aspects related to the interviewer's characteristics, (b) aspects related to the respondent's characteristics, (c) the conditions and context of the research, and (d) characteristics related to the research tool (questionnaire). The latter category is mainly related to the questionnaire's design, clearness of the definitions, terms used, format, etc. Category c) considers the environmental conditions of the interview (e.g., place, presence of other persons), as well as the collection methodology used, the standardization of the interview conditions, the training and supervision of the interviewers, and also the monitoring and observation of these variables by the interviewers and researchers (Durrant et al. 2010; Groves and Lyberg 2010; Marchese 2011; Blom et al. 2011).

The interviewer effect is operationalized for VLV research by three sets of variables regarding the interviewer, respondent, and context, respectively. For the fourth component—the questionnaire—we consider the Trail Making Test (Reitan 1958; Bowie and Harvey 2006), which has two parts: TMT-A, in which the participants are asked to link numbers, and TMT-B, in which the participants have to alternate numbers and letters. More concretely, each participant was asked to

---

[10]Note that we applied this model to the non-answers for the question on monthly household income, but we only found a limited gender effect (a female interviewer had somewhat more non-responses, on average); quite obviously, when the interaction was positive (when the interviewer evaluated the respondent as cooperative), the non-answers were halved. For the sake of parsimony, we remained with the simple model shown in Table 10.

Table 11 Trail Making Test process in VLV, 2011

Steps in the cognitive tests	TMT-A		TMT-B	
	n	%	n	%
Refused TMT short	157	5.1	28	1.0
Failed TMT short	84	2.7	242	8.9
Refused TMT	8	0.3	10	0.4
Failed TMT	99	3.2	607	22.2
Passed TMT	2732	88.7	1845	67.5
With time indicated	2130		1742	
No time indicated	602		103	
Total	3080	100	2732	100

complete a short version of the TMT-A as an exercise (and the interviewer noted "fail" or "pass") and then to pass the full version (the interviewer noted "fail" or "pass" and had to note the duration). Then, the same had to be done for TMT-B. Table 11 simply shows the resulting process of selection. Starting with 3080 participants, 5.1 % refused to complete the first exercise; this initial rejection was the strongest. Only 8, 28, and 10 participants refused at one of the next three steps. While only a small proportion (6 %) failed the TMT-A short or extended and could not continue, the TMT-B appeared to be much harder, with around 30 % failing. Such situations were not uncommon for both the participants and the interviewers. Anecdotally, all of the fieldwork leaders remember collaborators who were all specifically trained but who, after some interviews, expressed concern. Although they explained to the participants that it was not at all a medical examination and that the result was not important, some people who failed were greatly affected and sometimes started to cry. Additionally, the incident with the immigrants is reported in the Kaeser chapter, in this volume. Moreover, we also see on Table 11 that when the test was passed with success, the interviewers forgot to note the duration in no <22 % of the cases for the TMT-A and 5.6 % for the TMT-B. This shows that managing the cognitive tests was also a cognitive exercise for the surveyors, who did not completely deal with the explanations and the interactions with the person, the stopwatch, and the computer.[11]

In Table 12, we analyze the initial refusal through logistic regressions, then the four situations in which participants failed to pass the tests, and finally the two situations in which the interviewer forgot to note the time, all situations described in Table 11. Refusals to complete the cognitive tests were more frequent when the interviewer was experienced. Indeed, this effect suggests that those who had already completed several interviews and faced people who were shocked and/or sad to have failed were not unhappy when a sample member refused to answer their questions

---

[11]A confirmation of the difficulty to manage the tasks for the interviewers is that out of the 900 initial missing duration information in the CAPI, more than 300 could be completed thanks to annotations on the exercise sheet. The interviewer simply forgot to introduce the result in the computer.

Table 12 Logistic regressions on the risk of refusal, failures, and missing time information in the Trail Making Test, VLV

		TMT-A			TMT-B		No time	
		Refusal 1st step	Fail short	Fail extended	Fail short	Fail extended	TMT A	TMT B
		Exp(B)						
Interviewer	Woman	1.34	2.24*	1.96*	1.16	1.00	1.89***	2.50*
	Age	1.00	1.01	1.00	0.99	0.98***	1.01*	0.99
	Experience	1.49*	0.85	0.90	1.49*	1.49***	0.91	1.05
	Performance	1.00	1.00	1.02*	1.01	1.01***	1.00	1.00
	Primary education	0.99	1.04	–	0.94	0.75	0.29***	0.34*
	Secondary education	1.10	2.30	–	1.72	0.58*	0.63*	0.59
Respondent	Age	1.09***	1.07***	1.03*	1.06***	1.03***	0.96***	1.00
	Woman	1.57*	1.38	1.20	1.25	1.15	0.82*	1.04
	Primary education	0.73	–	1.02	0.97	1.83	0.82	0.67
	Secondary education	0.51	–	0.48	0.92	1.19	1.03	0.76
	Higher education	0.47	–	0.37	0.37*	0.91	1.09	0.62
	Cooperative	0.42**	0.69	0.81	0.66	0.89	0.69*	2.22
	Canton	1.10	0.97	0.97	0.92*	0.97	0.85***	0.87*
	Fragile-dependent	1.21	1.22	1.35	1.08	1.21*	0.79**	0.61*
	Depressive	2.23***	2.04*	1.45	1.59*	1.16	1.00	2.23
	Swiss	0.59	0.50*	0.98	0.59*	0.92	1.13	2.02*
Context	Time treatment	1.00	0.99	1.00	1.00	1.00	1.00	1.00
	Private residence	0.44***	0.98	1.74	1.05	0.83	0.88	0.73
	Other people present	1.27	2.69**	1.49	1.25*	0.94	0.71*	1.05
	Intervention	1.04	0.73	0.72	1.18	1.18	1.32	1.14
	Constant	0.00	0.00	0.00	0.00	0.09	11.20	0.05
	Sig. chi-square	0.000	0.000	0.000	0.000	0.000	0.000	0.018
	R² Cox & Snell	0.062	0.033	0.019	0.055	0.055	0.068	0.019
	R² Nagelkerke	0.187	0.153	0.071	0.123	0.082	0.104	0.056
	N observations	3080		2839		2462	2732	1845

Note: *p < 0.10; **p < 0.05; ***p < 0.01

and sent implicit messages carrying this feeling. From the respondents' point of view, older persons and women were more reluctant and more often used their freedom to say "no," as did people in the French-speaking cantons. Unsurprisingly, depressed persons tended to reject those tests. Inversely, Swiss natives—especially in the German-speaking cantons—were less inclined to refuse; quite obviously, this was also the case for the participants whom the interviewer evaluated as cooperative. Regarding the context, quite expectedly, the interview in the participant's private lodging was much more favorable to response than when in a tea room or another place.

When we consider the experience of failing, we see a sequence suggesting that the first questions created both a selection and a dynamic. Indeed, for the short and extended versions of the TMT-A, the participant failed more often if the participant was older or, whatever his/her gender, if the participant had to pass the test in front of a young female interviewer. Then, for the TMT-B, the age of the respondent had an impact—which is quite normal—but the impact of the interviewer's sex disappears, while another characteristic emerges. Indeed, people failed more often when the interviewer was experienced. Once again, this apparently strange result supports the hypothesis of a disaffiliation among the survey collaborators who adhered less and less to those questions. The other protective or risk factors are more obvious (high education, depression, or frailty) and not the topic of this chapter (see Ihle et al. 2015, for an in-depth analysis), but it is worth noting that the context of the interview is not that important by comparison. The presence of another person in the room has a negative effect on the probability of succeeding in the short versions of the TMT-A and TMT-B, but not for the two extended versions.

As we have seen, the situations in which the interviewer forgot to note the time taken by the participant to successfully complete one of the tests were much more frequent for the TMT-A than for the TMT-B, which once again suggests that the collaborator had too many things to manage at the same time and was stressed when reaching this part of the face-to-face questionnaire. The results are somewhat complicated, but three points emerge. First, information on time was more often missing when the interviewer was a woman and older, while interviewers with low level of education more strictly followed the instructions and were, hence, more reliable for that task. Second, the probability of forgetting to record the test time diminished when the participant was old, female, and frail, which could indicate more attention from the surveyor to the persons showing those characteristics. Third, the opposite was true for the TMT-B when the person suffered from depression, which apparently perturbed the interviewer. Still, the more obvious positive impact of the respondent's cooperative attitude suggests that the atmosphere—the climate of the social interactions between the interviewer and the participant—has a real effect.

5 Conclusion

This contribution addresses the complicated challenge of surveying vulnerabilities and vulnerable persons in a context of decreasing participation rates for surveys, especially in Switzerland and among the elderly. Vivre-Leben-Vivere (VLV) has been a laboratory in which various experiences have been accumulated. It is structured through the frame offered by the total survey error approach, resulting in several lessons of general interest.

The first challenge is related to the costs, a point that must not be definitively neglected, since most social science surveys are funded by public money and reveal resource inequalities within a society. From that point of view, outdated frame information is related to unavoidable problems specific to the elderly (like death) or not (mobility, discrepancy between de jure and de facto addresses). They are costly in financial terms, but for VLV, they also affected the motivations of some interviewers, resulting in non-contacts after many contact attempts. The survey collaborators were required to be resilient, to receive many kind but also aggressive refusals, to insist, and to travel through cities and the countryside, through the plains and the mountains, always with the risk of only finding a closed door or just a postal box. And of course, they had to be paid.

The second challenge is related to the refusals by the sample members who do not want to participate. Here, we face a real problem that moreover appears to be continuously growing. The reasons deserve more attention. Does the constantly increasing refusal rate result from reactions to over-solicitations by survey and market institutes or from a crisis of confidence with respect to research, combined with tendencies to socially withdraw, tendencies which can be related to socio-emotional processes associated with ageing and to the perceptions of the elderly in our societies? All of these aspects were apparent in the causes of refusal observed during the VLV fieldwork. This issue still needs to be more systematically addressed before the challenge becomes impossible to take up. Specifically, in the Vivre-Leben-Vivere survey, notwithstanding a participation rate of only 35 %, no fewer than 45 % of the files were obtained by repeated phone calls, home visits, and resorting to proxies. It is an enormous proportion, and it seems difficult to imagine going beyond this, at least with this mode of data collection.

However, "do low survey response rates bias results?" (Rindfuss et al. 2015). This is a third challenge that also includes the ability to include vulnerable persons in the sample of respondents. Based on the collected data, having quite simple but sound tools make it possible to identify states of vulnerability, in terms of evidence, latency (overexposure to risk), and absence on several dimensions. These indicators have been used to test the survey procedures. The results show contrasting effects linked to widely varying situations and a heterogeneity that is a fundamental characteristic of the aged population. Among the "young old," obstinacy in phone calls allowed the most dynamic to be surveyed, particularly men. In the intermediary areas between the so-called 3rd and 4th ages (75–84), home visits were somewhat effective in including people that the questionnaire analysis is revealing now as facing latent states of vulnerability. And among those at the most advanced ages, whose health is also the most affected, the approach by proxies effectively incorporated those who are evidently vulnerable, especially women. In the second stage, the prevalence of poverty, functional health problems, and depression in the VLV data was compared with other data sources. Overall, we can conclude that Vivre-Leben-Vivere faced the challenge and that vulnerable elderly are well-represented in its sample of respondents. The low participation rate has not biased the results, at least from our research perspective. Once again and specific to a survey on old adults, home visits and, even more, the recourse to proxies explain this success.

We should fairly consider the recent criticisms made against the proxy method, but also bear in mind that its contribution to studies on the aged is undeniable. More thought should be given to the ethical conditions of its use in the future, since we obviously face a tension between strict respect for what must be an informed consent and the scientific, social, and political relevance of the research. Groves and Lyberg (2010) noted with insistence that relevance is a difficult to assess, although essential, component in the identification of what contributes to the "quality" of a survey. To stay away from this tension, an option may be to refrain from collecting information on subjective measures and to collect only "objective" data on health and material conditions.

A fourth challenge, which is rarely directly related to the preceding one, concerns item non-response, or the refusal by the participants to answer certain questions. It is a reasonable hypothesis to assume negative impacts of both latent and manifest states of vulnerability on such risks. At the same time, saying "no" is also a proper use of the participant's individual agency and consequently can express the inverse of personal vulnerability. Consequently, estimating the resulting impact on the measurement errors can be delicate. And indeed, the evidence in the VLV data is mixed, both in the self-administered and face-to-face questionnaires, with some situations that reveal dis-affiliation, dis-adjustment, or withdrawal, and others revealing a self-conscience and capacity to decide. Typically, as far as poverty is concerned, non-response to the questions on household monthly income come disproportionately from the oldest old and women, who are groups at risk, but also from people with high levels of education, who are just the opposite. When we come to the assessment of cognition, we reach a point at which the survey's legitimacy and scientific objectives appear to be contested by the main collaborators—the interviewers. They expressed their doubts on the basis of their fieldwork experience when very concretely dealing with this part of the questionnaire, and the required devices (exercise sheets, stopwatch, computer), at the same time as trying to give clear instructions, and preserving proper social interactions with the respondent. Situations of failure that affected the participants also affected the interviewers' attitudes, once again with contrasting effects: better attention to frail people but less to depressed persons. Obviously, the climate of the interviews, the quality of the interactions, and more generally the means of maintaining adherence to the survey objectives, and the civic engagement of each participant (both those who answer as well as those who question) must remain central concerns.

References

Baer, N., Schuler, D., Füglister-Dousse, S., & Moreau-Gruet, F. (2013). *Depressionen in der Schweizer Bevölkerung. Daten zur Epidemilogie, Behandlung und sozial-beruflichen Integration.* Neuchâtel: Schweizerisches Gesundheitsobservatorium (OBSAN Bericht 56).

Bak, C. K., & Larsen, J. E. (2014). Social exclusion or poverty individualisation? An empirical test of two recent and competing poverty theories. *European Journal of Social Work, 18*(1), 1–19.

Baltes, M. M., & Lang, F. R. (1993). Everyday functioning and successful aging: The impact of resources. *Psychology and Aging, 12,* 433–443.

Baltes, P. B., & Mayer, K. U. (1999). *The Berlin Aging Study: Aging from 70 to 100.* New York: Cambridge University Press.

Berrut, S., & Junker, C. (2008). *D'une génération à l'autre. Evolution des causes de décès en Suisse de 1970 à 2004.* Neuchâtel: Office fédéral de Statistique.

Bétemps, C., Bickel, J.-F., Brunner, M., & Hummel, C. (1997). *Journal d'une enquête. La récolte de données dans le cadre d'une recherche sur échantillon aléatoire.* Lausanne: Réalités sociales.

Bickel, J.-F. (2014). La participation sociale, une action située entre biographie, histoire et structures. In I. Mallon, C. Hummel, & V. Caradec (Eds.), *Vieillesses et vieillissements* (pp. 207–226). Rennes: Presses universitaires de Rennes.

Blom, A., De Leeuw, E., & Hox, J. (2011). Interviewer effects on nonresponse in the European social survey. *Journal of Official Statistics, 27*(2), 359–377.

Börsch-Supan, A. (coord.). (2005). *Health, ageing and retirement in Europe. First results from the survey of health, ageing and retirement in Europe.* Mannheim: MEA.

Börsch-Supan, A., Hank, K., Jürges, H., & Schröder, M. (2008). *Longitudinal data collection in continental Europe: Experiences from the survey of health, ageing and retirement in Europe (SHARE).* Mannheim: Research Institute for the Economics of Aging.

Bourdelais, P. (1997). *L'âge de la vieillesse. Histoire du vieillissement de la population.* Paris: O. Jacob.

Bowie, C. R., & Harvey, P. D. (2006). Administration and interpretation of the Trail Making test. *Nature Protocols, 1,* 2277–2281.

Bundesamt für Statistik. (2012). *Gesundheit von Betagten in Alters- und Pflegeheimen. Erhebung zum Gesundheitszustand von betagten Personen in Institutionen* (2008/2009), Neuchâtel.

Bundesamt für Statistik. (2014). *Die funktionale Gesundheit von älteren Menschen in Privathaushalten,* Neuchâtel.

Cavasso, B., & Weber, G. (2014). The effects of the great recession on the wealth and financial distress of 65+ Europeans. In A. Börsch-Supan, M. Brandt, H. Litwin, & G. Weber (Eds.), *Active ageing and solidarity between generations in Europe* (pp. 27–36). Berlin: De Gruyter.

Cheshire, H., Oftedal, M. B., Scholes, S., & Schroeder, M. (2011). A comparison of response rates in the English Longitudinal Study of Ageing and the Health and Retirement Study. *Longitudinal and Life Course Studies, 2*(2), 127–144.

Dannefer, D. (2001). Age stratification. In N. J. Smelser & P. Baltes (Eds.), *Encyclopedia of the social and behavioral sciences* (pp. 278–283). Oxford: Pergamon.

Dannefer, D. (2003). Cumulative advantage/disadvantage and the life course: Cross-fertilizing age and social science theory. *The Journals of Gerontology Series B: Psychological Sciences and Social Sciences, 58*(6), 327–337.

De Leeuw, E. (2008). Self-administered questionnaires and standardized interviews. In A. Pertti, L. Bickman, & J. Brannon (Eds.), *Handbook of social research methods* (pp. 313–327). London: Sage Ltd.

De Luca, G., & Peracchi, F. (2005). Survey participation in the first wave of SHARE. In A. Börsch-Supan & H. Jürges (Eds.), *The survey on health, aging, and retirement in Europe–methodology* (pp. 88–101). Mannheim: Mannheim Research Institute for the Economics of Aging.

Diener, E., Emmons, R. A., Larsen, R. J., & Griffin, S. (1985). The satisfaction with life scale. *Journal of Personality Assessement, 49*, 71–76.

Durrant, G. B., Groves, R. M., Staetsky, L., & Steele, F. (2010). Effects of interviewer attitudes and behaviors on refusal in household surveys. *Public Opinion Quarterly, 74*, 1–36.

Duvoisin, A., Baeriswyl, M., Oris, M., Perrig-Chiello, P., & Bickel, J.-F. (2012). *Pro Senectute : visibilité et usages d'une association bientôt centenaire. Au service des vulnérables ?* Genève: CIGEV.

Fillit, H. M., Rockwood, K., & Woodhouse, K. (Eds.). (2010). *Brocklehurst's textbook of geriatric medicine and gerontology*. Amsterdam: Elsevier.

Gabriel, R. (2015). *Inequalities within progress? Social stratification and the life course among the elderly population in Switzerland between 1979–2011*. PhD in Socioeconomics, University of Geneva.

Gabriel, R., Oris, M., Studer, M., & Baeriswyl, M. (2015). The persistence of social stratification? A life course perspective on old-age poverty in Switzerland. *Swiss Journal of Sociology, 41*(3), 465–487.

Girardin, M., Spini, D., & Ryser, V.-A. (2008). The paradox of well-being in later life: Effectiveness of downward social comparison during the frailty process. In E. Guilley & C. J. Lalive d'Epinay (Eds.), *The closing chapters of long lives* (pp. 129–142). New York: Nova Science Publishers.

Groves, R. M. (2011). Three eras of survey research. *Public Opinion Quarterly, 75*(5), 861–871.

Groves, R. M., & Couper, M. P. (1998). *Nonresponse in household interview surveys*. New York: Wiley.

Groves, R. M., & Lyberg, L. (2010). Total survey error, past, present, and future. *Public Opinion Quarterly, 74*(5), 849–879.

Groves, R. M., Fowler, F. J., Jr., Couper, M. P., Lepkowski, J. M., Singer, E., & Tourangeau, R. (2004). *Survey methodology*. New York: Wiley.

Guggisberg, M., Müller, B., & Christin, T. (2012). *Pauvreté en Suisse: concepts, résultats et méthodes. Résultats calculés sur la base de l'enquête SILC 2008 à 2010*. Neuchâtel: Office fédéral de Statistique.

Guilley, E., & Lalive d'Épinay, C. (Eds.). (2008). *The closing chapters of long lives. Results from the 10-year Swilsoo study on the oldest old*. New York: Nova Science Publishers.

Ihle, A., Oris, M., Fagot, D., Baeriswyl, M., Guichard, E., & Kliegel, M. (2015). The association of leisure activities in middle adulthood with cognitive performance in old age: The moderating role of educational level. *Gerontology* (in press).

Joye, D., Pollien, A., Sapin, M., & Ernst Stähli, M. (2012). Who can be contacted by phone? Lessons from Switzerland. In: M. Häder, S. Häder, & M. Kühne (Eds.), *Telephone surveys in Europe: Research and practice* (pp. 85–102). Heidelberg: Springer.

Katz, S., Ford, A. B., Moskowitz, R. W., Jackson, B. A., & Jaffe, M. W. (1963). Studies of illness in the aged. The index of ADL: A standardized measure of biological and psychological function. *JAMA, 185*(12), 914–919.

Köhler, M., Kliegel, M., for the AgeCoDe Study Group, et al. (2011). Malperformance in verbal fluency and delayed recall as cognitive risk factors for impairment in instrumental activities of daily living. *Dementia and Geriatric Cognitive Disorders, 31*, 81–88.

Lalive d'Épinay, C., & Spini, D. (2008). *Les années fragiles: La vie au-delà de quatre-vingts ans.* Québec: Les Presses de l'Université Laval.

Lalive d'Épinay, C., Bickel, J.-F., Maystre, C., & Vollenwyder, N. (2000). *Vieillesses au fil du temps. 1979–1994: Une révolution tranquille.* Lausanne: Réalités sociales.

Lawton, M. P., Moss, M., Hoffman, C., Grant, R., Ten Have, T., & Kleban, M. H. (1999). Health, valuation of life, and the wish to live. *Gerontologist, 39,* 406–416.

Lessler, J. T., & Kalsbeck, W. D. (1992). *Nonsampling error in surveys.* New York: Wiley.

Ludwig, C., Cavalli, S., & Oris, M. (2014). 'Vivre/Leben/Vivere': An interdisciplinary survey addressing progress and inequalities of aging over the past 30 years in Switzerland. *Archives of Gerontology and Geriatrics, 59*(2), 240–248.

Malter, F. (2013). Fieldwork monitoring in the survey of health, ageing and retirement in Europe (SHARE). *Survey Methods: Insights from the Field.* Retrieved from http://surveyinsights.org/?p=1974

Marchese, O. (2011). *Questionnaires, enquêteurs et enquêtés.* Document de travail Conservatoire nationale des Arts et Métiers, France.

Marpsat, M., & Razafindratsima, N. (2010). Survey-methods for hard-to-reach populations. Introduction to the special issue. *Methodological Innovations, 5*(2), 3–16.

Masotti, B., & Oris, M. (2015). Il ricorso ai servizi domiciliari e il ruolo della famiglia nella quarta età. In: F. Giudici, S. Cavalli, M. Egloff, & Masotti (Eds.), *Fragilità e risorse delle persone anziane residenti in Ticino* (pp 87–109). sl, Ufficio di statistica.

Michel, J.-P., Guilley, E., Armi, Fr., & Robine, J.-M. (2005). Les multiples dimensions de la fragilité. In: Ph. Thomas et C.H. Thomas (dir.), *Traité de psychogériatrie* (pp. 230–239), Med-Line.

Nicolet, M., & Oris, M. (forthcoming). Mesures et capture de la vulnérabilité dans une enquête sur les conditions de vie et de santé des personnes âgées. L'expérience de VLV (Vivre-Leben-Vivere) en Suisse. In Conférence Universitaire de Démographie et d'Etude des Populations, *Les Populations vulnérables,* Bordeaux, CUDEP.

Nolan, B., & Marx, I. (2009). Economic inequality, poverty, and social exclusion. In S. Wiemer, B. Nolan, & T. M. Smeeding (Eds.), *The Oxford handbook of economic inequality* (pp. 315–341). New York: Oxford University Press.

Oris, M., & Lerch, M. (2009). La transition ultime. Longévité et mortalité aux grands âges dans le bassin lémanique. In: *Transitions dans le parcours de vie et construction des inégalités* (pp 407–432). Lausanne: Presses polytechniques et universitaires romandes.

Paugam, S. (2000). *Le salarié de la précarité.* Paris: Presses Universitaires de France.

Peytchev, A., Baxter, R., & Carley-Baxter, L. (2009). Not all survey effort is equal. Reduction of nonresponse bias and nonresponse error. *Public Opinion Quaterly, 73*(4), 785–806.

Pilgram, A., & Seifert, K. (2009). *Vivre avec peu de moyens. La pauvreté des personnes âgées en Suisse.* Zurich: Edition Pro Senectute.

Reitan, R. (1958). Validity of the Trail Making Test as an indicator of organic brain damage. *Perceptual and Motor Skills, 8,* 271–276.

Rindfuss, R. R., Choe, M. K., Tsuya, N. O., Bumpass, L. L., & Tamaki, E. (2015). Do low survey rates bias results? Evidence from Japan. *Demographic Research, 32,* 797–828.

Roberts, C., Vandenplas, C., & Ernst Stähli, M. (2014). Evaluating the impact of response enhancement methods on the risk of nonresponses bias and survey cost. *Survey Research Methods, 8*(2), 67–80.

Robine, J.-M., & Jagger, C. (2004). Allongement de la vie et état de santé de la population. In G. Caselli, J. Vallin, & G. Wunsch (Eds.), *Démographie : analyse et synthèse* (Population et société, Vol. VI, pp. 51–84). Paris: INED.

Scholes, S., Medina, J., Cheshire, H., Cox, K., Hacker, E., & Lessof, C. (2009). *Living in the 21st century: Older people in England. The 2006 English longitudinal study of ageing. Technical Report,* National Center for Social Research.

Sen, A. K. (1999). *Development as freedom.* Oxford: Oxford University Press.

SKOS/CSIAS. (2013). *Armut und Armutsgrenze – Grundlagenpapier der SKOS.* Bern: SKOS/CSIAS.

Snijkers, G., Hox, J. J., & De Leeuw, E. D. (1999). Interviewers' tactics for fighting survey nonresponse. *Journal of Official Statistics, 15*, 185–198.

Tourangeau, R., Edwards, B., Johnson, T., Wolters, K., & Bates, N. (Eds.). (2014). *Hard-to-survey populations*. Cambridge: Cambridge University Press.

Van Oyen, H., Nusselder, W., Jagger, C., Kolip, P., Cambois, E., & Robine, J. M. (2013). Gender differences in healthy life years within the EU: An exploration of the "health-survival" paradox. *International Journal of Public Health, 58*(1), 143–155.

Vaupel, J. W., Manton, K. G., & Stallard, E. (1979). The impact of heterogeneity in individual frailty on the dynamics of mortality. *Demography, 16*(3), 439–454.

Wang, R. I., et al. (1975). A brief self-assessing depression scale. *Journal of Clinical Pharmacology, 15*(2–3), 163–167.

Wanner, P., Gabadinho, A., & Pecoraro, M. (2008). *La situation économique des actifs et des retraités*. Berne: Office fédéral des Assurances sociales.

Adapting Quantitative Survey Procedures: The Price for Assessing Vulnerability? Lessons from a Large-Scale Survey on Aging and Migration in Switzerland

Laure Kaeser

1 Capturing Vulnerable Populations: A Dilemma for Large-Scale Quantitative Surveys

This chapter aims at understanding the issues of capturing vulnerable populations in large-scale quantitative surveys. We limit ourselves to a specific group, elderly migrants, who nevertheless illustrate a global challenge. Surveying vulnerability requires being able to gain access to vulnerable individuals or groups. Vulnerability is defined as: "A lack of resources, which in a specific context, places individuals or groups at a major risk of experiencing (1) negative consequences related to sources of stress; (2) the inability to cope effectively with stressors; and (3) the inability to recover from the stressor or to take advantage of opportunities by a given deadline" (Spini et al. 2013).

These populations are often hard to reach for surveyors; according to the definition, it is primarily a lack of resources, within a specific context, that places certain groups at a major risk of not being represented by large-scale surveys. Such a deficiency translates into problems of availability (being homeless or away from home during data collection period), absence of identification with the survey goals and uses (refusing to participate, misunderstanding the survey questions, refusing to be contacted, etc.), inability to answer to survey questions (not speaking the local language, not reading properly, mental handicap, etc.) or special group features such as ethnic or religious minority groups, or drug users (Schiltz 2005; Riandey and Quaglia 2009; Marpsat and Razafindratsima 2010).

L. Kaeser (✉)
NCCR LIVES, IP 213, Geneva, Switzerland

Centre for the Interdisciplinary Study of Gerontology and Vulnerability,
University of Geneva, Geneva, Switzerland
e-mail: laurekaeser@gmail.com

© The Author(s) 2016
M. Oris et al. (eds.), *Surveying Human Vulnerabilities across the Life Course*,
Life Course Research and Social Policies 3, DOI 10.1007/978-3-319-24157-9_3

   Thus, the dilemma in survey construction arises when a target vulnerable population to be analyzed cannot be reached using standard survey design. Indeed, adapting standard procedures may help to improve access to the targeted vulnerable population; however, these changes may lead to inaccurate comparisons with other population subgroups.

   To discuss this dilemma, this chapter deals with the data collection process of the large-scale survey on aging *Vivre/Leben/Vivere: Old Age Democratization? Progress and Inequalities in Switzerland* (VLV). VLV aims at analyzing life and health conditions and trajectories of the population aged 65 and over living in the Swiss Confederation. VLV also includes a focus on ageing populations with a migrant background. Researchers at the Center for the Interdisciplinary Study of Gerontology and Vulnerability in Geneva were responsible for designing the study and analyzing the data. They were also responsible for conducting the data collection, which took place in 2011 and 2012.

   VLV is a quantitative survey that in many ways reflects the above-mentioned methodological challenges. It is based on two samples: the main sample of people over 65 years old living in five cantons, and an oversample of elderly migrants living in the cantons of Basel and Geneva (see the Sect. 3 for more details on the research design). The VLV research team strictly defined contact and interviewing procedures and standardized the data collection for all selected sample units. Since the research objectives included studying elderly people with a migrant background,[1] it was initially decided to use the same research design for them as for the main sample precisely to avoid *a priori* differences. Nevertheless, elements of vulnerability made them hard to reach for reasons explicitly explained below. To avoid this potential failure, the team decided to adapt some of the standard procedures, but this was not without giving up some benefits of standardization. This chapter tells the story of VLV's successes and failures, with the aim of highlighting the tension between scientific requirements and realities on the ground in the context of surveying vulnerability.

   To do so, this chapter explains why the case of elderly migrants is relevant to discussing the dilemma of capturing vulnerability within large-scale surveys. Then it questions the need to adjust standard procedures of a quantitative survey, and the impact of doing so, to access elderly migrants. Finally, we show the need for a constant dialogue around the scientific requirements and the realities of fieldwork in order to avoid an under-representation of vulnerable groups in surveys, which can also be viewed as a form of discrimination. For example, Elcheroth and his colleagues have argued that, "Systematic bias in survey response also intrigues because it appears to betray a democratic ideal that is frequently projected onto surveys: one person, one voice. The substantive concern about processes that

---

[1] Immigrant is defined as an individual born in another country than the one he/she lives in and who has crossed a border (or several borders) since his/her birth. He/she may be citizen of his/her birth country or another country, in particular of his/her country of residence (Definition of the French National Institute of Demographic Study).

produce social exclusion, and that reproduce it in particular by way of exclusion from social surveys, goes hand-in-hand with the pragmatic concern to enhance the representativeness of surveys, not least in order to break societal and scientific cycles that render certain minorities invisible to the public eye (and leave the public indifferent to their fate)" (Elcheroth et al. 2011: 4).

2   Surveying Elderly Migrants as an Illustration of Surveying Vulnerability

Many studies on survey methodology underline the difficulties in obtaining a representative sample of the target population. Results may be inferred to the whole (sub)population thanks to sampling methods, which determine the quality of the sample representativeness (Tabutin 2006; Gerville-Réache et al. 2011). Nevertheless, even if the sampling method promises representativeness, some subpopulations are hard to reach for availability, access, or monitoring reasons. This may lead to differences between the original sample and the size and profile of the responding sample (Groves and Couper 1998; Elcheroth et al. 2011).

Groves and Couper (1998) identify several reasons explaining participation in surveys: individual characteristics such as social and/or psychological components (including attitudes, norms and values); demographic variables (age, marital status, household structure, education, income, place of residence); and from a heuristic perspective, features of the research design (data collection mode, number of contact attempts, period of data collection); the interviewers' characteristics (sex, age, experience); and interactions between interviewers and respondents. VLV decided to deal with the elderly migrants in almost the same way as the other elderly sample members. Because of their life course, however, elderly migrants differ from the overall population in a number of specific ways. Their particular characteristics may interfere with their participation in the survey. These points are detailed below.

In Switzerland, most elders of foreign origin arrived in the second half of the twentieth century. They mainly came from Italy in the 1950s, from Spain in the 1960s, and from Portugal and former Yugoslavia in the 1980s and early 1990s (Piguet 2004). After World War II, the main goal of Swiss migratory policy was to get temporary workers responding to the needs of a growing economy without competing with Swiss natives. Immigrants experienced severe legal restrictions (including the interdiction of family reunification, seasonal status) and a lack of integration policies until the early 1990s. A part of the Swiss population also openly expressed hostility against immigrants during the campaign for the so-called Schwarzenbach initiatives[2] against "foreign overpopulation." In this context, painful professional and health trajectories have been part of individual migration

---

[2]Schwarzenbach's initiatives (originating from the name of the initiator, representative of the "Action nationaliste," a conservative political party) were initiatives against the "foreign over-

stories. As a consequence, elderly migrants are overrepresented among the most disadvantaged groups of the retired population in Switzerland (Bolzman et al. 2004).

Small-scale studies in the cities/cantons of Geneva and Basel (Bolzman et al. 2001, 2004) have highlighted special features of the living conditions of elderly people coming from abroad compared to the overall population. Most of them worked in low-skilled jobs (e.g. construction, industry, cleaning). Their income is on average lower than that for Swiss natives because of an earlier retirement age (explained by bad health status due to the demanding nature of the work and higher risk of unemployment) and/or a shorter contribution period to the retirement funds (e.g. due to carrying out professional activity in two or more countries). Those with the worst health status were active in the construction sector; half of whom receive benefits from disability insurance (Bolzman et al. 2004).

Nowadays, elderly migrants have either chosen to, or must, spend the last stage of their lives in their host country. They are on average younger than the Swiss population but the share of elderly migrants within the total population aged 65 and over is increasing steadily.[3] People originating from Italy, Germany, France, Austria, and Spain are the most numerous. But the proportion of each nationality in relation to the total foreign population varies over time. This evolution reflects the various migration movements during the last century. Italians constitute the most important group among elderly migrants, representing around 40 % of the foreign population aged 65 and over. This share has not varied much over time, while by contrast, other nationalities are constantly on the rise, especially those from southern Europe, including more recent migration flows such as those originating in Portugal or Turkey. In contrast, there has been a large decrease in the number of Northern Europeans in the foreign aged population of Switzerland.

When surveying these groups, including those coming from the south of the continent, numerous obstacles induced by their life trajectories and current living conditions may engender their underrepresentation in the responding sample. Scientific literature reveals that there are various barriers that make people with a migrant background hard to reach by standard survey fieldwork procedures. Not speaking the survey language is one factor. But having living conditions that make someone uneasily reachable by standard procedures or having a system of beliefs and values that make the questions not understandable constitute major difficulties as well (Feskens et al. 2006; Lipps et al. 2011; Elcheroth et al. 2011; Laganà et al. 2011). Moreover, analysis of reasons for inclusion and exclusion of national minority groups from Swiss large-scale surveys confirms the relation between nonresponse

---

population" submitted twice to the vote of the Swiss population in the 1970s. Finally refused, they deeply impacted the foreign populations living in Switzerland at that time.

[3]In 1995, the resident foreign population aged 65 and over represented 6.0 % of the total resident population of that age. This share grew to 10.5 % by 2010. This increase would be even more striking if people of immigrant origin who became Swiss citizens were taken into account. As for the total resident population 65 and over, there was an increase of 21 % from 1995 to 2010, while the foreign population increased 55 % in the same period of time (Swiss Federal Statistical Office 2012).

rate and ethno-social affiliations (Lipps et al. 2011; Elcheroth et al. 2011; Laganà et al. 2013). These studies conclude that the underrepresentation of national minorities results in bias even after controlling for socioeconomic status. Though weak for people speaking the same language and from neighboring countries, this problem becomes extreme for people originating from former Yugoslavia, Albania, Turkey, and outside Europe (Elcheroth et al. 2011; Lipps et al. 2011). In the case of VLV and referring to the work of Groves and Couper (1998), elderly migrants' characteristics such as their age, language, overrepresentation in low socioeconomic and health status groups, low level of education and ambivalent position in several cultural contexts may impair their representation within a large-scale survey. However, Elcheroth and his colleagues argue that, "The inclusion/exclusion of minority groups in/from general social surveys might be one of the most challenging and understudied issues in contemporary survey research" (Elcheroth et al. 2011: 1).

It is also important to keep in mind that migration issues represent a challenge for social science surveys precisely because of their socio-political dimension. From a broad perspective, the methodological challenges are underpinned by the necessity for public actors, especially those defining social policies, to get reliable statistics to understand the evolution of social problems and their subsequent needs (Rossini 2013: 92). In the case of VLV, surveying elderly migrants specifically questions the need for public policies to get a more detailed picture of the life conditions, resources, and requests of these growing populations. Thus, surveying migrants also constitutes a challenge for surveys on aging to access a growing population among the most vulnerable retired persons. Various papers published in Switzerland and elsewhere in Europe have stressed the improvement in the living conditions, health status, and well-being of the new cohorts reaching retirement age (Von Dem Knesebeck et al. 2007; Lalive d'Epinay et al. 2000). However, if these findings are well established for elderly persons in general, much less is known about the population of migrant workers who are now retired. In this light, being able to represent elderly migrants within a large-scale survey is a challenge in terms of generating knowledge for the orientation of policies targeted at the aging population.

Including elderly migrants in the general VLV research design implied several adaptations of standard procedures, and these adjustments reflect the dilemma mentioned in the introduction. In summary, the VLV experience of attempting to survey elderly migrants raised the following questions:

- Which were the specific obstacles that prevented elderly migrants from participating in the VLV survey with the standard fieldwork procedures and which elements of vulnerability do these obstacles underline?
- Which adaptations succeeded in overcoming these obstacles and improving the access to elderly migrants?
- If their inclusion in the survey was better in quantitative terms (higher response rate), what was the impact of the adjustments to standard procedures on the data quality? In other words, was the representativeness of the responding sample of elderly migrants affected by the adaptations of the procedures implemented in the middle of the fieldwork?

Once again, this chapter examines the need to adapt standard survey procedures in order to facilitate the participation of elderly immigrants, who make up an important part of the most vulnerable groups within the aging population. We developed an original methodological framework based on quantitative and qualitative data to empirically address this issue.

3   A Mixed Method Design for Analyzing VLV's Ability to Survey Elderly Migrants

Our analyses are based on the VLV field research. Scholars from various disciplinary backgrounds (medicine, psychiatry, psychology, sociology and demography) designed the VLV study and delegated the data collection to researchers from the Center for Interdisciplinary Gerontology and the study of vulnerabilities (hereafter referred to as "the VLV team"). The survey was conducted in 2011 and 2012 in five Swiss cantons: Geneva, Valais (restricted to the Central Valais area), Bern (restricted to the Mittelland, Oberland, and Seeland areas), Basel (including Basel-Stadt and Basel-Land) and Ticino. In each canton, 20–30 external interviewers were hired to contact the respondents and conduct the interviews, and two to three members of the VLV team managed the interviewers and monitored the fieldwork. The main target sample consisted of 3600 individuals and was randomly selected in the cantonal population records, and stratified by age (65–69; 70–74; 75–79; 80–84; 85–89; 90 and above) and sex, for a total of 720 respondents in each canton, either community dwelling or living in nursing homes. The contact procedure was done either by phone or a visit at home in case of no landline phone. Then, the survey was conducted in two phases. First, the respondents received a self-administered questionnaire and a life-event calendar. Second, an interviewer conducted a face-to-face interview with an average duration of 2 h (Ludwig et al. 2014).

To address the increasing diversity of the elderly population, an important subproject of VLV was set up to investigate the living conditions and the life trajectories of elderly migrants compared to the national population. In addition to the main sample, VLV researchers decided to oversample the migrant population. Oversamples stratified by sex were planned in the cantons of Geneva and Basel based on people aged between 65 and 79, with 120 individuals by nationality. In Geneva, the oversample included natives from Portugal, Spain, and Italy. In Basel, it was originally intended to interview people from Italy and former Yugoslavia. These choices of groups and sites were determined by the distribution of these populations relative to the national population and other ethnic-minority groups.

Nevertheless, obstacles such as a low response rate quickly emerged (see below) and began to compromise the data collection. Therefore, the VLV team decided to adjust some features of the research design with varying success. To identify causes of exclusion of elderly migrants within VLV, we collected and analyzed quantitative and qualitative data. Scholars using qualitative approaches regularly undertake a reflective and critical exercise relating to the production of data, especially on issues related to strategies for negotiating and gaining access to carry out fieldwork. Such a critical exercise may also constitute an introduction to data analysis: types of access to the fieldwork and reception of the survey may be indicative of certain characteristics of the target population (Mauger 1991; Bonnet 2008). Moreover, even if they are used less in survey research, qualitative data remain of great interest for understanding what is being examined with survey practices. Indeed, "Ethnographic approaches to interviewer experiences and interviewer respondent interactions should provide a more fine-grained understanding of the micro-process by which certain types of respondents are excluded from survey participation, on the basis of reciprocal expectations, perceptions, and communicative practices" (Elcheroth et al. 2011: 11).

A qualitative approach gives a better understanding of the perception of the survey by elderly migrants. During the fieldwork, it also gave suggestions to researchers about how to adapt the procedures to improve the response rate and survey practices. Three bodies of text were analyzed. First, researchers in charge of the data collection kept logbooks of oral reports from interviewers responsible for the oversamples. The analysis of these field stories complemented data from the VLV fieldwork monitoring by giving interpretations of the reasons for non-response (refusal and non-contact). Second, a content analysis of strategic discussions within the VLV team examined the effects of the procedures for elderly migrants compared to the rest of the sample. Finally, a focus group with the interviewers in charge of the oversamples was created to better understand the perception of the VLV approach procedures and the way to conduct interviewing among these populations.

On the quantitative side, access to the research field was analyzed with respect to effects on the representativeness of the population covered by the study (Groves 2006; Marpsat and Razafindratsima 2010). Thus, we analyzed refusal, non-response, and contact rates of elderly migrants compared to the main sample. The monitoring of VLV, which collected results on contact attempts, made these classical analyses in survey methodology possible (Groves and Couper 1998). We also conducted statistical tests on the final sample to verify if the adjustments of procedures introduced biases. Thus, combining qualitative and quantitative approaches helps to shed light on VLV data production and its adaptation strategies.

4 Varying Effects of Adjusting Procedures to Survey Elderly Migrants

It is worth remembering that the VLV team made the initial decision to not construct *a priori* differences between elderly migrants and the rest of the sample by applying the same contact and interviewing procedures to both. This is a crucial starting point since this choice resulted in underestimating risks related to equal treatment of these populations. Nevertheless, it was not a completely strict approach.

Four subsidiary measures were implemented from the start: first, oversampling people originating from Italy, Spain, Portugal and former Yugoslavia; second, translations of survey materials; third, recruitment of bilingual interviewers; and fourth, promotion of the survey in migrant communities. These decisions were built upon the experiences of the previously mentioned surveys of elderly migrants in Switzerland for which the representativeness of the final samples of respondents had been ensured. This fieldwork highlighted two elements of vulnerability faced by aging immigrants: the lack of language proficiency and the distrust of the administrative aspects of the survey. The four measures taken dealt with these problems and were assumed to not interfere with the initial objective, which was to apply the same research design to native and non-native elderly persons. This approach was designed to facilitate access to fieldwork and overcome any language barriers. Bilingual interviewers were trained the same way as the other interviewers; the entire material was translated without any modification, and the same contact and interviewing procedures were used. However, these four measures had varying effects, as described in the following.

Since elderly migrants only represent a small part of the elderly population and as it was assumed that they would probably have a lower response rate than the overall main sample, oversamples were planned to make sure that the final sample size would be large enough to permit reliable quantitative analysis. Four oversamples were foreseen, each with 120 respondents. However, in the end, as Table 1 shows, the planned objectives for the oversample were not achieved.

The motivation for translating the survey materials was based on the hypothesis that some elderly migrants would not have been able to understand the question-naires in French or German. There are several reasons for a lack of language proficiency in these subpopulations (e.g. lack of time, low level of education, demanding jobs, etc.), all of which may create daily obstacles to accessing services for these people. It also may lead to a major risk of under-representation in the survey of people who feel less comfortable speaking, or feel unable to answer questions in the local language. Contact letters, life event calendars, and instructions (see Fig. 1), self-administered and face-to-face questionnaires were all translated into Portuguese, Spanish, Italian, Albanian, and Serbo-Croatian.

In Geneva, 87 % of the Portuguese respondents in the oversample, 81 % of the Spanish respondents in the oversample, and 90 % of the Italian respondents in the oversample responded in their native language. These results highlight how crucial the translation option is for reaching elderly migrants. High proportions of those

Table 1 Final oversamples obtained by random procedures (planned effectiveness: 120 by nationality and canton)

	Geneva		Basel	
	Portugal	Spain	Italy	Former Yugoslavia
Random oversamples	61	41	46	5

Planned effectiveness: 120 by nationality and canton

UNIVERSITÉ DE GENÈVE

VIVRE
LEBEN
VIVERE

Calendario de vida

EJEMPLO

La Sra. Claire Dupont tiene 86 años y creció en Evolene. A los 16 años, se va a trabajar a Zermatt. Ahí conoce a Henri. Se casan dos años más tarde. Después de tener cinco hijos, empieza un trabajo como secretaria. En 1972, se le detecta un cáncer de seno, situación que la obliga a disminuir su tiempo de trabajo. Poco después del fallecimiento de su esposo, se somete a una cirugía del corazón. Debido a estos acontecimientos, la Sra. Dupont se ve obligada a vender su casa y a mudarse. Actualmente vive en un EMS en Sion.

Año	Edad	Residencia	Familia / Pareja	Actividad		Salud	Nacionalidad	Edad	Año
					Carga				
1925	0	Evolène VS					Suiza	0	1925
1926	1							1	1926
1927	2		Nace hermana					2	1927
1928	3							3	1928
1929	4							4	1929
1930	5		Nace hermano					5	1930
1931	6							6	1931
1932	7			Escuela obligatoria				7	1932
1933	8		Nace hermana					8	1933
1934	9							9	1934
1935	10							10	1935
1936	11							11	1936
1937	12			Escuela para las tareas domésticas				12	1937
1938	13							13	1938
1939	14			Ayuda en la granja				14	1939
1940	15							15	1940
1941	16	Zermatt, VS		Señora de la limpieza	100			16	1941
1942	17			limpieza				17	1942
1943	18		Conoce Henri					18	1943
1944	19							19	1944
1945	20							20	1945
1946	21	Nendaz, TI	Matrimonio	Hogar	0			21	1946
1947	22		Nace Paul					22	1947
1948	23							23	1948
1949	24		Nace Anne					24	1949
1950	25							25	1950
1951	26							26	1951
1952	27							27	1952
1953	28		Nace Gabriel					28	1953
1954	29		Nace Emile					29	1954
1955	30							30	1955
1956	31							31	1956
1957	32							32	1957
1958	33							33	1958
1959	34		Nace Yvonne					34	1959
1960	35							35	1960
1961	36							36	1961
1962	37							37	1962
1963	38							38	1963
1964	39							39	1964
1965	40			Secretaría	50			40	1965
1966	41							41	1966
1967	42							42	1967
1968	43							43	1968
1969	44							44	1969
1970	45		Fallecimiento padre					45	1970
1971	46							46	1971
1972	47				30	Cancer de seno		47	1972
1973	48		Fallecimiento suegra					48	1973
1974	49							49	1974
1975	50		Fallecimiento madre					50	1975
1976	51				50			51	1976
1977	52							52	1977
1978	53		Abuela					53	1978
1979	54							54	1979
1980	55							55	1980
1981	56							56	1981
1982	57							57	1982
1983	58							58	1983
1984	59							59	1984
1985	60							60	1985
1986	61							61	1986
1987	62			Jubilación				62	1987
1988	63							63	1988
1989	64							64	1989
1990	65					Accidente de auto		65	1990
1991	66							66	1991
1992	67							67	1992
1993	68		Fallecimiento hermano					68	1993
1994	69							69	1994
1995	70							70	1995
1996	71							71	1996
1997	72							72	1997
1998	73							73	1998
1999	74		Fallecimiento Henri			Cirugía del corazón		74	1999
2000	75	Sion						75	2000
2001	76							76	2001
2002	77							77	2002
2003	78							78	2003
2004	79							79	2004
2005	80		Conoce Stefano					80	2005
2006	81							81	2006
2007	82							82	2007
2008	83							83	2008
2009	84	EMS, Sion, VS				Fractura de cuello del fémur		84	2009
2010	85					fémur		85	2010
2011	86							86	2011
Año	Edad	Residencia	Familia / Pareja	Actividad	Carga	Salud	Nacionalidad	Edad	Año

Fig. 1 Example of the VLV life event calendar translated into Spanish

who chose to answer in their mother tongue included people who would have been able to answer in the local language but who felt more comfortable and confident when answering in their native language.

Nevertheless, this measure also has some side effects. For scientific translations, two professional translators should translate the survey material with constant dialogue with researchers (Harckness 2003). There was at least one member of the VLV team who was a native speaker in Portuguese, Italian and Spanish. But this was not the case for Albanian and Serbo-Croatian, resulting in some uncertainty and insecurity in trusting the validity of the translations. There was confusion between Serbian and Croatian and two translations had to be done without being reviewed by a researcher from the VLV team. Moreover, translations into Albanian, Serbian, and Croatian were incorrectly evaluated by the interviewers in charge of the Yugoslavian oversamples leading to "on-the-fly" corrections by the interviewers. To conclude, such translation procedures consume time and money. Results may also imply negotiating within the team on the priorities to give to translations among other survey needs, considering human and financial resources. This may explain why many surveys do not translate their questionnaires and run the risk of not reaching immigrants who did not get the opportunity to master the local language enough to understand relatively complex questionnaires.

For contact and interviewing procedures in native and local languages, bilingual interviewers were hired. The same interviewers conducted the initial contact, follow-up of the respondent files, and face-to-face interviews. The VLV team in Basel and Geneva recruited people with graduate degrees. Preference was given to second-generation immigrants from the same country as the target populations but this was kept as an option. Language and interviewing competences were prioritized and we did not pay much attention to cultural proximity. As an example, the first wave of Geneva interviewers included first-generation migrants from Latin America. However, those Latin American collaborators reported signs of rejection from Spanish and Portuguese elderly. These interviewers complained about being judged as less legitimate, or less well-integrated newcomers by the respondents, i.e. the former generations of immigrants. Some respondents did not understand, and sometimes did not accept, being interviewed by people from Latin America. Interviewers from the second generation also spoke about some signs of social distance, of a generational gap; "You cannot understand what we went through" was the kind of sentence often heard during contact or interviewing. Finally, recruiting interviewers with a university degree and being a member of the Albanian and Serbo-Croatian communities in Basel proved to be difficult. For the Serbo-Croatian interviews, this difficulty was greater during the contact procedure if the respondent was not from the same community of origin because of resentments from the war in ex-Yugoslavia in the 1990s. This led to a high degree of mistrust toward the interviewers and, most of the time, to refusal to participate as well.

The last measure mentioned was to promote the study among migrant communities. This was designed to reduce distrust. Letters were sent to immigrant associations. Information also circulated among mass media (radio and newspapers), churches, grocery stores, bars, where Portuguese, Spanish, or Italians often went. The impact of such a promotion is hard to measure:

> It's hard to give an opinion of the efficiency of the promotion. Honestly, I'm not sure it was really effective. Out of all the people I interviewed, I had two people who said they had heard of us. Once at the church and once at the Casa Benefica. (148, Portuguese interviewer).

But some were reassured that the survey was serious:

> I got some feedback from the respondents. They had seen the poster at the Spanish consulate and also at the church .... People talking about that said that it reassured them, that it was not fraudulent [approval of other interviewers]. That it was not a rip-off. (159, Spanish interviewer)

These measures confirm the aforementioned elements of vulnerability: a lack of proficiency in local language and distrust toward survey features provide evidence of social distance between the VLV research design and the target populations. Despite measures to overcome these obstacles, the response rate remained low and other, unexpected obstacles started to appear.

5 VLV Research Design Confronted with Realities on the Ground

Portuguese and Spanish oversamples in Geneva were the first two projects launched. Despite the measures initially taken, it appeared that elderly migrants were harder to reach than expected because of various reasons explained below. After a few weeks, the response rate remained low; after 6 weeks, it was only 2 % for Portuguese and 8 % for Spanish. The Italian oversample was launched in Basel a few weeks later and experienced the same difficulties in motivating people to participate. The former Yugoslavian oversample launched at the same time as the Italian one was doing worse; after experiencing many difficulties with translations and interviewer recruitment, the VLV team was confronted with a quasi-systematic refusal from former Yugoslavian elders.

The low response rate of elderly immigrants was due to higher non-contact rate and a higher refusal rate than for the main sample. We calculated the final response, refusal, and contact rates according to the standards of the American Association for Public Opinion Research.[4] The response rate refers to the number of people who wholly or partially completed the questionnaires. It was 36 % for the VLV main

---

[4] Standard definitions of the American Association for Public Opinion Research (2010):

- Response rate $= (I+P)/(I+P) + (R+NC+O) + (UH+UO)$
- Refusal rate $= R/((I+P)+(R+NC+O) + UH + UO))$
- Contact rate $= (I+P)+R+O/(I+P)+R+O+NC+ (UH + UO)$

I = completed interview; P = partial interview; R = refusal and break-off; NC = Non-contact; O = Other; UH = Unknown Household; UO = Unknown other.
For additional information, please refer to the following Web site:
http://www.aapor.org/Standard_Definitions2/4232.htm

Table 2 Response, refusal, and contact rates by nationality		Italians	Portuguese	Spanish
	Response rate	0.15	0.22	0.18
	Refusal rate	0.66	0.37	0.59
	Contact rate	0.81	0.59	0.76

Oversample—Geneva—Individuals reached by snowball procedures not included

sample in Geneva (Guichard et al. 2012), illustrating the difficulties of running a survey in Switzerland, a country where low rates of participation in surveys are increasingly commonplace (see the chapter of Oris et al. in this volume). The rate was even lower for the oversample populations. It was particularly low for the Spanish and Portuguese (see Table 2). Spanish and Italians tended to be easier to reach but had a higher refusal rate, whereas Portuguese were less reachable but more inclined to complete the questionnaires.

The contact rate refers to the proportion of all cases contacted including those who refused to participate. Compared to the Italians and Spanish, the Portuguese were much harder to contact. Having or not having a landline phone may explain this: more than 37 % of the Portuguese oversample did not have a landline phone, compared to 23 % for the Italians and Spanish. As a reminder, in the case of no landline phone, the instruction was to do a visit at home. The success rate for such a procedure was low in Geneva for the main sample. For the oversamples, the visit procedure turned out to be unfruitful because elderly migrants are generally away from home for several weeks due to travelling back-and-forth between their home country and Switzerland. This procedure was gradually given up because it was time and money consuming. According to the reports of the Portuguese interviewers and members of the community, many Portuguese migrants choose to go back and forth between Switzerland and Portugal. These people spend only a few weeks of the year in Switzerland, which makes them hard to reach, whereas this way of living might be less financially advantageous for the Italians and Spanish.

Once a person is reached by phone or by a visit at home, there are still many barriers to overcome before he or she accepts to participate. Many were suspicious of guaranteed anonymity and confidentiality: "What is the guarantee that you will not give my name to the authorities?" Some expressed feelings of resentment against Switzerland: "What's the point of that? Things will never change ... I worked all my life in Switzerland and I receive a wretched pension." Others equated the university with the authorities and feared controls: "Your questionnaire is far too intrusive." Many didn't have time for an appointment either because they were working to supplement their pension or because of travel between their country of origin and Switzerland: "I don't have time, I'm about to go back to Portugal for three months." Finally, the length and difficulty of the questionnaire scared many people. Its complexity led to the fear of not being able to correctly answer or understand the questions despite the translation. Clearly, a lower level of education compared to the overall population or cases of illiteracy may contribute to reluctance to answer a long questionnaire. For some, especially people from former Yugoslavia, reviewing their life course using the life event calendar involved remembering traumatizing events related to war or dictatorship. Some family members of respondents reproached this intrusiveness: "My father has had nightmares since the visit of your interviewer."

To conclude this section, VLV monitoring shows that there are specific reasons for elderly migrants to not participate in the VLV survey and that these reasons are strongly related to their living conditions and past lives. Traveling between countries of origin and Switzerland, high suspicion toward VLV, and resentment against what reminded them about the difficulties of their past life created risks of not gaining access to elderly migrants that were largely underestimated by the VLV team. The response rate was lower than for the oversamples than for the main sample, and it was hard to reach such a level. After a few weeks of fieldwork, elements of vulnerability appeared to be so prominent for elderly migrants that they started compromising the success of the VLV subproject on migration. It became urgent to start thinking about a different approach for dealing with these difficulties.

6 Adapting the Research Design to Reduce Social Distance

Our analyses of reasons for non-response reflects the social distance between the VLV research design and the population covered by the survey. Social distance refers to the idea of a social space structured by characteristics such as age, gender, origin, or social status (Bonnet 2008). In this sense, the survey reveals social disparity each time that the respondents have a status, in particular social status, lower than the interviewer. The survey also constitutes a space of "symbolic violence" when the interviewer or researchers unilaterally impose the rules of the game—goals and use of data—without possible negotiation or complete understanding from the respondents (Bourdieu and Balazs 1993). Elderly migrants did not tend to identify themselves with the goals of the VLV survey; or more explicitly, we did not succeed in convincing them to. In other words, VLV remained an institutional project far from their interests. Once this was recognised, the goal of the VLV team became to reduce this social distance by innovating with the contact and interviewing procedures, but we also had to give up some goals.

Since the oversamples of the elderly coming from Portugal and Spain living in Geneva were the first to be contacted, they were used for innovating new contact and interviewing approaches and to create good practice exchanges with the VLV team in Basel. People from former Yugoslavia living in Basel were reluctant to participate, and completed interviews were rare. Considering the difficulties related to translations and interviewer recruitment, but also more importantly, the reasons of refusal that included war trauma, the VLV team decided maximizing their response rates should not be done at the expense of ethical considerations and ended this field-work. It was replaced by an Italian oversample in Geneva, since Italians represent 40 % of immigrants 65 and over. Since Portuguese, Spanish, and Italian oversamples knew difficulties, but not to the same degree as former Yugoslavians, the VLV team decided to overcome the obstacles by respecting ethical and scientific requirements.

The first step for these oversamples was to change the interviewers' profile to reduce social distance between interviewers and respondents. At the beginning, being bilingual was the only criterion for recruitment. A preference was given to second-generation immigrants originating from the same country as the target population and to people with a university degree. To break the deadlock, being a first-generation immigrant from the same country—or even better the same region—as the target populations, having a good network within the immigrants' communities, not necessarily having an academic profile but an experience with the elderly were the new recruitment criteria. Most of the interviewers with the previous profile were discouraged and gave up. The VLV team assigned new cases to the most effective interviewers. Interviewers with the new profile had 1 month to convince new respondents. New interviewers worked in close collaboration with the field officer to ensure quality but also to maintain their motivation. It had also been decided to not self-administer questionnaires but that the interviewers would be ready to do the entire VLV questionnaires with the respondents to prevent the obstacle of complete or partial illiteracy.

Despite the new criteria, three out of seven interviewers did not obtain an acceptable response rate. Beyond personal reasons for not fulfilling the requirements, a high level of motivation seems to be the primary factor in a high contact rate (tenacity despite the difficulty in reaching the respondents) and a low refusal rate (capacity to convince and inspire confidence):

> It was mainly to make a step towards my community, which I do not frequent a lot. It was a way to meet people and see the problems they face … see how people cope with their living conditions. I thought it was good for them and so I was motivated to convince them of the value of the survey. I knew that, once we met, it was always a nice encounter. And I could also somehow bring a little more, give some information, the address of an association or other social information. (148, Portuguese interviewer)

> I work alongside my studies. I did it for this reason. I was interested. It was an interdisciplinary survey; it ties into my studies, even a lot. Then I realized it was really interesting for them [the Spanish elders] actually. For the community. And it inspired me a lot, not only to earn one's living. (159, Spanish Interviewer)

Adding a snowball sample to the oversample was an added measure to increase the number of cases available for analysis. Respondents had to be between 65 and 79 with Spanish or Portuguese nationalities. Since it was difficult to reach these populations, the VLV team decided to include people with dual nationality. The total sample (original oversample and snowball sample) was stratified by sex. Respondents were recruited among interviewers' networks, immigrant associations, and Spanish and Portuguese churches. Each respondent was asked if he or she knew someone interested in completing the questionnaires. Since it was also hard to reach Italians, the VLV team conducted the same snowball procedure for them.

Some 13.8 % (18 out of 130 individuals) of Iberian interviews come from the snowball procedure, which only had a small effect on the number of individuals from Spain in the final sample. The competence of the new Iberian interviewers to convince respondents on the phone played a more important role in explaining the increase in response rate. A snowball procedure through the respondents' network did not work because of the length and the content of the questionnaires:

> Some people who completed the questionnaires told others what it was really about, the questions and so on, and then some refused, three-quarters of people refused because they had heard how it is . . . They heard that we wanted to know about their possessions in their origin country. They wondered if their children would get in trouble because of that (156, Portuguese interviewer).

In Geneva, the number of snowball questionnaires accounted for 36.4 % (43 out of 118 individuals) of the final Italian sample of respondents. As noted above, this fieldwork was launched at the end of the Iberian oversample to compensate for the failure of the ex-Yugoslavian effort. Recruitment of interviewers for the Italian oversample was based on the same procedures and profiles as for the new Iberian generation of interviewers. Five Italian collaborators started to recruit respondents from the original contact list. They also had 1 month to show their ability to convince and complete interviews. Even within this short period, contacts were decreasing too quickly. Recruitment by snowball was quickly launched.

Interviewers frequently reported difficulties for elderly migrants to be tested on cognitive resources. The latter started with a vocabulary test in French (for Geneva) and German (for Basel) that had not been translated because of equivalence problems. This test requires an excellent knowledge of vocabulary. Some respondents had a feeling of failure and were highly frustrated after this section of the questionnaire. They felt like they were being tested on their ability to speak the local language, at the same time as most of them were responding in their mother tongue to the questionnaires. This may also mirror some discussions on local language exams to test one's integration in Switzerland. Whatever the cause, it was embarrassing for the interviewers who reported people crying or furious, interrupting the procedure and refusing to continue with the survey, or staying passive until the end of the interview. The VLV team decided to give up this section for the Portuguese and Spanish respondents to prevent a break in the snowball sampling, and to not show disrespect toward the respondents.

At the end of a complicated and difficult experience, it was confirmed that reducing the social distance between research designers, interviewers, and potential respondents helped to include elderly migrants in the survey, though with varying success depending on the adaptations and the targeted populations. The question remains as to what kind of sample we get at the end of such a process.

7 Cost-Benefit Analysis of Adapting Standard Procedures to Represent Elderly Migrants

Adapting procedures may improve access to hard-to-reach groups within large-scale surveys, but the impact of such adjustments may not be neutral regarding the quality of final samples. In the case of including elderly migrants within VLV, such adaptations were crucial to avoid the failure of the subproject on migration, but this also involved taking some risks. The challenge was to negotiate a trade-off between biasing results by modifying contact and interviewing procedures, and not getting a final sample large enough for further analyses. To know if the rewards made the effort worthwhile, a cost-benefit analysis of the impacts of such adjustments was necessary.

The most obvious cost is the loss of comparison with former Yugoslavians because of ending the fieldwork in Basel. This comparison was worthwhile because of the specific characteristics of this group. Their arrival in Switzerland was more recent than Italians and Spanish. Some former Yugoslavians came to Switzerland to seek asylum, which is not the case for the other groups of old immigrants who arrived as adults and grew old in Switzerland. They are not EU citizens and this difference in legal status may give rise to different practices compared to other elderly migrants such as not spending extended periods of time alternately in Switzerland and the country of origin. One of the good practices in surveys is to maximize cooperation or response rates within the limits of ethical treatment of human subjects. This last criterion played a major role for former Yugoslavians regarding the above-mentioned trade-off.

On the other hand, such a loss was compensated by an oversample of Italians in Geneva. Having Italian oversamples in Geneva and Basel allows comparison of immigrants from the same origin but who immigrated to different regions of Switzerland, which differ in their population composition, linguistic dimension, size of urban area, and integration policies. Such comparisons should give rise to analysis of the impact of these differences on immigrant living conditions at retirement.

Even if the response rate of elderly people with foreign origins remains lower than that of the main sample (see Table 2), increase in participation to the survey was an important benefit of the adjustments to the standard procedures, especially with the recruitment of new interviewers. This benefit can only be measured for the Portuguese and Spanish fieldwork because they were the first two populations for which innovating contact and interviewing procedures were introduced after having noted the difficulties of the standard procedures for these groups. Indeed, only these two projects allow a comparison between first and second wave interviewers. The following graph shows the coincidence between the increase in the response rate for the Spanish and Portuguese oversamples and the recruitment of new collaborators (Fig. 2).

It is not possible to run the same analysis to observe the effect of new recruitment for the Italian oversamples in Basel and Geneva, since they immediately benefited from the experience acquired. Nevertheless, Italian oversamples also strongly profited from the snowball approach. Indeed, 55.1 % (43 out of 78 individuals) of the Italian oversample in Geneva came from the snowball approach, 54.5 % (55 out of 101 individuals) in Basel. Adjusting VLV contact procedures by introducing this technique based on a positive appreciation of the social relations within the communities contributed to more than half of the final Italian oversamples.

The reader will have noticed that the initial objective of 120 respondents by nationality and canton was not achieved despite the implementation of new contact

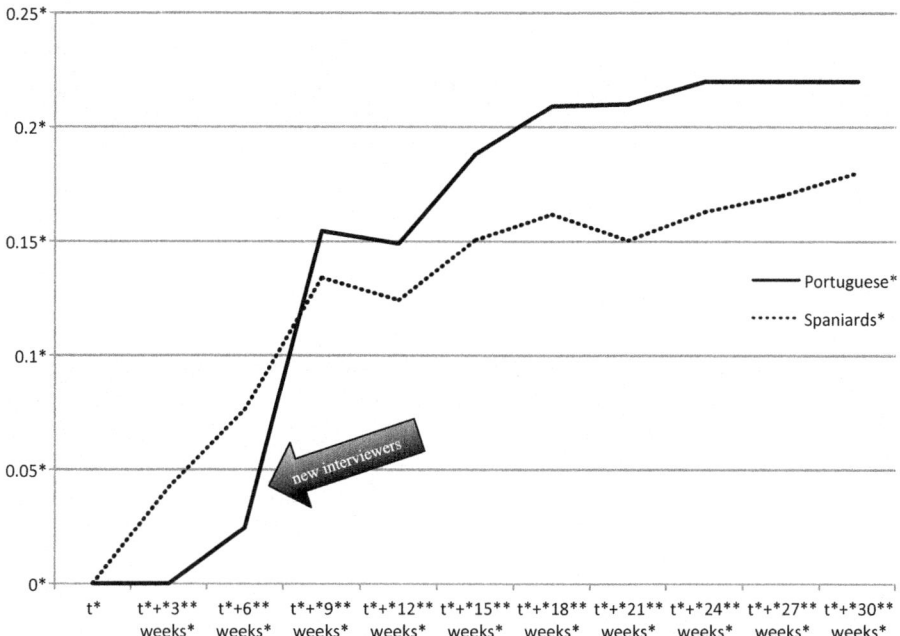

Fig. 2 Evolution of the response rate throughout fieldwork. Spanish and Portuguese oversample—Geneva—snowball sample not included

and interviewing procedures. The decision was made to take into consideration elderly migrants from the main sample as well, meaning elderly of foreign origins who were randomly selected to be part of the main fieldwork in Geneva and Basel (see Oris et al. in this volume). From a quantitative perspective, the final samples of elderly migrants are the result of several methodological choices that led to the sample composition showed in Table 3. The objective of 120 respondents by nationality and canton was achieved for Italians, but not for Portuguese and Spanish. Some researchers proposed to merge these two groups into a single Iberian sample. Nevertheless, from a theoretical point of view, this is not pertinent considering their different migratory trajectories, the evolution of migratory and integration policies, and living conditions in their host countries. In the end, the final overall immigrant sample contains 366 individuals from Italy, Spain, and Portugal between 65 and 79.

Considering the various components of the final oversamples, one may question the impact of the different contact procedures (snowball or random sample) on the representativeness of the files delivered to the researchers. Do the respondents obtained by snowball significantly differ from those randomly obtained? This question is not relevant for the Portuguese oversample since only two participants were part of the snowball sample, however, a significant share of the Spanish and Italians were recruited through this procedure. To establish if those two subpopulations significantly differ from each other, we ran chi-square tests (or

Table 3 Composition of the VLV final samples of elderly migrants

		Geneva			Basel
		Italy	Portugal	Spain	Italy
Oversample	Random	35	61	41	46
		30 %	97 %	61 %	39 %
	Snowball	43	2	16	55
		36 %	3 %	24 %	47 %
Main sample		40	0	10	17
		34 %	0 %	15 %	14 %
	Total	118	63	67	118

Fisher's exact test in the case of small n in the cross-tables) to test the null hypothesis of no significant association between the age group, sex, level of education, and last occupational status of respondents and the method of sampling (random/snowball). The p-values of each test are above 0.05, so we accept the null hypothesis and conclude that there is no significant bias as far as the above-mentioned variables are concerned. To conclude, the adjustments of contact approaches do not appear to have distorted the quality of the final samples and allow a sample large enough to run some descriptive and multivariate analyses.

The initial objective was reached since elderly migrants are largely overrepresented in the VLV database. For example, Spanish migrants are three times more numerous in our database (for the 65–79 year-olds) than they are in the residential population. Consequently, weighting issues do arise, and attention should be paid as to how weights are assigned. Furthermore, manipulating the database with care remains crucial considering the impossibility to reach many of them. When analyzing and interpreting the data, one has to be conscious of what the database contains and what it does not. The file does not include individuals who left Switzerland to spend their retirement in their country of origin (though it was not the goal of VLV to gain access to such groups), individuals who did not identify themselves to the goals and uses of VLV, and individuals who were not in Switzerland at the time of the survey. Moreover, with such complicated questionnaires, the biggest risk for VLV was to reach only highly skilled persons who are the exceptions among elderly migrants from Italy, Spain, and Portugal living in Switzerland. Nevertheless, the focus group with the interviewers in charge of the oversamples demonstrates that the risk did not materialize for VLV:

> I had many respondents who only did primary school, or almost nothing. Because at that time it was normal, education was not mandatory in Spain, in Franco's time … A lot dropped out of school to help their family or to help in the fields … For illiterate respondents, it was not a big deal for us because we were with them all the time throughout the questionnaire, we were there for that purpose, and then it was easy. (159, Spanish interviewer).

Further analysis on socioeconomic and health conditions confirm these words: elderly migrants in the VLV database generally have a low level of education, a low skilled status, and suffer from worse health status and economic situations than the overall population of the same age (Kaeser and Bolzman 2013).

8   Capturing Vulnerability: A Delicate Balance Between Scientific Requirements and Realities on the Ground

The VLV experience underlines the dilemma of large-scale surveys aimed at capturing vulnerability: not having tailored contact and interviewing procedures but running the risk of failing to capture vulnerability; or introducing specific procedures but running the risk of impairing the comparison. VLV's team faced this tension through an active dialogue between scientific requirements and realities on the ground to adapt survey procedures pragmatically and carefully.

To create conditions that favor such a dialogue, it is first necessary to take into account the components and reasons why target groups might be vulnerable. It is fundamental to get to know as much as possible about the groups' specificities before launching the fieldwork, and to create contact and interviewing procedures in accordance with the different components of the target groups. Most important, it is crucial to take time throughout the fieldwork to establish and maintain a pragmatic dialogue within the research team to understand what happened on the ground and to respect scientific requirements of research designers at the same time. Such a balance is key to reducing social distance between research designers, interviewers and respondents, and to assessing vulnerability without impairing the quality of the data.

As we have seen, social distance between the target populations and the survey may be expressed through age, socioeconomic status, social and cultural capital, and other factors. It may lead to an asymmetric relation between the interviewers—representing the monopole of symbolic violence brought about by the formality of the survey—and the respondents. The VLV experience confirms that the interviewers play a major role in reducing this gap. They are more than a neutral conduit for the transmission of standardized questionnaires. They constitute intermediaries because of their "double affiliations to the world of researchers and to the world of respondents"[5] (Bessière and Houseaux 1997: 103). When they are aware, they can manage the intrinsic ambivalence of the survey situation to produce more positive and fewer negative outcomes. This is a reminder that research designers need to communicate, train, manage, and inform interviewers not only before but also throughout the fieldwork according to the goals and uses of the survey to create reflexivity from the collaborators on their practices and roles.

Admittedly, the price may be a time- and money-consuming survey, the necessity to be flexible, getting off the beaten track, and even sometimes giving up some comparisons as was the case for the VLV's cognitive tests. Nevertheless, this is

[5] Author's own translation.

often necessary if one claims to better understand vulnerability. Not taking this major issue into account means running the risk of getting into a vicious circle: being vulnerable puts oneself at risk of not being reached by a large-scale survey, and not being represented in large-scale surveys may amount to being ignored by scientific and political agendas. Providing resources to assess vulnerability is not only a methodological engagement; this is also a major social issue about giving a voice to the voiceless.

Acknowledgements This communication results from research works executed within the framework of the National Centre of Competence in Research LIVES and the SINERGIA Project CRSII1-129922, which are financed by the Swiss National Science Foundation. The author is grateful to the Swiss National Science Foundation for its support. The author is warmly thankful to Prof. Michel Oris for his significant support and contribution during the data collection and for having carefully reviewed this chapter, and to Dr. Floriane Demont and Dr. Guy Elcheroth for their scientific support during the writing process. Finally, the author thanks the interviewers—especially the ones in charge of the elderly migrants' sample—and the staff of the centre for the interdisciplinary study of gerontology and vulnerability who highly contributed to the VLV data collection.

References

Bessière, C., & Houseaux, F. (1997). Suivre des enquêteurs. *Genèses, 29*, 100–114.

Bolzman, C., Fibbi, R., & Vial, M. (2001). *Les loisirs des personnes âgées immigrées: pratiques, besoins, demandes*. Genève: Institut d'études sociales.

Bolzman, C., Poncioni, R., Vial, M., & Fibbi, R. (2004). Older labour migrants' wellbeing in Europe: The case of Switzerland. *Ageing and Society, 24*(3), 411–429.

Bonnet, F. (2008). La distance sociale dans le travail de terrain: compétence stratégique et compétence culturelle dans l'interaction d'enquête. *Genèses, 4*(73), 57–74.

Bourdieu, P., & Balazs, G. (1993). L'interrogatoire. In P. Bourdieu (Ed.), *La Misère du monde* (pp. 927–939). Paris: Éditions du Seuil.

Elcheroth, G., Fasel, N., Gianettoni, L., Kleiner, B., Laganà, F., Lipps, F., Penic, S., & Pollien A. (2011, September). Minorities in general social surveys: What we can learn from the Swiss case and why the black box should be opened wider. *FORS Position Paper Series*.

Feskens, R., Hox, J., Lensvelt-Mulders, G., & Schmeets, H. (2006). Collecting data among ethnic minorities in an international perspective. *Field Methods, 18*(3), 284–304.

Gerville-Réache, L., Couallier, V., & Paris, N. (2011). Echantillon représentatif (d'une population finie): Définition statistique et propriétés. *Archive ouverte pluridisciplinaire HAL*, n° hal-00655566.

Groves, R. (2006). Nonresponse rates and nonresponse bias in household surveys. *Public Opinion Quarterly, 70*(5), 646–675.

Groves, R. M., & Couper, M. P. (1998). *Nonresponse in household interview surveys.* New York: Wiley.

Guichard, E., Nicolet, M., Monnot, C., Joye, D., & Oris, M. (2012). *Surveying the elderly in Switzerland.* Conference organized by the NCCR-LIVES, Lausanne.

Harckness, J. (2003). Questionnaire translation. In J. A. Harkness, F. J. R. Van de Vijver, & P. P. Mohler (Eds.), *Cross-cultural survey methods* (pp. 35–56). Hoboken: Wiley-Interscience.

Kaeser, L., & Bolzman, C. (2013). *The well-being of immigrant elders.* Conference organized by the Research Committee on Migration of the International Sociological Association, Tel-Aviv.

Laganà, F., Elcheroth, G., Penic, S., Kleiner, B., & Falsel, N. (2011). *National minorities and their representation in Swiss surveys (II): Which practices make a difference?* (FORS working paper series, paper 2011-3). Lausanne: FORS.

Laganà, F., Elcheroth, G., Penic, S., Kleiner, B., & Fasel, N. (2013). National minorities and their representation in Swiss surveys (II): Which practices make a difference? *Quality and Quantity, 47*(3), 1287–1314.

Lalive d'Epinay, C., Bickel, J. F., Maystre, C., & Vollenwyder, N. (2000). *Vieillesses au fil du temps. 1979–1994: Une révolution tranquille.* Lausanne: Réalités sociales.

Lipps, O., Laganà, F., Pollien A., & Gianettoni L. (2011). National minorities and their representation in Swiss surveys (I): Providing evidence and analyzing causes for their under-representation, *FORS Working Paper, (2),* 1–20.

Ludwig, C., Cavalli, S., & Oris, M. (2014). "Vivre/Leben/Vivere": An interdisciplinary survey addressing progress and inequalities of aging over the past 30 years in Switzerland. *Archives of Gerontology and Geriatrics, 58*(2), 240–248.

Marpsat, M., & Razafindratsima, N. (2010). Les méthodes d'enquêtes auprès des populations difficiles à joindre: introduction au numéro spécial. *Methodological Innovations Online, 5*(2), 3–16.

Mauger, G. (1991). Enquêter en milieu populaire. *Genèses, 6,* 125–142.

Piguet, E. (2004). *L'immigration en Suisse. Cinquante ans d'entrouverture.* Lausanne: Presses polytechniques et universitaires romandes.

Riandey, B., & Quaglia, M. (2009). Surveying hard-to-reach groups. In P. Bonnel, M. Lee-Gosselin, J. Zmud, & J. L. Madre (Eds.), *Transport survey methods: Keeping up with a changing world* (pp. 127–144). Bingley: Emerald.

Rossini, S. (2013). De la mesure des politiques sociales. In J. M. Bonvin, P. Gobet, S. Rossini, & J. P. Tabin (Eds.), *Manuel de politiques sociales* (pp. 91–117). Lausanne: EESP et Réalités sociales.

Schiltz, M. A. (2005). Faire et défaire des groupes: L'information chiffrée sur les "populations difficiles à atteindre". *Bulletin of Sociological Methodology, 86,* 30–54.

Spini, D., Hanappi, D., Bernardi, L., Oris, M., & Bickel, J. F. (2013). Vulnerability across the life course: A theoretical framework and research directions. *LIVES Working Paper,* 2013 (27).

Tabutin, D. (2006). Les systèmes de collecte des données en démographie. In G. Caselli, J. Vallin, & G. Wunsch (Eds.), *Démographie, analyse et synthèse. Vol. VIII. Observation, méthodes auxiliaires, enseignement et recherche* (pp. 13–64). Paris: National Institute of Demographic Study.

Von dem Knesebeck, O., Wahrendorf, M., Hyde, M., & Siegrist, J. (2007). Socioeconomic position and quality of life among older people in 10 European countries: Results of the SHARE study. *Ageing and Society, 27*(2), 269–284.

Vulnerability Following a Critical Life Event: Temporary Crisis or Chronic Distress? A Psychological Controversy, Methodological Considerations, and Empirical Evidence

Pasqualina Perrig-Chiello, Sara Hutchison, and Bina Knöpfli

1 Introduction

Vulnerability is a multifaceted concept that is widely used, but not uncontested in science and practice. Scholars and practitioners from different disciplines, including social sciences, psychology, medicine, ethics, environmental sciences, and economy, use the term vulnerability to refer to conditions of human exposure to hazards, risks, and stresses. Vulnerability has – like similar concepts such as health, ageing, or resiliency – basically a "mobile" and flexible character. As a travelling concept it moves among disciplines, times, contexts and cultures, and changes its content by this translocation (Bal 2002). This creates a multidisciplinary picture, which sheds light on the various specific aspects of a concept or topic. Each discipline has its own reasons and methods to conceptualize and benchmark vulnerability, and consequently concepts, measures, and methods differ widely across disciplines. The multidisciplinary character and use of the term account, however, for the fact that there is little if any consensus with regard to a reliable and coherent conceptualization and operationalization of vulnerability (Morawa 2003).

P. Perrig-Chiello (✉) • B. Knöpfli
NCCR LIVES, IP 212, Chavannes-près-Renens, Switzerland

Institute of Psychology, University of Bern, Bern, Switzerland
e-mail: pasqualina.perrigchiello@psy.unibe.ch

S. Hutchison
NCCR LIVES, IP 212, Chavannes-près-Renens, Switzerland

Swiss Federal Institute for Vocational Education and Training (SFIVET), Bern, Switzerland

© The Author(s) 2016
M. Oris et al. (eds.), *Surveying Human Vulnerabilities across the Life Course*,
Life Course Research and Social Policies 3, DOI 10.1007/978-3-319-24157-9_4

Difficulties in defining vulnerability in a comprehensive and interdisciplinary[1] way have additionally prompted discussions surrounding its utility as a qualifying and discriminant concept in research and practice (Ruof 2004). For example it has been argued that labelling individuals as *vulnerable* risks viewing them as different, marginalized, and pitiable (Danis and Patrick 2002). In addition and above all, the label vulnerable may also be associated with the more or less implicit assumption that this is a stable and enduring characteristic, which again bears a further risk, namely the perpetuation of a negative state.

Although acknowledging these caveats, in our mind vulnerability remains a useful concept, provided that attempts are made to contextualize it distinctly (a) within the canon of different disciplines, and (b) within the status quo of a specific discipline by clearly delineating the theoretical base, the methodological approach and the associated implications and limitations. Along these lines the aims of the present contribution are, to show:

1. The challenges of contextualizing vulnerability conceptually and theoretically in psychological research by giving an overview of the status quo of research with regard to the question of whether vulnerability following a critical life event, namely the break-up of a long-term partnership, is a temporary crisis or rather a chronic strain (Sect. 2 of this chapter).
2. The impact of these challenges on designing an empirical study to answer the research questions around this controversy and a possible way to solve it methodologically, as it was done in the research project *"Vulnerability and Growth. Developmental dynamics and differential effects of the loss of an intimate partner in the second half of life*[2] (Sect. 3 of this chapter).
3. First results of this project focusing on two questions: (1) Is there empirical evidence that psychological vulnerability due to marital breakup is a temporary state? (2) What distinguishes psychologically highly vulnerable individuals from the least vulnerable ones in terms of psychosocial resources? (Sect. 4 of this chapter).

---

[1]In contrast to "multi-disciplinarity," which means an addition of different disciplinary perspectives, "inter-disciplinarity" refers to a common problem definition, a coordination of methods and a common way of presenting and implementing the results provided by exponents of different disciplines (Perrig-Chiello and Darbellay 2002).

[2]The project is part of the National Centre of Competence in Research LIVES "Overcoming Vulnerability over life course", supported by the Swiss National Science Foundation (project Nr. 125770) awarded to the first author.

2 Vulnerability Following a Critical Life Event from a Psychological Perspective

2.1 Contextualizing Vulnerability in the Status Quo of Psychological Research

The construct of vulnerability has been characterized by extensive theoretical and empirical research in various fields of psychology, but especially in clinical, health, and social psychology. Unsurprisingly, there is not one common definition of vulnerability in psychology, but different attempts at defining it. One broad and overarching definition delimits vulnerability as an individual belief system to be susceptible to harm, negative outcomes and unprotected from unpredictable danger or misfortune. Accompanying this lowered sense of control is an affective component consisting of feelings of anxiety, fear and apprehension (Perloff 1983). In the same line, but more specifically, vulnerability has been conceptualized in clinical psychology as a disturbance of self-concept or interpersonal relationships, which can trigger maladaptive attitudes and detrimental behaviors. Psychological vulnerability is thought to comprise a set of emotions and cognitions that pro- mote harmful reactions to stress, such as perceived helplessness and maladaptive coping behaviors. In turn, these maladaptive reactions to situations or critical life events can negatively affect psychological, physical, and social well-being (Sinclair and Wallston 2010). Vulnerability is conceptualized as resulting from an interaction between the resources available to individuals (such as personality, cognitive competence, social networks), and the life challenges they face. There is empirical evidence that psychological vulnerability results from developmental problems (early life experiences), personal incapacities, disadvantaged social status, inadequacy of interpersonal networks and support, and the complex interactions of these factors over the life course.

In line with this, in developmental psychology vulnerability has been primarily studied in childhood and youth, and to a much lesser extent in later adulthood or from a life course perspective. In the literature this fact is not only mirrored in considerable research gaps, but also in various theoretical controversies as well as in inconsistent findings. One major controversy focuses on the question of whether biographical transitions, and especially critical life events – such as marital breakup, unemployment, or serious illness – entail psychological vulnerability in the form of temporary dysfunctional reactions to acute stress, or rather if they produce a permanent state of vulnerability marked by persistent negative affect, sense of hopelessness, bad subjective health, etc. Furthermore, although a large consensus exists that psychological adaptation (i.e. the process of overcoming the state of vulnerability and adapting back to the state before the event) depends on available intra- and interpersonal resources (such as personality, resiliency, social support) as well as on external circumstances (e.g. predictability of the event), the differential impact of these variables and possible interactions are still not well understood. This applies especially to separation and divorce after a long-term partnership, since most research has been carried out with younger age groups (Pudrovska and Carr 2008).

2.2 Vulnerability Following Critical Life Events: State or Trait?

In the literature two major paradigms can be identified that deal with psychological adaptation to critical life events such as marital breakup. Whereas the *state approach* assumes that there are direct effects on psychological well-being caused by marital dissolution, the *trait approach* claims that psychological adjustment to marital breakup is primarily based on stable personality traits. Both paradigms are characterized by various theoretical approaches and controversies, which are delineated in the following sections.

2.2.1 State Approach: Does Marital Dissolution Cause Temporary or Chronic Psychological Vulnerability?

The current debate regarding the state approach is whether spousal breakup is a temporary stressor (or crisis) or rather a chronic strain. If marital breakup represents a crisis, people should adapt to their new life circumstances and recover from the negative impacts on psychological, physical and social well-being after a certain time. The chronic strain model in contrast assumes that marital breakup has the potential to create further stressors such as economic difficulties, which perpetuate the negative consequences over time (Amato 2000).

Empirical research has revealed mixed findings: Some study results support the crisis approach, others the chronic strain approach. Using three-wave panel data, Booth and Amato (1991) found that the increased level of psychological distress and unhappiness of divorced or permanently separated individuals declines within the 2 years following the event to then reach the level of the continuously married. In contrast, study results by Mastekaasa (1995) suggest that divorced individuals reported short-term (0–4 years after divorce) as well as long-lasting (4–8 years after divorce) increases in the amount of subjective distress compared to the stably married. More recent research studies could also not solve this controversy. Findings from a longitudinal study by Lucas (2005) showed that life satisfaction decreases after a divorce and then gradually rebounds in the 5 years following the event. However, the individuals also reported long-lasting changes: The level of life satisfaction 6 years after the divorce was significantly lower than the one reported during marriage. The author concludes that some individuals may not be able to adapt completely. Another longitudinal study over 12 years (Johnson and Wu 2002) found, consistent with the chronic state approach, that the level of psychological distress during and after the divorce does not decline until the individuals enter into a new marriage or cohabiting relationship. In contrast, the results of the study of Clark et al. (2008), which are based on observations in 20 waves of German panel data, show a rapid adaptation to divorce. There is even evidence that both women and men who divorced 5 or more years ago are currently significantly more satisfied with their lives compared to their level of life satisfaction 2–4 years before the event. Another longitudinal research by Clark and Georgellis (2013) investigated life satisfaction and mental well-being of divorcees in 16 waves of British panel data. The results also support the crisis theory and showed, with the exception of unemployment, a complete and rapid adaptation within 2 years to life events including divorce. Focusing on middle-aged individuals, Hughes and Waite (2009) found that some health dimensions such as depression seem to respond both rapidly and intensely to changes in marital status, whereas others such as chronic physical health problems develop slowly over a long period of time. In line with these results, Lorenz et al. (2006) conclude in their study with divorced women that the increase of depressive symptoms can be interpreted as a temporary reaction to acute stressors caused by divorce. Furthermore, a decade after the event, divorcees reported a significantly higher amount of physical illness than their married counterparts. The authors interpret the difference in physical illness as a possible cumulative response to chronic stress.

The crisis model assumption is based on the hedonic treadmill model of Brickman and Campbell (1971). According to this perspective, individuals are affected by emotionally significant events, but usually adapt back to a neutral set point or baseline of subjective well-being (Diener et al. 2006). Although this approach has meanwhile been modified, e.g. taking into consideration that the baseline set-points may be positive rather than neutral (Diener et al. 2006), it has been supported by results that show that objective circumstances account for surprisingly little variance in reports of subjective well-being (Clark et al. 2008). The basic concept of adaptation to divorce implies a model of marital dissolution as a crisis where psychological distress is low before the event, increases as the breakup approaches and then declines following the event. Furthermore it suggests that the psychological distress following marital dissolution represents short-time secondary stressors, such as the acute pain of the loss, economic difficulties or changes in the social network (Booth and Amato 1991). In the same line, but more specifically, the divorce-stress-adjustment perspective (Amato 2000) views marital breakup as a process that sets into motion numerous stressful events. Severity and duration of negative outcomes resulting from these stressors depend on the presence of a variety of moderating or protective factors such as individual and interpersonal resources. Of all forms of social support, a new intimate relationship may be the most important factor to foster adjustment to divorce (Amato 2000). For example, Wang and Amato (2000) demonstrated that individuals with a new intimate relationship reported more positive appraisals of life and better overall adjustment than those who stayed single. Another factor that may have an impact on psychological adaptation to marital breakup is the initiator status, that means, which spouse takes the initiative to separate. Being the initiator enables the individual to control the event, which thus may lead to better adaptation after separation (Wang and Amato 2000). The study of Wang and Amato (2000) showed that initiators report a better overall adjustment than non-initiators, however, only short-term effects (on average 16 months after the divorce) were investigated. The relevance of the initiator status has been confirmed by the study of Hewitt and Turrell (2011). Women and men who self-initiated or jointly initiated the separation reported better well-being and mental health than non-initiators. Again, the results refer to short-term effects within 2 years after separation. Another possible and often discussed determinant of psychological adaptation is marital history (e.g. couples' perception of marital quality), however its role is controversially discussed in literature. While some studies suggest that persons from low-distress marriages have more difficulties in adapting than those from high-distress ones (Amato and Hohmann-Marriott 2007), other studies could not replicate these findings (Waite et al. 2009).

An important aspect of the debate is furthermore whether men and women differ in the process of adaptation to marital dissolution. Do women exhibit more vulnerability than men to impacts of divorce or vice versa? Simon (2002) showed in her longitudinal analyses that women have lower adjustment to divorce with regard to depression (higher depression rates), whereas the benefit of remarriage among persons who were previously divorced or separated was greater for men regarding health behavior (lower alcohol consumption). Men's and women's vulnerability to distress after marital breakup may be shaped by cultural and gender-typical norms for emotional display (Simon 2002). Analyzing data from 16 waves of the German Socio-Economic Panel Study, Andreß and Bröckel (2007) found that women reported significantly higher life satisfaction than men within the first 2 years after the separation. However, Strohschein et al. (2005) did not find any gender differences in the short-term effects of marital breakup.

To sum up it can be said that there is empirical evidence that whereas some individuals adapt rapidly to marital breakup, others remain vulnerable over a longer period of time. However it is not clear what exactly accounts for these individual differences. The topic of the large heterogeneity of reactions to loss has been tackled by a major research strand, the trait approach, which focused on personality factors as determinants of psychological adaptation to critical life events. This approach is highlighted in the following section.

2.2.2 Trait Approach: The Role of Personality in the Psychological Adjustment to Marital Disruption

The trait approach goes beyond the question of whether a critical life event such as marital disruption entails a chronic stress or if it is merely a temporary crisis. The trait approach focuses on individual differences due to personality-inherent characteristics (mostly assessed with the Big Five framework for personality traits, namely openness, conscientiousness, extraversion, agreeableness, and neuroticism). In the literature there is increasing empirical evidence that personality dimensions play a central role in coping with marital breakup. Pudrovska and Carr (2008) show in their study that recently divorced women who reported high levels of extraversion and openness, low levels of neuroticism and who applied advantageous coping strategies (such as problem- and positive emotion-focused coping), had a better adjustment regarding mental health. These results are confirmed by a study of Clark and Georgellis (2013), which shows that women with higher levels of extraversion were more satisfied with life after divorce. Diener et al. (2006) indicate in their revision of the hedonic treadmill-model that individual differences in well-being baseline levels are partly due to personality-based influences. The authors list three different lines of research that support this view. First, subjective well-being shows moderate stability over long periods of time and even in the face of changing life circumstances. Second, behavioral genetic studies suggest that well-being is moderately hereditary. Finally, several research studies show that personality factors strongly correlate with well-being variables. Diener et al. (2006) conclude that personality factors may predispose individuals to reach different levels of adjustment after a marital dissolution.

In addition to the Big Five personality traits, another personality dimension that has been discussed as a protective factor for negative adjustment to critical life events is resilience. Resilience pertains to the ability of adults to maintain relatively stable, healthy levels of psychological and physical function in the face of a highly disruptive event (Bonanno 2004). The available empirical evidence suggests that individual differences in psychological resilience predict accelerated recovery from stressful events (Ong et al. 2006). However, there is little literature that devotes attention to the role of resilience in psychological adaptation to the stressful event of marital dissolution.

A further debate that concerns the adjustment to marital breakup from a trait-approach is the relevance of the social selection hypothesis (Avison 1999). This hypothesis claims that individuals with certain patterns of personality and social characteristics are, to some extent, predestined for divorce. However, Gähler (2006) could not confirm that the effects of permanent selection explain the lower well-being after a divorce. Amato (2010) concludes in his review article that most of the results support the notion that marital breakup negatively affects the mental and physical health and that selection processes may play only a limited role.

Taken together, we can state that a considerable amount of psychological research exists with regard to psychological vulnerability after critical life events such as marital breakup. However, the status quo of research is marked by large inconsistencies. These inconsistencies concern mainly questions about the role of time passed since the event, and whether people recover or if they rather remain in a state of vulnerability. There seem to be large inter-individual differences in psychological adaptation to such critical life events, which are not fully understood. In particular the question of whether psychological vulnerability (if temporary or stable) is an inevitable outcome of marital breakup or not, has hardly been studied. Against this background, in the next section we attempt to shed light on the open questions around these controversies and research gaps by presenting possible methodological ways to answer them.

3   Vulnerability After Marital Breakup: An Empirical Study

3.1   *Outline of the Research Project, Aims and Research Questions*

Based on the shortcomings and research gaps mentioned above, the present project aimed at studying predictors of psychological adjustment to marital breakup due to separation, divorce or widowhood after a long-term partnership. The reason for focusing on long-term partnership is twofold: On the one hand it can be assumed that a marital breakup after a long shared life is particularly destabilizing and has a high potential of vulnerabilization. On the other hand – in the case of divorce – this is a contribution to close a significant research gap, since most research on marital breakup has been done with younger individuals having under-age children.

In this survey with two age groups (one in middle, the other in old age), four different loss-groups (one within the last 12 months, a second 12–24 months ago, a third 24–60 months ago, and a fourth with 5 or more years since marital breakup or spousal loss), and a group of age-matched married people serving as controls, a multi-method and an interdisciplinary approach[3] was used. Two assessments were planned, a first one in 2012, and a second one in 2014. The convenience of the design with the four marital disruption-groups lies in the possibility to gain some empirical evidence concerning the role of time passed since the breakup for psychological adaptation, despite the limitations of cross-sectional data. Of course, these results will have to be confirmed by longitudinal data (gathered in wave 2).

In this contribution we will present cross-sectional data focusing on the following aims:

(a) First we want to shed light on the short and middle-term outcomes of marital breakup in persons aged 40–65 years, which were on average married for 19 years prior to the divorce. For this sake we will compare four marital breakup groups (separated and/or divorced persons): one with a split within the last 12 months, another with a split 12–24 months ago, a further one with a separation that happened 24–60 months ago, and a last one who separated more than 5 years ago. The criterion for group classification is explicitly the time of separation, and not of divorce as it has been largely done in previous research, and which in our view is a shortcoming, since the time between separation and divorce can vary in a substantial way and renders a comparison rather difficult. These groups will be compared with a group of married age-matched people, continuously married (controls) regarding various well-being outcomes. This

---

[3] An outline of the study design and methods (sampling, psychometric quality of variables) is given in Hutchison et al. (2013). Working Report, NCCR LIVES.

approach should allow a first estimation with regard to the role of time passed since the critical life event for psychological adaptation and recovery (and in the negative case for lasting vulnerability). Considering the mixed findings on the issue, particular attention will be paid to gender effects.

(b) Second, extreme group analyses with regard to various indicators of psychological vulnerability (depression, hopelessness, life satisfaction, feeling of having overcome the loss) should allow insights concerning the question of to what extent highly vulnerable individuals differ from marginally vulnerable ones in terms of socio-demographic variables (education, financial situation), personality variables (Big Five traits, resilience), divorce circumstances (initiator-status), and post-divorce situation such as time passed since separation or being in a new intimate relationship.

3.2   Theoretical Base of the Study and Hypotheses

As a theoretical framework for investigating these research issues we propose a modified and extended view of the crisis-versus-chronic-stress model and the model of divorce-stress-adjustment (Lorenz et al. 2006; Amato 2000). Marital *separation* is viewed as a biographical turning point that can be expected or unexpected, initiated or endured, but which in any case has a high probability of creating turmoil and stress. The phase after separation can be viewed as a biographical transition, when routines of everyday life are shattered, people have to reorganize their lives, and take on new roles (phase of destabilization and reorganization). There is empirical evidence that after this phase of increased psychological vulnerability, a majority of people begin to adapt to the new situation, develop a new routine, and overcome this phase of psychological vulnerability around 2–3 years after the critical life event (Booth and Amato 1991; Clark and Georgellis 2013). This period is followed by a phase of stabilization when the majority of people is expected to get back to their habitual baseline-level of well-being prior to the turning point (after 3–5 years) (Dupre et al. 2009). A minority however is expected not to recover and to remain vulnerable. Whether the separation turns out to be a temporary crisis (after which people recover from their vulnerability) or whether it becomes a chronic stressor (mourning the loss of the partner, chronic depression and hopelessness) depends on the one hand on the available individual resources. We assume that individuals – based on their intra- (personality, resilience) and interpersonal resources (having children, relatives, friends, a new relationship) develop strategies, which allow them to adapt their life perspectives to the new situation in order to bring continuity to their lives and to assure their well-being. Socio-demographic variables such as gender, education and financial resources may also be important for adaptation to the new situation. On the other hand, besides these factors, the separation circumstances (predictability) may also play an important role for psychological adaptation. We know from the literature that not only initiator-status and having a new relationship have an impact on well-being outcomes, but also the anticipation of the separation and the time passed since separation (Amato 2010). Specifically, we expect:

1. Significant differences between the marital-breakup-groups with regard to certain indicators of psychological vulnerability, namely depression, life satisfaction, hopelessness, feeling of having overcome the break-up, but also subjective health, depending on the time passed since marital breakup: Individuals with a separation within the last 12 months are expected to be more vulnerable than those who experienced the breakup 12–24 months ago, and these again more than those with a separation that happened 2–5 years ago, and these finally more than those with a breakup more than 5 years ago. The latter group is expected to have adapted to the new situation, and therefore should not differ from the age-matched married control group. Considering the mixed findings in the literature with regard to gender differences, we do not have specific hypotheses on this issue.
2. That the central variables discriminating between highly vulnerable versus marginally vulnerable individuals are primarily personality traits (Big Five, resilience), separation circumstances (initiator-status), the time passed since separation, and being in a new relationship. Socio-demographic variables such as education and financial situation are expected to play a minor or inconsistent discriminating role.

3.3   Methodological Outline of the Study

3.3.1   Study Context and Participants

Our analyses are based on data of the first wave collected in spring 2012 in the context of the study described above.[4] To generate the sampling frame the Swiss Federal Office of Statistics (SFOS) supplied a quota sample stratified into cells of equal size by age group (5-year groups), gender (50:50), and marital status (separated/divorced, widowed, married). Quota sampling is the method of choice when the proportion of men and women with a special characteristic (such as recent divorce or bereavement) is relatively low. This is the case for recently divorced or widowed individuals in Switzerland (of a population of 7,954,662 Swiss residents in 2011, about 17 % were divorced and 12 % widowed, compared to 44 % married individuals (SFOS 2013). To allow for statistically significant comparisons among men and women and age groups, some groups (divorce at older age, bereavement among men) are over-represented. A total of 6890 persons between 40 and 89 years old (1551 separated/divorced, 1365 widowed, 3974 married), residing in German- or French-speaking Switzerland were contacted by mail and asked to participate in a survey about continuity and change in intimate relationships in the second half

---

[4]The project has been approved by the ethical committee of the University of Berne.

of life. Participants had the choice between filling out a paper-pencil questionnaire or using an online version. Non-respondents were re-contacted twice. Overall, the return rate for the sample supplied by the Federal Office of Statistics was 32 % ($n = 2236$). Due to ethical concerns, the SFOS was unwilling to supply a sample of persons who had experienced a divorce or bereavement in the past 2 years, so an alternative sampling strategy was used to recruit these participants. Specifically, we recruited a convenience sample using advertisements and appeals in newspapers and radio shows. All interested individuals were contacted with essentially the same invitation letter as the SFOS-sample. Eighty-seven percent of the directly recruited participants (n = 620) returned a filled-out questionnaire. For the research presented here, we will focus on individuals who had experienced a divorce and were between 40 and 65 years old ($n = 980$; average duration of ex-partnership = 19 years), and a control group of continuously married individual ($n = 348$, average duration of marriage: 28 years). Since we do not dispose of the baseline well-being measures before the critical event, the inclusion of continuously married controls is crucial in order to contextualize the results from the divorced and bereaved individuals.

An essential criterion of comparability of both groups is that they should be age-matched. As can be seen from Table 1, the married and the marital breakup group did not differ with regard to age. However the separation/divorce group contained a significantly higher ratio of women than the control group (62 % versus 54 %, $\phi = -.070, p = .011$). This can be explained by the fact that men are less likely to disclose than women regarding close relationships (Derlega et al. 2008). Table 1 gives a description of the socio-demographic variables of both groups.

There was also a significant group difference in education and financial situation, with more persons in the marital breakup group having higher educational degrees ($\chi2(6) = 20.43, p = .002$), and reporting a better financial situation ($\chi2(2) = 17.98$, $p < .001$). In the marital breakup group, a significantly higher percentage of men than women reported being in a new relationship at the time of the data collection (60 % versus 35 %, $\phi = -.247, p < .001$).

3.3.2   Variables and Measures

The questionnaire comprises mainly standardized test instruments and some original items developed by the research team. It was pretested in German and translated into French, followed by a back-translation and a pretest of the French version.

Psychological Outcome Variables: Indicators of Vulnerability

- *Depression* was measured with the German short version of the Center of Epidemiologic Studies Depression Scale (CES-D), which is called ADS-K (Hautzinger and Bailer 1993; French version by Fuhrer and Rouillon (1989)). This scale consists of 15 items (answers on a 4-point scale: 0 = *not at all* to 3 = *all the time*) and displays good internal consistency (Cronbach's alpha .80 in

Table 1 Characteristics and comparison of marital breakup group and continuously married controls

	Marital breakup group ($n = 980$)			Continuously married controls ($n = 348$)			Comparison divorced/married
	Women	Men	U-Test (z)/Chi²/ Phi	Women	Men	U-test (z)/Chi²	U-test (z)/Chi²/ Phi
N	608 (62 %)	371 (38 %)		189 (54 %)	159 (46 %)		−.070*c
Age: M (*SD*)	51.3 (*6.9*)	52.6 (*7.0*)	−2.79**a	51.6 (*7.6*)	52.7 (*8.3*)	−1.30 ns¹	−.36 nsa
Education (in %)			37.02***b			13.39*b	20.43**b
Primary school	4.1	3.8		3.8	6.4		
Second. school	1.6	1.9		5.4	3.8		
Professional formation	37.7	30.4		43.5	33.1		
Secondary II	14.2	6.2		14.5	9.6		
Higher prof. form.	30.3	33.9		22.6	26.1		
University	11.4	22.5		8.1	18.5		
Other	0.7	1.4		2.2	2.5		
Financial situation (%)			10.37**b			.68 nsb	17.98***b
More than enough m.	9	16		18	20		
Enough money	77	69		73	74		
Not enough money	14	15		9	6		
Time since separation in months: M (*SD*)	60.9 (*60.5*)	79.4 (*72.1*)	−3.87***a	–	–	–	–
In new relationship? (%)			−.25***c				
Yes	35	60					
No	65	40					

*$p < .05$, **$p < .01$, ***$p < .001$
[a]Mann-Whitney test
[b]Chi-squared test
[c]Phi

the present sample). Comparisons with the full version show that the short form is almost as accurate in correctly classifying depressed individuals as the long version (Hautzinger and Bailer 1993). The scores reported in this chapter are the mean of all ADS-K items.

- *Hopelessness* was measured with the German version of Beck's Hopelessness Scales (Krampen 1994; French version by Bouvard et al. 1992). Specifically, we used the 10-item short version H-RA (answers on a 6 point scale: 1 = *very much untrue* to 6 = *very much correct*), which had good internal consistency in the sample used (Cronbach's alpha .81). The hopelessness scores were calculated by taking the mean of all hopelessness items.
- *Life satisfaction* was assessed with the Satisfaction with Life Scale (Diener et al. 1985; German version by Schumacher (2003); French version by Blais et al. (1989)). This instruments consists of five items (answers on a 7-point scale: 1 = *completely disagree* to 7 = *completely agree*) which all load onto one factor. The instrument displayed good internal reliability (Cronbach's alpha .89). We report the mean of the five items.
- *Subjective health* was assessed with a single item question from the Swiss Household Panel. The question was phrased as follows: *How are you doing healthwise at the moment?* There were five answer options ranging from "very good" to "very badly".
- *Time needed to get over the breakup* (*feeling of having overcome the loss*) was also assessed with an original single-item question worded "*How long did it take you to get over this separation?*". There were six answer options: "There hasn't passed enough time yet to get over it"; "Less than 1 year"; "2–3 years"; "4 years and more"; "I'll probably never get over this separation".
- In addition to these established scales, we also inquired about whether the participants *mourned the loss* of their partner with an original single item question. The question was worded as follows: "Do you mourn this relationship?" with the answer options "yes, very much", "sometimes", "no", and "no, rather the opposite".

Personality

- *Personality* was assessed with the BFI-10 (Big Five Inventory, German version by Rammstedt and John (2007), French version by Plaisant et al. (2010)). The BFI-10 consists of two items for each of the five personality dimensions. Each item can be scored on a scale from 1 = *disagree strongly* to 5 = *agree strongly*. Even though this is a short version of the original BFI-44, the authors state that it does "retain significant levels of reliability and validity" (Rammstedt and John 2007).
- *Resilience* was measured with the short version of the Resilience Scale (RS-11) (original version by Wagnild and Young (1993); German short version by

Schumacher et al. (2005)). Resilience is defined as a personality trait with protective properties against stress. The RS-11 is a unidimensional scale with 11 items (answer options range from $1 = I \ don't \ agree$ to $7 = I \ agree \ completely$, and correlates strongly with the full version of the Resilience Scale ($r = .95$) (Schumacher et al. 2005). In our sample it demonstrated excellent internal consistency (Cronbach's Alpha .91).

Separation Circumstances

- *Initiator status* was measured with an original item asking "In the end, who initiated the separation?". Answer options included "I myself", "my ex-partner", "both of us".
- *Marriage length*: Participants were asked, how many years they had been married (original item).
- *Time since separation and new partnership*: Time since separation (original item) was calculated by subtracting the date of separation from the date of filling out the questionnaire (resulting time in months). A second question inquired whether the participant was currently in a (new) relationship (original item).

Socio-demographic Variables

- We also inquired about participants' age, sex, and education (6-point ordinal scale), as well as about their financial situation (original item). For this last information, participants could check one of three options: "I have more than enough money to meet my needs", "I have enough money to meet my needs", and "I don't have enough money to meet my needs".

3.3.3 Analytical Strategy

In a first step, we calculated one-way analyses of variance to compare the breakup groups (divided in 4 time subgroups) with the married controls regarding the outcome variables life satisfaction, depression and hopelessness. In a second step, we focus on the separated or divorced individuals to investigate by two-way analyses of variance the role of time since separation and gender for psychological adaptation to the event. In a third step, extreme group comparisons within the breakup sample were run to explore what discriminates highly affected individuals from minimally affected ones in terms of life satisfaction, depression, hopelessness, and never feeling to have overcome the breakup. Group differences were tested by Mann-Whitney U- tests for interval variables and Chi-squared tests as well as the measure Phi for categorical variables.

3.4 Results

3.4.1 Psychological Vulnerability After Marital Breakup: Crisis or Chronic Strain? Cross-Sectional Group Comparisons

To gain insight into whether our data fits better a crisis or a chronic strain model, subgroups were created with regard to the time since *separation* (0–12 months, 13–24 months, 25–60 months, more than 60 months), and the variables *life satisfaction, depression, and hopelessness* were then charted for these time groups. Additionally, the scores of the continuously married controls of the same age group were outlined to gain a comparison.

Depression: As can be seen in Fig. 1, people do seem to recover with time – however, the depression scores of the married controls are still significantly lower than any of the separation groups ($F(4,900) = 36.37$, $p < .001$, all post hoc Bonferroni tests $p < .001$). Among the separation groups, the most recently separated participants have significantly higher scores than the other separation groups (post hoc Bonferroni, $ps < .001$), while the scores of people with a separation longer than 12 months ago do not differ significantly (post hoc Bonferroni, $ps > .05$). None of the groups reaches a clinical level of depression according to the ADS-K manual (Hautzinger and Bailer 1993). However, the most recently separated have higher depression scores than 75 % of the population. For the other separation groups, the depression scores range between 59 and 49 % with the controls situated in the 30th percentile, i.e. only 30 % of the general population have lower depression scores compared to them.

Life satisfaction: The married controls have significantly higher scores in life satisfaction than all breakup groups ($F(4,1057) = 41.22$, $p < .001$, post hoc Bonferroni tests $p < .001$). However the separation groups did not differ significantly from one another (post hoc Bonferroni all $ps > .05$) (Fig. 2).

Hopelessness: Here there is only one significant group difference, namely between the married controls and the most recently separated group ($F(4,1060) = 3.06$, $p = .016$, post hoc Bonferroni $p = .006$, all other post hoc tests $p > .05$): the

Fig. 1 Depression scores of breakup groups by time since separation and of married controls (possible range: 0–3)

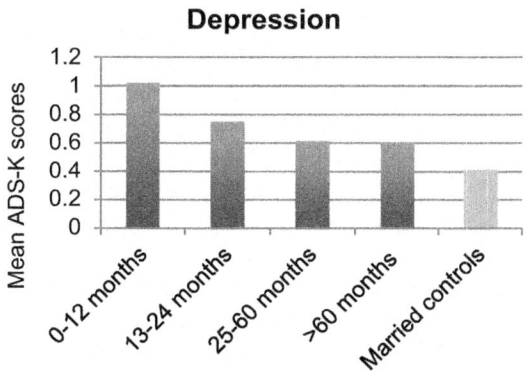

Fig. 2 Life satisfaction scores of breakup groups by times since separation and of married controls (possible range: 1–7)

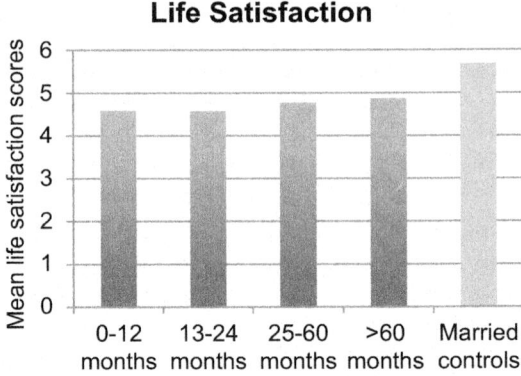

Fig. 3 Hopelessness scores of breakup groups by times since separation and of married controls (possible range: 1–6)

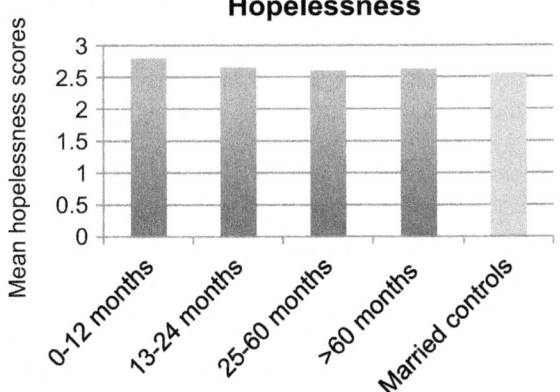

latter scored significantly higher in hopelessness. There were no other significant group differences (Fig. 3). The scores of all groups are average according to norm values (PR 50; Krampen 1994).

In a second step, we focused on the divorced/separated sample and investigated whether there is an interaction between time of adaptation and gender on psychological adaptation. We calculated separate two-way analyses of variance with the factors gender and time since separation (4 levels) and psychological adaptation in terms of depression, life satisfaction, and hopelessness as dependent variables.

The ANOVA with the *dependent variable depression* yielded a significant main effect for both gender ($F(1, 615) = 17.46$, $p < .001$), and time since separation ($F(3, 615) = 14.79$, $p < .001$). The interaction did not reach statistical significance ($p = .450$). Women displayed higher depression scores than men in all four groups of time since separation. Post hoc tests (with Bonferroni correction) for time since separation, showed that the group who had experienced a breakup within the last 12 months had significantly higher depression scores than all other groups (all $ps < .01$). The three groups who reported a separation longer than 12 months ago did not differ significantly from one another (all $ps > .05$).

In the ANOVA with the *dependent variable life satisfaction*, only the factor gender had a statistically significant effect on reported life satisfaction ($F(1, 706) = 12.18, p = .001$). Neither time since separation nor the interaction were significant ($p > .05$). Men reported higher life satisfaction than women in all time breakup groups.

Similar to the results for life satisfaction, in the ANOVA with *dependent variable hopelessness* only the factor gender reached significance ($F(1,709) = 13.56, p < .001$). Women had higher hopelessness scores than men in all time breakup groups.

Taken together, the results show that the first year after marital breakup is characterized by pronounced psychological vulnerability, but afterwards there is a significant improvement with regard to depression and hopelessness, but not for life satisfaction. Even though people seem gradually to recover from marital separation in the course of time, they nevertheless do not reach the low level of depression nor the higher level of life satisfaction of the married controls. Focusing on the breakup group, the data reveal a strong gender effect for all three dependent variables. Divorced or separated women have higher depression as well as higher hopelessness scores and lower scores in life satisfaction than men independently of the time passed since separation.

3.4.2 Extreme Group Comparisons: What Distinguishes Highly Vulnerable Individuals from Marginally Affected Ones?

To determine what distinguishes individuals who are severely affected by marital breakup in terms of life satisfaction, depression, hopelessness, and never feeling to have overcome the breakup from those who are the least affected, we contrasted divorced individuals scoring in the top quartile in those measures with those scoring in the bottom quartile. The resulting two groups were compared regarding the following variables: Intra-personal resources, namely personality variables (Big Five dimensions, resilience) and subjective health, furthermore marital breakup circumstances such as time since separation (time coded into four groups, 0–12 months, 13–24 months, 25–60 months, more than 60 months), length of marriage (in years having been married), initiator-status, and finally social (new relationship) and economic resources (financial situation, education). We used Mann-Whitney U-tests for interval variables (Big Five dimensions, resilience, subjective health, length of marriage), and Chi-squared tests and Phi coefficients for categorical variables (time groups, financial situation, education, initiator status and current relationship status).

Participants who scored in the *top quartile of depression* (n = 252) differed from those in the bottom one (n = 245) as follows: They

- had lower scores in resilience ($U = 11,862.0, p < .001$);
- had lower scores in conscientiousness ($U = 24,237.0, p < .001$), and extraversion ($U = 22,166, p < .001$), higher scores in neuroticism ($U = 11,477.0, p < .001$)

and marginally lower scores in openness ($U = 27,886.0, p < .10$). However, there were no significant difference with regard to agreeableness ($p = .215$);

- reported worse health ($U = 10,319.0, p < .001$);
- were more likely to have experienced a separation in the past 12 months ($\chi2(3) = 22.195, p < .001$);
- were marginally less likely to have initiated the separation ($\chi2(2) = 5.430, p < .10$);
- were less likely to be currently in a relationship (phi $= .291, p < .001$);
- were less likely to have more than enough money to meet their needs ($\chi2(2) = 51.399, p < .001$), and to have a lower level of education ($p = .05$).

There was no significant difference regarding how long they had been married previous to the divorce ($U = 14,341.0, p = .990$).

Participants who scored in the *top quartile of hopelessness* (n = 234) differed from those in the bottom one (n = 246) significantly as follows: They

- had lower scores in resilience ($U = 6536.00, p < .001$);
- had lower scores in conscientiousness ($U = 20,374.00, p < .001$), agreeableness ($U = 19,462.00, p < .001$) openness ($U = 19,258.00, p < .001$), and extraversion ($U = 15,352.50, p < .001$), and higher scores in neuroticism ($U = 9592.50, p < .001$);
- reported worse health ($U = 9154.5, p < .001$);
- were less likely to currently be in a relationship (phi $= .263, p < .001$);
- had a lower level of education ($\chi2(6) = 38.310, p < .001$), and were more likely to not have enough money to meet their needs ($\chi2(2) = 51.654, p < .001$).

The groups did not differ significantly in terms of who had initiated the separation ($\chi2(2) = 4.534, p = .104$), and neither considering the time passed since the separation ($\chi2(3) = 4.219, p = .239$), nor regarding how long they had been married prior to the divorce ($U = 14,410.0, p = .796$).

People in the *bottom quartile of life satisfaction* (n = 260) differed from to those in the top one (n = 280) as follows: They

- had lower resilience scores ($U = 12,898.0, p < .001$);
- had lower scores in agreeableness ($U = 27,697.00, p < .001$), conscientiousness ($U = 29,900.50, p < .001$), openness ($U = 29,890.00, p < .001$), and extraversion ($U = 23,227.50, p < .001$), and higher scores in neuroticism ($U = 17,583.50, p < .001$);
- reported worse health ($U = 13,203.50, p < .001$);
- were less likely to be currently in a relationship (phi $= -.325, p < .001$);
- had a lower level of education ($\chi2(6) = 31.827, p < .001$), and were less likely to have enough money to meet their needs ($\chi2(2) = 102.268, p < .001$).

The groups did not differ significantly in terms of who had initiated the separation ($\chi2(2) = 1.177, p = .56$), neither considering the time passed since the separation ($\chi2(3) = 3.934, p = .269$), nor with regard how long they had been married previous to the divorce ($U = 17,567.0, p = .479$).

Feeling of overcoming the breakup: As a further indicator of vulnerability, we compared participants who stated that they would never get over the divorce (N = 119) with those who stated that they had needed less than 1 year (N = 255) to get over the divorce. As could be expected, participants in the first group differed from the second one as follows: They

- were more hopeless ($U = 7363.0$, $p < .001$), had higher depression scores ($U = 4478.0$, $p < .001$), and lower life satisfaction ($U = 6980.0$, $p < .001$);
- had lower scores in resilience ($U = 9571.5$, $p < .001$);
- were less extroverted ($U = 12,296.0$, $p = .002$), scored lower in agreeableness ($U = 12,545.0$, $p = .006$) and conscientiousness ($U = 13,254.0$, $p = .044$), and higher in neuroticism ($U = 9227.5$, $p < .001$). There was no difference in openness (U = 14,926.5, $p > .05$);
- reported worse health ($U = 9974.5$, $p < .001$), and had a lower education ($p < .05$);
- were more likely to have experienced a separation in the past 12 months ($U = 5940.0$, $p = .008$);
- reported significantly more frequently that their ex-partner (and not they themselves) had initiated the separation ($\chi2(2) = 38.890$, $p < .001$);
- had been married significantly longer before the divorce ($U = 9772.5$, $p < .001$);
- were less likely to be currently in a new relationship (phi = .262, $p < .001$);
- were financially worse off ($\chi2(2) = 11.432$, $p = .003$).

The comparison of highly vulnerable individuals with those who are the least affected shows in an impressive way the crucial importance of intra-personal resources, i.e. of personality traits. In all four indicators high vulnerability was associated with elevated scores in neuroticism, low scores in extraversion and conscientiousness, and to a lesser degree with low agreeableness and openness. High psychological vulnerability is also clearly associated with lower scores in resilience. These findings are in line with our expectations, according to which personality traits account predominantly for psychological adaptation after marital breakup. A further common feature in all four well-being indicators was subjective health: Highly vulnerable individuals consistently rated their health worse than the least affected. A new relationship also plays an important and consistently discriminating role. Highly vulnerable persons are significantly less likely to have a new partner, and this holds for the most depressed, hopeless, and dissatisfied people independently of how long their ex-marriage was, how much time has passed since the breakup, and whether they had initiated the divorce or not. This rather unexpected result clearly relativizes the importance of length of ex-marriage and time passed since separation (important for depression and feelings of not being able to overcome the separation, but not for life satisfaction and hopelessness), and moreover it underlines again the crucial role of personality. Furthermore the consistent and strongly discriminant role of financial situation and education was rather unexpected. The most vulnerable individuals were less educated and complained significantly more about a precarious financial situation than the least affected group.

4 Conclusions and Further Considerations

In this contribution the concept of vulnerability has been first discussed within the canon of different disciplines, and then contextualized in psychological research, where it has been mainly studied with regard to adverse life events. Based on these insights we aimed in a first step at giving a brief overview of the status quo of research on psychological vulnerability by focusing on the impact of marital breakup in the second half of life. In a second step we wanted to make an empirical contribution to close some gaps in research on psychological adaptation to divorce, and to shed light on specific controversies. One major issue refers to the question of whether vulnerability after marital breakup is a temporary crisis or rather a chronic strain. In this chapter we wanted to present two possible methodological options to tackle this question: First, comparing a sample of almost 1000 middle aged persons, who were married on average 19 years, and who experienced a marital split-up within the last 5 years (4 time groups), with a group of age-matched married controls with regard to various indicators of psychological vulnerability (depression, hopelessness, life satisfaction). Second by comparing within the divorced group of the most vulnerable individuals (with regard to depression, hopelessness, life satisfaction) with those who were the least affected. This comparison focused on intra-personal resources, divorce circumstances, and post-divorce situation, and socio-economic resources. Based on a modified and extended perspective of the crisis-versus-chronic-stress model we hypothesized that time would play a significant role in recovering from this critical life event, but that at the same time there would be large inter-individual differences in psychological adaptation dependent on the diverse resource constellations of individuals.

Our results underline the crucial importance of both *time and personal resources* for psychological adaptation to marital breakup. The first year after marital separation is indeed characterized by an increased psychological vulnerability. Even though there is a gradual improvement of well-being with time passing, separated or divorced persons (even those with a marital breakup more than 5 years ago) do not reach the levels of the continuously married controls. These results are in line with our expectation that the time directly after a breakup is marked by a general decrease of psychological and physical well-being. However, in contrast to our hypothesis, divorced or separated people having experienced the breakup 5 years or longer ago still differ significantly from the never-divorced married individuals with regard to life satisfaction and depression. We can therefore conclude that our data support a crisis as well as a chronic strain model. Nevertheless it has to be said, that due to the lack of data we cannot conclusively answer the question, whether divorced people reached their baseline well-being before the event. Neither can we exclude that there is a selection effect, i.e. that the divorced individuals had already a lower level of habitual well-being before marital breakup.

Our data show further that psychological vulnerability after marital separation is more pronounced in women, who have higher depression as well as hopelessness and lower life satisfaction scores than men in all separation groups. This result stands in contrast to many findings, according to which men would have a more difficult time after a marital breakup and exhibit less improvement over time (Baum 2003; Hetherington 1993; Wallerstein and Lewis 2004). As we already pointed out, the effect of gender has been discussed in a very controversial way in literature, since some of the studies found no gender differences (Kim and McKenry 2002; Johnson and Wu 2002), whereas others found either women or men to be more affected (Simon 2002). Due to the fact that men are underrepresented in this study, it could be that the most vulnerable are those that are missing. It is indeed known from literature that men are less likely to disclose than women regarding close relationships (Derlega et al. 2008). Against this background a cautious interpretation of gender differences is indicated.

The findings of our extreme group comparisons confirm those of the time-group-comparisons with regard to the central role of *personality traits* for overcoming a critical life event. As expected personality, particularly neuroticism, extraversion, conscientiousness, and resilience, was a discriminant variable between both groups with regard to all indicators of psychological vulnerability. These results confirm existing research – especially with regard to the negative impact of neuroticism (Hetherington and Kelly 2002; Pudrovska and Carr 2008) – and extend it by showing the important role of resilience, which was seldom investigated in this context. However, and partially in contrast to our expectation, *initiator-status* played a limited role as discriminant variable between highly and marginally affected individuals, namely only with regard to depression and feelings of overcoming the loss, but not for life satisfaction and hopelessness. This result demonstrates the importance of specifying psychological vulnerability by distinguishing among its different dimensions. Whereas life satisfaction and hopelessness (not having a perspective and plans for the future) are primarily cognitive dimensions, depression and feelings of being able to overcome the loss or not are more emotional ones. It could be that most people confronted with marital separation adapt first and foremost to the situation in a rational and volitional way (by adjusting their life satisfaction and future perspectives). They diverge however much more with regard to the mainly emotional adaptation, since feelings can be much less voluntarily influenced than thoughts and beliefs. In other words: Emotions are much less controllable than cognitions, especially when the critical life event was not anticipated and initiated. It has been reported in literature that people who initiate a marital breakup generally are better off because they have an increased sense of control over this critical life event since they anticipate and instigate it (Wang and Amato 2000).

The importance of *time passed since separation* for psychological adaptation was underlined in the extreme-group comparisons and revealed a differentiated view. It seems that time is an important factor for adjusting life satisfaction and future perspectives, but not for depression. As was stated above, life satisfaction and future perspectives can be considered rational dimensions of well-being and are therefore more susceptible to change than the emotional ones such as depression, which can be viewed as more stable and less modifiable. Rather surprising was furthermore that *length of marriage* played only a marginal role as a discriminating variable between low and high psychological vulnerability. This result suggests that people exiting from a long-term marriage adapt quite well on a rational level, but that they have more problems on the emotional one, at least with regard to feelings of being able to overcome the breakup. By contrast, better psychological adaptation was consistently associated with being in a *new relationship*. This result, which confirms our expectation, is also in line with findings by Johnson and Wu (2002), who found in their longitudinal study that psychological distress due to marital breakup declines only upon remarriage or the formation of a cohabiting relationship. In fact, a new romantic partnership and remarriage have also been found to increase adjustment in various other studies (Amato 2000; Quinney and Fouts 2003; Wang and Amato 2000; Locker et al. 2010).

Finally, our results suggest that the *financial situation* – and highly correlated with it, *education* – play a much greater role as discriminant variables between highly and minimally vulnerable individuals than expected. Having a higher education and enough money to meet one's own needs were important discriminant variables for all four indicators of psychological vulnerability. Our results confirm other research where the factors associated with favorable post-divorce adjustment include having higher income and getting remarried (Wang and Amato 2000; Johnson and Wu 2002). These results could be confirmed by further multivariate analyses (latent profile analysis) where five classes of differently affected individuals were compared (Perrig-Chiello et al. 2014).

Taken together our study results underline the vulnerabilizing impact of marital breakup, but at the same time they reveal significant individual differences in psychological adaptation due to personal resources (personality), social resources (new partnership), economic resources, and, last but not least, time. Furthermore our data strongly suggest that there is not a generalized psychological vulnerability after marital breakup, but that the emotional dimensions such as depression or feelings of not overcoming the loss are more affected than the more rational ones such as life satisfaction. Even though our study makes a substantial contribution to extend existing knowledge on marital separation, one limitation has to be considered. Since our data are cross-sectional we cannot give a conclusive answer with regard to the question of whether marital separation can lead to enduring vulnerability or not. As we stated in the introduction, our results should be considered as a first estimation of the role of time passed since the critical life event for psychological adaptation and recovery (and in the negative case for lasting vulnerability), and should be validated by longitudinal measurements. The planned future waves of this study will hopefully help in progressing this issue.

References

Amato, P. R. (2000). The consequences of divorce for adults and children. *Journal of Marriage and the Family, 62*(4), 1269–1287. doi:http://dx.doi.org/10.1111/j.1741-3737.2000.01269.x.

Amato, P. R. (2010). Research on divorce: Continuing trends and new developments. *Journal of Marriage and Family, 72*(3), 650–666. doi:http://dx.doi.org/10.1111/j.1741-3737.2010.00723.x.

Amato, P. R., & Hohmann-Marriott, B. (2007). A comparison of high- and low-distress marriages that end in divorce. *Journal of Marriage and Family, 69*(3), 621–638. doi:10.1111/j.1741-3737.2007.00396.x.

Andreß, H.-J., & Bröckel, M. (2007). Income and life satisfaction after marital disruption in Germany. *Journal of Marriage and Family, 69*(2), 500–512. doi:http://dx.doi.org/10.1111/j.1741-3737.2007.00379.x.

Avison, W. R. (1999). Family structure and processes. In A. V. Horwitz & T. L. Scheid (Eds.), *A handbook for the study of mental health: Social contexts, theories, and systems* (pp. 228–240). New York: Cambridge University Press.

Bal, M. (2002). *Travelling concepts in the humanities*. Toronto: University of Toronto Press.

Baum, N. (2003). The male way of mourning divorce: When, what, and how. *Clinical Social Work Journal, 31*(1), 37–50.

Blais, M. R., Vallerand, R. J., Pelletier, L. G., & Briere, N. M. (1989). The satisfaction scale: Canadian-French validation of the satisfaction with life scale. *Canadian Journal of Behavioural Science/Revue Canadienne des Sciences du Comportement, 21*(2), 210–223. doi:http://dx.doi.org/10.1037/h0079854.

Bonanno, G. A. (2004). Loss, trauma, and human resilience: Have we underestimated the human capacity to thrive after extremely aversive events? *American Psychologist, 59*(1), 20–28. doi:http://dx.doi.org/10.1037/0003-066X.59.1.20.

Booth, A., & Amato, P. (1991). Divorce and psychological stress. *Journal of Health and Social Behavior, 32*(4), 396–407. doi:http://dx.doi.org/10.2307/2137106.

Bouvard, M., Charles, S., Guerin, J., Aimard, G., & Cottraux, J. (1992). Study of the hopelessness scale: Validation and factorial analysis. *L'Encephale: Revue de Psychiatrie Clinique Biologique et Therapeutique, 18*(3), 237–240.

Brickman, P., & Campbell, D. T. (1971). Hedonic relativism and planning the good society. In M. H. Appley (Ed.), *Adaptation level theory: A symposium* (pp. 287–302). New York: Academic Press.

Clark, A. E., & Georgellis, Y. (2013). Back to baseline in Britain: Adaptation in the British Household Panel Survey. *Economia, 80*(319), 496–512. doi:10.1111/ecca.12007.

Clark, A. E., Diener, E., Georgellis, Y., & Lucas, R. E. (2008). Lags and leads in life satisfaction: A test of the baseline hypothesis. *Economic Journal, 118*(529), F222–F243.

Danis, M., & Patrick, D. (2002). Health policy, vulnerability, and vulnerable populations. In M. Danis, C. Clancy, & L. Churchill (Eds.), *Ethical dimensions of health policy* (pp. 310–334). New York: Oxford University Press.

Derlega, V. J., Winstead, B. A., & Greene, K. (2008). Self-disclosure and starting a close relationship. In S. Sprecher, A. Wenzel, & J. Harvey (Eds.), *Handbook of relationship initiation* (pp. 153–174). New York: Psychology Press; US.

Diener, E., Emmons, R. A., Larsen, R. J., & Griffin, S. (1985). The satisfaction with life scale. *Journal of Personality Assessment, 49*(1), 71–75. doi:10.1207/s15327752jpa4901_13.

Diener, E., Lucas, R. E., & Scollon, C. N. (2006). Beyond the hedonic treadmill. Revising the adaptation theory of well-being. *American Psychologist, 61*(4), 305–314. doi:http://dx.doi.org/10.1037/0003-066X.61.4.305.

Dupre, M. E., Beck, A. N., & Meadows, S. O. (2009). Marital trajectories and mortality among U. S. adults. *American Journal of Epidemiology, 170*, 546–555.

Fuhrer, R., & Rouillon, F. (1989). The French version of the CES-D (Center for Epidemiologic Studies-Depression Scale). *European Psychiatry, 4*(3), 163–166.

Gähler, M. (2006). "To divorce is to die a bit …": A longitudinal study of marital disruption and psychological distress among Swedish women and men. *The Family Journal, 14*(4), 372–382. doi:http://dx.doi.org/10.1177/1066480706290145.

Hautzinger, M., & Bailer, M. (1993). *Allgemeine Depressions Skala*. Manual. Göttingen/Deutschland: Beltz Test GmbH.

Hetherington, E. M. (1993). An overview of the Virginia longitudinal study of divorce and remarriage with a focus on early adolescence. *Journal of Family Psychology, 7*(1), 39–56. doi:http://dx.doi.org/10.1037/0893-3200.7.1.39.

Hetherington, E. M., & Kelly, J. (2002). *For better or for worse: Divorce reconsidered*. New York: W. W. Norton.

Hewitt, B., & Turrell, G. (2011). Short-term functional health and well-being after marital separation: Does initiator status make a difference? [Research Support, Non-U.S. Gov't]. *American Journal of Epidemiology, 173*(11), 1308–1318.

Hughes, M. E., & Waite, L. J. (2009). Marital biography and health at mid-life. *Journal of Health and Social Behavior, 50*, 344–358.

Hutchison, S., Perrig-Chiello, P., Höpflinger, F., Morselli, D., van Rhee, E., & Spini, D. (2013). *Vulnerability and growth. Developmental dynamics and differential effects of the loss of an intimate partner in the second half of life*. IP12: Study outline and first results. LIVES Working Paper. doi:http://dx.doi.org/10.12682/lives.2296-1658.2013.23.

Johnson, D. R., & Wu, J. (2002). An empirical test of crisis, social selection, and role explanations of the relationship between marital disruption and psychological distress: A pooled time-series analysis of four-wave panel data. *Journal of Marriage and Family, 64*(1), 211–224. doi:http://dx.doi.org/10.1111/j.1741-3737.2002.00211.x.

Kim, H. K., & McKenry, P. C. (2002). The relationship between marriage and psychological well-being: A longitudinal analysis. *Journal of Family Issues, 23*(8), 885–911. doi:http://dx.doi.org/10.1177/019251302237296.

Krampen, G. (1994). *Skalen zur Erfassung von Hoffnungslosigkeit (H-Skalen)*. Göttingen: Hogrefe.

Locker, L., Jr., McIntosh, W. D., Hackney, A. A., Wilson, J. H., & Wiegand, K. E. (2010). The breakup of romantic relationships: Situational predictors of perception of recovery. *North American Journal of Psychology, 12*(3), 565–578.

Lorenz, F. O., Wickrama, K., Conger, R. D., & Elder, G. H., Jr. (2006). The short-term and decade-long effects of divorce on women's midlife health. *Journal of Health and Social Behavior, 47*(2), 111–125. doi:http://dx.doi.org/10.1177/002214650604700202.

Lucas, R. E. (2005). Time does not heal all wounds. A longitudinal study of reaction and adaptation to divorce [Research Article]. *Psychological Science, 16*(12), 945–950.

Mastekaasa, A. (1995). Marital dissolution and subjective distress: Panel evidence. *European Sociological Review, 11*(2), 173–185.

Morawa, A. H. E. (2003). Vulnerability as a concept of international human rights law. *Journal of International Relations and Development, 6*(2), 139–155.

Ong, A. D., Bergeman, C. S., Bisconti, T. L., & Wallace, K. A. (2006). Psychological resilience, positive emotions, and successful adaptation to stress in later life. *Journal of Personality & Social Psychology, 91*(4), 730–749.

Perloff, L. S. (1983). Perceptions of vulnerability to victimization. *Journal of Social Issues, 39*(2), 41–61. doi:http://dx.doi.org/10.1111/j.1540-4560.1983.tb00140.x.

Perrig-Chiello, P., & Darbellay, F. (2002). *Qu'est-ce que l'interdisciplinarité?* Lausanne: Réalités Sociales.

Perrig-Chiello, P., Hutchison, S., & Morselli, D. (2014). Patterns of psychological adaptation to divorce after a long-term marriage. *Journal of Social and Personal Relationships*, 1–20, doi:10.1177/0265407514533769.

Plaisant, O., Courtois, R., Reveillere, C., Mendelsohn, G., & John, O. (2010). Factor structure and internal reliability of the French Big Five Inventory (BFI-Fr). Convergent and discriminant validation with the NEO-PI-R. *Annales Médico-Psychologiques, 168*(2), 97–106. doi:http://dx. doi.org/10.1016/j.amp.2009.09.003.

Pudrovska, T., & Carr, D. (2008). Psychological adjustment to divorce and widowhood in mid- and later life: Do coping strategies and personality protect against psychological distress? *Advances in Life Course Research, 13*, 283–317. doi:http://dx.doi.org/10.1016/S1040-2608(08)00011-7.

Quinney, D. M., & Fouts, G. T. (2003). Resilience and divorce adjustment in adults participating in divorce recovery workshops. *Journal of Divorce & Remarriage, 40*(1–2), 55–68. doi:http:// dx.doi.org/10.1300/J087v40n01_04.

Rammstedt, B., & John, O. P. (2007). Measuring personality in one minute or less: A 10-item short version of the Big Five Inventory in English and German. *Journal of Research in Personality, 41*(1), 203–212. doi:10.1016/j.jrp.2006.02.001.

Ruof, M. C. (2004). Vulnerability, vulnerable populations, and policy. *Kennedy Institute of Ethics Journal, 14*(4), 411–425. doi:10.1353/ken.2004.0044.

Schumacher, J. (2003). SWLS – Satisfaction with life scale. In J. Schumacher, A. Klaiberg, & E. Braehler (Eds.), *Diagnostische Verfahren zu Lebensqualität und Wohlbefinden* (pp. 305–309). Göttingen: Hogrefe.

Schumacher, J., Leppert, K., Gunzelmann, T., Strauß, B., & Brähler, E. (2005). Die Resilienzskala – Ein Fragebogen zur Erfassung der psychischen Widerstandsfähigkeit als Personmerkmal. *Zeitschrift für Klinische Psychologie, Psychiatrie und Psychotherapie, 53*(1), 16–39.

SFOS Swiss Federal Office of Statistics. (2013). *Bevölkerungsstand und -struktur – Detaillierte Daten.* http://www.bfs.admin.ch/bfs/portal/de/index/themen/01/02/blank/data/01.html. Accessed 15 Feb 2014

Simon, R. W. (2002). Revisiting the relationships among gender, marital status, and mental health. *American Journal of Sociology, 107*(4), 1065–1096. doi:http://dx.doi.org/10.1086/339225.

Sinclair, V. G., & Wallston, K. A. (2010). Psychological vulnerability predicts increases in depressive symptoms in individuals with rheumatoid arthritis. *Nursing Research, 59*(2), 140–146. doi:10.1097/NNR.0b013e3181d1a6f6.

Strohschein, L., McDonough, P., Monette, G., & Shao, Q. (2005). Marital transitions and mental health: Are there gender differences in the short-term effects of marital status change? *Social Science & Medicine, 61*, 2293–2303.

Wagnild, G. M., & Young, H. M. (1993). Development and psychometric evaluation of the resilience scale. *Journal of Nursing Measurement, 1*(2), 165–178.

Waite, L. J., Luo, Y., & Lewin, A. C. (2009). Marital happiness and marital stability: Consequences for psychological well-being. *Social Science Research, 38*(1), 201–212. doi:10.1016/j.ssresearch.2008.07.001.

Wallerstein, J. S., & Lewis, J. M. (2004). The unexpected legacy of divorce: Report of a 25-year study. *Psychoanalytic Psychology, 21*(3), 353–370. doi:http://dx.doi.org/10.1037/0736-9735. 21.3.353.

Wang, H., & Amato, P. R. (2000). Predictors of divorce adjustment: Stressors, resources, and definitions. *Journal of Marriage and the Family, 62*(3), 655–668.

A Survey of Couples Facing Breast Cancer in Women

Linda Charvoz, Nicolas Favez, Sarah Cairo Notari, Bénédicte Panes-Ruedin, and Jean-François Delaloye

1 Introduction

Breast cancer is a reality for 5000 women in Switzerland every year (Ligue Suisse contre le Cancer 2005). This form of cancer is the most prevalent one among women (one woman out of eight will present a breast cancer) and represents the principal cause of mortality among women under 60. Consequences of the disease are not restricted to somatic health; facing diagnosis and medical treatment represents a source of severe stress with a possible impact on social and emotional functioning (Manne et al. 2004). Women have to cope with somatic symptoms (pains, loss of appetite, nausea, tiredness, for example) and emotional consequences (anxiety, depression, anger, helplessness, for example), difficulties related to their body image and sexual identity, and with the uncertainty about the prognosis as well as their marital and familial future (Zimmermann and Heinrichs 2008). Breast cancer may thus be considered as a critical life event. Moreover, it is associated with chronic strain (worries, long-term treatment) and daily hassles: daily life has to be partly reorganized to allow the women to follow their medical treatment, so that couple, family and work relationships are affected.

When women are married or in a committed relationship, breast cancer represents a critical event for their partners as well. Some of them report high level of physical and psychological distress, which can be even higher than the

L. Charvoz (✉) • N. Favez • S. Cairo Notari
NCCR LIVES, IP 11, Geneva, Switzerland

Section of Psychology, University of Geneva, Geneva, Switzerland
e-mail: linda.charvoz@eesp.ch

B. Panes-Ruedin • J.-F. Delaloye
NCCR LIVES, IP 11, Chavannes-près-Renens, Switzerland

Unit of Senology, CHUV, University of Lausanne, Lausanne, Switzerland

© The Author(s) 2016
M. Oris et al. (eds.), *Surveying Human Vulnerabilities across the Life Course*,
Life Course Research and Social Policies 3, DOI 10.1007/978-3-319-24157-9_5

level of distress reported by women. Partners worry because they do not know whether the women will survive the disease. Moreover, they fear the consequences of their partners dying from the illness, such as loneliness (Kayser and Scott 2008; Northouse 1989). In addition, breast cancer specifically affects the couple relationship as it concerns a body part intimately related to sexual activity. For these reasons, there is now a consensus in the literature to consider breast cancer as an event involving couples as much as women alone.

1.1 The Couple Relationship as the Primary Resource of Social Support

Implications for the couple relationship can be seen from the woman's perspective. One way to cope with the stress related to the illness is indeed to receive support from significant others, especially from the partner (Ell et al. 1989; Manne et al. 2004; Pistrang and Barker 1995). Social support plays an important role in one's life at two inter-related levels (Cutrona 1996; Weiss 1974). First, at a general level, it allows the fulfillment of interpersonal needs in everyday life. In this perspective, social support is an ongoing resource that increases well-being and acts as a resiliency factor that lowers the probability that daily life events will be perceived as stressors by the individual. Second, at a more specific level, social support refers to the assistance that an individual receives during times of adversity when she has to face and cope with a critical event. In this perspective, social support is conceptualized as a moderator factor which influences the link between a critical event and an individual's health. In case of a somatic illness like cancer, support is sought especially from the partner (Ell et al. 1989; Manne et al. 2004; Pistrang and Barker 1995). Three types of supportive social interactions have been traditionally distinguished: emotional, instrumental and informational. The first one is of primary importance in stress situations: it refers to reassurance and love needs that a person will have when facing a challenging situation. In the case of a breast cancer, this is usually the first need women report that they expect from their partner. The second one refers to pragmatic help, like money or assistance in the realization of daily tasks. Women expect this kind of help both from their partners (daily shopping, household chores) and from the larger social circle or even from institutions (having money for the medical treatment). The latter refers to advice or information which is mainly expected from medical staff. Women's satisfaction with the social support they receive from their partners is an important predictor of the enhancement of their mood and quality of life (Giese-Davis et al. 2000; Helgeson and Cohen 1996). Moreover, women's perception of her partner as highly supportive predicts a better adjustment to the stress of the illness as it plays a buffering role against comorbid disorders such as depression or anxiety (Manne et al. 1999), and helps to maintain a good quality of life which is in turn predictive of better outcomes (e.g. more chances to get back into work after treatment) (Northouse et al. 2002; Schulz and Schwarzer 2004).

On their side, partners are in the difficult situation in which they have to manage a "double agenda": on the one hand, they have to cope with their own stress and on the other hand they have to be supportive to their wife (Zimmermann et al. 2007). When they face the distress of their wife, they report feeling helpless and often not knowing how to provide an adequate support (Zimmermann and Heinrichs 2006). Some of them lack the necessary resources, as they may be overwhelmed by the stress and consequently display inadequate social support: for example, emotional withdrawal, criticism, minimization of the effects of the disease, lack of empathy, avoidance of discussion related to cancer (Pistrang and Barker 1995; Wortman and Dunkel-Schetter 1987). Most of the time, partners do not receive support from the medical staff because attention is primarily given to the woman; existing psychosocial interventions are also mainly addressed to the woman, or to the couple as an "entity" but rarely to the partner him(her)self – when it is the case, it is most often to enhance their skills to help their wives (see for example Manne and Ostroff 2008). Data are indeed scarce about the way partners manage their own stress.

The importance of the help partners give to each other when facing an aversive event has been underscored by theoretical and empirical data about stress and coping. Bodenmann (2005) has coined the term "dyadic coping" to put the emphasis on the way partners communicate their needs to one another and how they respond to the others' needs. Dyadic coping is supposed to be implemented when individual coping is not efficient to regulate emotions associated with a stress situation; this is in essence a reciprocal process, which means that the help one partner may provide to the other depends to a certain extent on the help she or he will receive. A comprehensive study should then take into account not only the woman needs, but also the partners' needs, how both get connected and what are the reciprocal behaviors they use to communicate their needs and their support to each other.

However, social support is not only a matter of what someone "does" for someone else, but also a matter of what the recipient of the help will perceive as such. The literature in the domain of social support has shown that there is a difference between the received social support (the "objective" social support) and the perceived social support (the "subjective" social support). Perception of social support depends on several factors such as personality or psychological states; depression may for example make a person unable to perceive the help she receives as her vision of the world is negative, by definition. On the contrary, an "optimistic" person may over-evaluate the help she receives (Cutrona 1996; Cutrona and Suhr 1992; Schwarzer and Leppin 1989).

1.2 Methodological Challenges

Studying social support in couples implies several methodological challenges. In order to have a comprehensive picture of the couple facing a stressful event, it is necessary to draw on the one hand on "objective" data, i.e. what the person receives, and on the other hand on "subjective" data, i.e. the perception the person has about received support. Getting objective data has two implications: first, several sources of information have to be solicited; second, at least one of these sources has to be an "external informant", that means a third person who evaluates the relationship between the partners. To date, social support in the domain of women breast cancer has been measured mainly by self-reported questionnaires completed by the women and, much more rarely, by their partners – the behavior of their partners is thus most often reported by the women themselves. Second, while a lot of attention has been given to the effect of the different types of social support (emotional, instrumental, informational) and to the effect of individual variables like coping strategies in women on adjustment to the stress of the illness, much less is known about the mechanisms though which social support is communicated and perceived in couples. It is difficult to draw a synthesis from the data available in the literature, as methodologies have been diverse and vary between studies. For example, Gerits (2000) found contradictory findings between studies using different assessment methods in the domain of breast cancer. He reported that studies using questionnaires did not find a link between coping strategies in women and disease outcomes, while studies measuring these variables by interviewing the women did find significant links between these variables.

2 Objectives of the Chapter

The goal of this chapter is to present the advantages and limitations of the two main methods of assessment that are used in the domain of couple relationships: questionnaires and observation. The necessity to combine the different methods is discussed. Comments will be illustrated with a project conducted in Switzerland funded by the Swiss National Science Foundation that formed part of the National Centre of Competence in Research (NCCR) "LIVES – Overcoming Vulnerability: Life Course Perspectives". This project examined couples facing breast cancer using a mixed method approach. Indeed the studies reported above have shown that women do not cope alone with their illness, but within their marital relationship, and that mutual social support between partners has an impact on the patient's as well as partner's adjustment (Kayser 2005). It is of primary importance to gain and refine knowledge about the way each partner copes with the disease and the social support they provide one another, in order to help them to avoid inadequate adjustment to the illness and to identify variables which may be used to set up psychosocial and psychological interventions. Although it is known that interventions addressed to the patients or couples facilitate social support within the interactional relationship, several questions are left unanswered (Kayser 2005), such as: What kind of interventions should be delivered? What is the more relevant between an individual (woman and partner separately) or a couple-based intervention in a given situation? At what point during the illness and treatment would the intervention be most helpful for each partner?

3   Considerations About the Different Assessment Methods

The two main methods of questionnaires and observation have both advantages and limitations that we present below.

3.1   Questionnaires

Questionnaires make it possible to obtain self-reported data (a person assesses his/her own thoughts, emotions, behaviors, relations to other people) or hetero-reported data (a person evaluates another person's thoughts, emotions, behaviors, relations to other people). Hetero-reported data can be obtained by participants of a study (for example: husbands evaluate their wife's behaviors) or by external judges (for example: questionnaires are filled in by researchers or practitioners) (Favez 2010).

3.1.1   Advantages of Questionnaires

Questionnaires offer the advantages to be quickly completed and easy to use. Furthermore, they make it possible to assess thoughts, emotions, behaviors and relations through different temporal perspectives: a woman could then assess her couple relationship as it was in the past, as it is in the present and how she expects (or hopes) it to be in the future (Favez 2010). Questionnaires mainly make it possible to assess the subjective point of view of the person; as far as social support is concerned, they make it possible thus to assess the perceived support, which is of utmost importance as several studies have pointed out the more important role of perceived social support compared to the received social support by people facing cancer (Uchino 2004).

Furthermore, in the domain of marital relationships, Hahlweg et al. (2000) noted that partners provide additional pieces of information about their relationships' history and their manner of interacting with each other when they fill in the questionnaires. They have the opportunity to report data which are to a certain extent representative of the "objective" reality of the relationship. Accordingly, Kenny and Acitelli (2001) assumed that motive (willingness to have a good perception of the partner), opportunity (spouses have a lot of occasions to observe their partner) and information (possibility to share with the partner intimate feelings) should lead to accurate data about the partner and the relationship.

3.1.2 Disadvantages of Questionnaires

Questionnaires present however some disadvantages and limitations, one being the possible influence of social desirability on the one hand, or of a lenience effect when assessing the relationship on the other hand. In the domain of couple marital interactions, Murray et al. (1996) explained this phenomenon by talking about a strong idealization effect. According to the theory of Sillars (1985), some individuals could have a biased perception of the social support provided by their partner in order to protect their marital relationship. Indeed, tactfully interpreting the personality or the behaviors of the partner could, in some situations, avoid harming the relationship. Sillars (1985) noted that the familiarity between the partners (impression of knowing the partner), the behavioral interdependence (ways of communicating and interacting between partners that take place over time) and the propensity of the couple relationship to generate strong positive and negative emotions (which could lead to erroneous inferences about the partner's actions and intentions) could also be a source of biased perception of the partner's social support. More globally, and not restricted to positive evaluations, answers may be biased by a halo effect. In marital studies, Nye (1988) showed this effect in satisfied partners who attribute a great number of positive traits to their partner and a negative halo effect in unhappily married couples where each partners attribute a lot of negative traits to each other. This effect has also been described as a sentiment override: in short, there is a kind of global judgment about the relationship which causes partners to see the different variables pertaining to the relationship with the same affective valence. Finally, answers to a questionnaire on relationships are also influenced by attribution bias – which is close to the halo effect (Bradbury and Fincham 1990; Jacobson et al. 1985). For example, an inadequate behavior of one partner (a criticism, an accusation, contempt, etc.) is interpreted by the other partner in a happily married couple as an unstable and situational behavior, and an adequate behavior is perceived as stable and internal to the partner. In contrast, in an unhappily married couple, an inadequate behavior is seen as stable and internal to the partner and an adequate one is perceived as unstable and dependent of the situation.

Another limitation lies not in questionnaires themselves, but in the use of a research methodology relying only on questionnaires. There are indeed often high correlations between different questionnaires completed by the same person, when these questionnaires are addressing close concepts. For example, in the domain of marital interactions, high correlations are systematically found between social support perceived and provided by the partners and marital satisfaction (Bodenmann 2000). While these correlations may refer to genuine associations between different variables, they may also stem from an artifact that Gottman has named the "GLOP problem" (Gottman 1998). It refers to the fact that an association between two variables assessed by the same person may be explained by a third "hidden" variable; to continue with the above example, a low marital satisfaction and a low perception of the support provided by the partner may both be the result of a depressed mood in the informant. This artifact is all the more evident when couple relationships are assessed. In this case, the between-informants agreement is significantly lower than within-informants agreement (Rhoades and Stocker 2006). This means that the real degree of similarity between both partners tends to be lower than the degree of similarity reported individually by each partner. For example, a woman facing cancer could give an account of a high level of emotional support provided to and received from her partner, whereas her partner reports that both he and his partner provided one another with a low level of emotional support. In this example, one partner reports a high degree of emotional support in the couple and the other one a low level. The between-informants agreement is thus low. However, the within-reporter agreement is high because each partner perceives a same level of emotional support by him/herself and the partner.

In short, it is thus important to note that researchers have emphasized that questionnaires make it possible to collect subjective data (the informant's representation) and to a certain extent "objective" data, but they are also subject to biases so that additional methodology is warranted when the researcher is interested in getting an accurate picture of interactional variables. Direct observation of behavior is the usual alternative to questionnaires in studies on interactions.

3.2   Observational Data

Observational data allow the collection of "here and now" information (Favez 2010). This collection can be naturalistic or standardized. Naturalistic observational data are obtained in the participants' natural environment (at home, for example). Standardized observational data are obtained in a laboratory situation with a task given to the participants. In most cases, technical equipment is used to make a video or audio recording of the behaviors (verbal and/or nonverbal). Trained coders visualize and listen then to the video- or audiotaped sequences and code them using standard coding tools.

3.2.1   Advantages of Observational Data

Observational data allow homogeneity between trained coders using a standardized coding grid, which may be consider as an index of "objectivity". For example, in the domain of marital interactions, in order to evaluate emotional social support provided by partners, coders firstly have to define and conceptualize the emotional social support (What is it? What are the behavioral indicators of emotional social support? How is emotional social support expressed?). Researchers then have to define the measuring unit: do they want to observe behaviors, for example, a look from a partner to the other one (molecular units) or a chain or group of behaviors that form a construct, for example, consolation (molar units) (Favez 2010). Researchers are then trained to code. This homogeneity cannot be obtained when asking both partners to individually evaluate their own couple relationship.

Moreover, observational data make it possible to take into account interactional sequences – that is, how the couple is functioning in moment-to-moment interactions. For example, in the domain of marital interactions, Margolin and Wampold (1981) showed that distressed partners tend more often to show a "negative reciprocity" than nondistressed couples, i.e. a negative action by one partner (a criticism, for example) is followed by a negative reaction by the other partner and so on. On the other hand, nondistressed couples show a tendency for a partner to react positively (with humor, for example) to a negative action of the other; this is absent in distressed couples, and has been labeled as "negative reactivity". In a similar vein, observational data has highlighted some communication patterns such as the demand-withdraw pattern (Christensen and Schenk 1991). This pattern is character-ized in marital relationships by the motivation of one partner (usually the wife) to discuss some issues and to solve problems, and by the efforts of the other partner (usually the husband) to avoid the discussion and to withdraw from the interaction.

Furthermore, observational data make it possible to analyze whether the answer provided by one partner is optimally matched with the needs and demands of the other one (Cutrona and Russell 1990). For example, a woman facing cancer is afraid of the disease and feels the need to share these concerns with her partner, to be heard by him, to be reassured by being taken in his arms and so on. This woman needs some emotional social support from her partner. The partner responds to her demand by suggesting to phone to her doctor in order to have some information about the disease. He gives her instrumental social support. Although the support provided by the partner is theoretically positive, it is not adapted to the specific woman's need at this very moment; consequently it is evaluated by the patient as inadequate and ineffective.

Finally, observational data allow the detection of possible incongruences between messages emitted by different communication channels. Nonverbal and paraverbal communication play an important role in the way social support between partners is perceived. If one partner gives positive verbal social support to the other one ("I will be with you in order to face the cancer"), but pronounces this sentence, for example, with anger (paraverbal) or without looking at his partner (nonverbal), the woman will perceive the social support as negative.

3.2.2   Hesitations and Arguments for the Use of Observational Data in the Domain of Couple Interactions

Several questions regarding observational methods have been under debate, espe-cially concerning laboratory observation. The first one is about representativeness of the data: is it possible to get information about how the couple does in "real" life when they are asked to interact in an artificial setting with cameras around them? Studies show that couples indeed behave differently in laboratories and at home without the presence of an observer. When they are under observation, partners are kinder to each other than when they are at home alone and they engage in far shorter chains of negativity (Gottman 1979), but if high negative emotions are present between them they tend nevertheless to show up after a while. Gottman (1994) demonstrated that couples could simulate adequate communication during maximum the first 2 min of an interaction and then they fall in their typical communication patterns. Vincent et al. (1979) ultimately asked the couples to try either to fake good or fake bad in the lab during 10 min. Both groups of couples were unable to fake their nonverbal behaviors. Nonverbal behavior may be a better discriminator of distressed and nondistressed groups than verbal behavior alone. Heyman (2001) summarized that, even if interactions of distressed couples observed in a laboratory are not as negative as interactions filmed at home, some "differences in affect, behavior, physiology, and interactional patterns and processes" could be revealed. In general, observational data may generate "false negatives" (some couples may be able to "hide" their negative feelings), so it is possible that partners interact in a more adequate way in the laboratory than they do at home and researchers might overlook conflicts in the marital interactions. By contrast, "false positives" are very unlikely to be found (when negative emotions are displayed in the laboratory, they are representative of the objective state of the relation). All in all, this tends to show that observational data collected in a laboratory can be representative of everyday interactions, especially for couples with a high level of conflict and negative emotions.

Another question concerns the possible selection bias as there might be a difference between people who agree to be filmed and observed in the lab and people who do not. Data are scarce in this domain. In one research, Krokoff et al. (1988) did not find differences between couples who volunteered to participate in the videotaped sequences and couples who were randomly assigned to participate in these sequences.

Finally, there might be concerns about the consequences for people of participating in laboratory observations, especially in procedures in which couples are asked to talk about conflict issues, with the possible risk that the negative emotions elicited in the laboratory may spread into their everyday life. Here also, data are scarce; in one research, Fichten and Wright (1983) did not find any negative effects for couples participating in observational studies. Indeed these authors videotaped couples' interactions in a laboratory. Six months later, the level of marital satisfaction reported by the couples was the same as the level reported at the time of the observation. Moreover, almost half of these couples reported an improvement of their marital satisfaction due to participating in the study. As far as couples facing cancer are concerned, we hypothesized that taking part in a situation of observation could also have benefits for both partners. Indeed being in a lab could facilitate talking about the disease between partners and mobilize individual resources of both partners and couples' resources.

3.2.3 Disadvantages of Observational Data

Hahlweg and collaborators (2000) remind us that the collection of observational data in the domain of marital interactions is "costly and time consuming, particularly for microanalytic coding systems that require the accurate classification of small units of behavior" (p. 61). These authors describe the typical process in order to obtain valid data. The couples have first to come to the laboratory and be videotaped during a discussion. Several external observers have to be trained in order to code the interactions with a standard grid. These coders are regularly supervised and the inter-rater validity has repeatedly to be probed. In consequence, observational data requires important resources.

4 The Necessity to Mix the Methods

So, what is the best methodology in studying social support in couples? Should we choose between the two? The first thing to consider is the extent to which information brought by these methods is redundant or complementary. In the domain of marital interactions, moderate correlations are found between questionnaires and observational data. For example, Hahlweg et al. (2000) computed associations between conflict patterns reported by partners – self-reported data based on the Communication Patterns Questionnaire (CPQ; Heavey et al. 1996) – and conflict patterns rated by external observers – observational data that relied on the Coding System for Marital/Family Interaction (KPI; Hahlweg et al. 1984) – in a nonreferred sample group. They only found moderate correlations between the results of the two instruments. In general, there are consistently low to moderate associations between questionnaires and observation, even when the instruments are designed to assess the same psychological construct.

Based on the fact that questionnaires provide access to the representations of each partner and that observational data allow the observation of verbal, nonverbal and paraverbal interactions between both partners, it is now relatively well accepted that the information is complementary and that the best strategy is to use both when possible. This is all the more relevant as the results obtained by these methods may highlight discrepancies which are clinically informative. For example in studies examining social support among couples facing breast cancer, the healthy partner may seem very supportive during the video sequences, but appears rather contemptuous in the data collected by questionnaires. These discrepancies may be due to the healthy partner's personality (for example: a passive-aggressive personality), or to the healthy partner's willingness to preserve the other partner and the couple interaction and not show his partner any discouragement. In contrast, the healthy partner may report good evaluations of his own social support in questionnaires, but appear to be inadequate during the audio- or videotaped interactions. This phenomenon could appear when the healthy partner tries to answer in a socially desirable way (it is easier to guess the expected answers by filling in questionnaires that by participating in a videotaped interaction) or when the healthy partner is not aware of his behavior.

This low to moderate association may also be due to stereotypes. For example, Neff and Karney (2005) highlight the fact that in studies relying on self-reported data both spouses tended to report a better social support provided by the women than by the men. In contrast to this, gender differences were not reported in studies using observational data.

5   The Study "Women Facing Breast Cancer" of the LIVES NCCR

In order to overcome the artifacts produced by the use of different assessment methods, the study "Women facing cancer" uses a mixed-method approach as mentioned above. We present now the details of this study.

5.1   Method

5.1.1   Sample

Eighty-nine women with breast cancer were recruited at the Breast Centre of the University Hospital of Lausanne (Switzerland). Sixty were in a relationship (their partners also participated in the study) and 29 were single. The mean age for women in relationships was 54.70 (SD = 12.55) and 55.59 (SD = 12.66) for single women; partners were on average 56.21 years old (SD = 14.75). 60 % of the women in relationship were married. 65.5 % of single women were divorced or separated, 17.2 % were widows, and 17.2 % were single (i.e. never married).

5.1.2   Procedure

Women were informed of the study by the breast nurse during their hospitalization (1–2 weeks after the diagnosis). Criteria for study inclusion were as follows: (a) the patient had a diagnosis of breast cancer; (b) the patient had had breast cancer surgery; (c) the patient and partner were 18 years of age or older; (d) the patient and partner were French speaking. Eighty-nine women accepted to participate (58 %) and 65 women refused (42 %). The principal reasons for refusal were the following: no desire to be filmed (32 %), a lot of stress and a lack of energy (26 %), no desire to talk about these difficult moments (29 %), and various other reasons (13 %). Comparisons were made between study participants and nonparticipants. Results indicated no significant differences in terms of age, $t(152) = 0.05$, ns nor in terms of relationship status (in couple or single), $\chi 2(1, 154) = 0.01$, ns. Women and their partners were received around 2 weeks after the surgery for an interview with the breast nurse, a situation of observation and to fill in questionnaires (T1). Follow ups were planned to take place 3 months (T2), 12 months (T3) and 24 months (T4) after the surgery.

5.1.3   Questionnaires

Questionnaires were used in order to assess several individual and relational variables by both partners, such as general distress (Brief Symptoms Inventory-18; Derogatis 2001), marital satisfaction (Relationship Assessment Scale; Hendrick 1988) or social support in couple interactions (Dyadic Coping Inventory; Bodenmann 2008). These questionnaires were paper self-completion questionnaires. The study also contained hetero-reported data such as the evaluation by both partners of the other one's social support (Dyadic Coping Inventory, Bodenmann 2008) or cancer- related communication (Cancer-related Communication Problems within Couples Scale, Kornblith et al. 2006). Questionnaires were constituted of Likert-scales. Each partner individually filled in the questionnaire at home and returned it by mail to the Breast Center using the prepaid envelope. Finally, questionnaires about medical information, such as diagnosis, complications, and treatment were administered by the breast nurse.

One of the questionnaires, the Family Attitude Scale (FAS; Kavanagh et al. 1997; French version Vandeleur et al. 2013), aimed at assessing "expressed emotions". This is one of the constructs that has been studied through observations and self-reports and thus it may illustrate the complementary information brought by these two methods. Expressed emotions refer to the degree of criticism and hostility and emotional over-involvement in a family or a marital relationship (Brown and Rutter 1966). High Expressed Emotion (HEE) is defined when one partner makes a lot of negative comments about the other one and the couple relationship and Low Expressed Emotion (LEE) describes a low rate of such comments. Expressed emotions are known to be a significant predictor of negative psychological outcomes (Butzlaff and Hooley 1998; Lister 2011), high level of partner caregiver burden (Möller-Leimkühler and Jandl 2011) and relationship dissatisfaction (Kronmüller et al. 2011) across several diseases. The FAS is a 30-item questionnaire assessing the informant's expressed emotions through self-reported attitudes and behaviors towards another person – in our case, the partner. Items are rated on Likert scales from 4 (every day) to 0 (never), except for positive attitudes and behaviors which are reverse scored. The total score has a range of 0–120, with higher scores reflecting high expressed emotions. Examples of questions are: "I find myself saying nasty or sarcastic things to him/her", "He/she is easy to get along with", "I am sick of having to look after him/her". In our study, women obtained a mean score of 21.4 (*SD* = 14.6; *median* = 19; *range* = 1–76); partners got a mean score of 14.6 (*SD* = 9.2; *median* = 14; *range* = 0–35).

5.2   *Observational Data*

Two kinds of observational data were collected by the breast nurse in the lab of the Breast Centre of the University Hospital of Lausanne. Firstly, a semi-standardized interview aimed at collecting information from both partners about the way they reacted to the diagnosis, the sense they gave to the illness, how they informed (if they have) their families and friends, how they have been managing the illness, how the relationship has been affected at an emotional as well at a sexual level, how they have been supporting each other and where they could find support outside their relationship, how they see their future. The partners were invited to answer freely to these questions. The interview was videotaped. Two researchers coded the verbal, paraverbal and nonverbal contents of the interview with standardized coding grids for social support or for diagnosis integration. Inter-rater reliability was assessed in order to warrant the validity of the data.

Secondly, each partner was invited to complete a standardized task aimed at evaluating "live" expressed emotion: the Five Minute Speech Sample (FMSS; Magana et al. 1986). This task consists in a monologue by each partner who is asked to talk about his/her partner and their couple relationship during 5 min. The speech is audiotaped and the verbal and paraverbal content is coded for expressed emotions with a standardized coding grid provided by the authors (Magana et al. 1986). An expert in this coding system trained three coders. In order to establish interobserver reliability, the coders rated 15 videotapes (that means 30 FMSS-sequences) independently. Cohen's kappa coefficients were then computed. For the different coded categories (e.g.: critics, quality of the relationship, etc.), the coefficients were higher than 0.80 between each coder and the expert and higher than 0.80 among the coders.

5.3 Observed and Self-Reported Expressed Emotions; A Case Example

The woman is 70 and the man 74 years old. The partners have known each other for 52 years and have been married for 51 years. They have two children of 51 and 48 years old. They filled in the questionnaires and participated in the FMSS 2 weeks after the surgery (6 weeks after the woman received a diagnosis of breast cancer).

The woman obtained a score of 40 on the FAS. This score is high compared to the mean score of the sample (larger than one standard deviation above the mean). For example, she gave high scores to items such as "He makes me feel drained" and "He ignores my advice". In the FMSS, this woman made mainly positive comments about her husband ("He is just and right", "He is gentle and kind, he is very sensitive") and her happiness to be in a marital relationship with him ("We are always on the same wavelength", "I am happy [with him]", "I am lucky [with him]", "I can count on him", "We are well together", "I will never change [my partner]").

The man obtained a score of 21 at the FAS. This score is average with regard to the sample of the current study (within one standard deviation above the mean). He displayed zero score on some items like: "She is really hard to take", "I feel disappointed with her". By contrast, in the FMSS, he displayed a very high expressed emotions pattern with several criticisms toward his partner; the monologue began with the sentence: "She was a girl I knew among others. I was taken by surprise, so my father told me that I made a mistake that I will pay to the bitter end. I didn't know her. I quickly saw that I could manipulate her, that I could rule her with a rod of iron." The husband gave next some criticisms: "She is quite impulsive. Her brother says she is unreliable. She sometimes deserves ....[silent, sigh], she freaks out."

This example illustrates the necessity to assess this construct with several methods as the results are not the same depending on the method that was used: according to the questionnaire, the woman was high on expressed emotion while the man was low; according to the situation of observation, the woman was low on expressed emotions and the man was high. This certainly refers to a certain degree of ambivalence in their relationship; the mixed-method approach allowed us to note that both partners are ambivalent while a single method would have led us to conclude that one partner only is high on emotion and thus "responsible" for the negativity in the relation. Moreover, we would not have identified the same partner as the "negative one" depending on the chosen method. The mixed method also allows a more complex and comprehensive evaluation of a situation. In fact, each method measures a different aspect of this situation and grasps its nuances and subtleties.

6 Conclusion

A mixed-method approach is crucial in order to study couple interactions in general and interactions in couples facing cancer in particular. It makes it possible to combine data representative of the "subjective reality" of the partners (i.e. the representations they have of the relationship) and of the "objective reality" (how they actually act when they talk about each other or when they interact together). Unfortunately, observation is often overlooked in research mainly because of its cost and the difficulty to operationalize psychological constructs in behavioral indexes (Weiss and Heyman 2004). Gottman (1994) has nevertheless made a plea for observation, arguing that observational data have a special place for two reasons:

1. Partners are not aware of the different patterns of communication and behaviors that usually occur in their couple interaction. It is also difficult for them to accurately report behavioral interactions.
2. Self-reported data assess perceptions, in other words the subjective reality of an individual. Observational data allow researchers to avoid the confusion between perceptions and reality.

Even if observational data require time and energy (i) to obtain videotaped sequences, (ii) to elaborate a coding system and (iii) to code the sequences, this chapter shows that this effort is worthwhile.

References

Bodenmann, G. (2000). *Stress und Coping bei Paaren*. Göttingen: Hogrefe.

Bodenmann, G. (2005). Dyadic coping and its significance for marital functioning. In T. A. Revenson, K. Kayser, & G. Bodenmann (Eds.), *Couples coping with stress: Emerging perspectives on dyadic coping* (pp. 33–50). Washington, DC: American Psychological Association.

Bodenmann, G. (2008). *Dyadisches Coping Inventar (DCI). Test manual*. Bern: Huber.

Bradbury, T. N., & Fincham, F. D. (1990). Attributions in marriage: Review and critique. *Psychological Bulletin, 107*, 3–33.

Brown, G., & Rutter, M. (1966). The measurement of family activities and relationships. A methodological study. *Human Relations, 19*(3), 241–263.

Butzlaff, R. L., & Hooley, J. M. (1998). Expressed emotion and psychiatric relapse. *Archives of General Psychiatry, 55*, 547–552.

Christensen, A., & Schenk, J. L. (1991). Communication, conflict, and psychological distance in nondistressed, clinic, and divorcing couples. *Journal of Consulting and Clinical Psychology, 59*, 458–463.

Cutrona, C. E. (1996). *Social support in couples*. Thousand Oaks: Sage.

Cutrona, C. E., & Russell, D. W. (1990). Type of social support and specific stress: Toward a theory of optimal matching. In B. R. Sarason, I. G. Sarason, & G. R. Gregory (Eds.), *Social support: An interactional view* (pp. 319–366). Oxford: Wiley.

Cutrona, C. E., & Suhr, J. A. (1992). Controllability of stressful events and satisfaction with spouse support behaviors. *Communication Research, 19*, 154–176.

Derogatis, L. R. (2001). *Brief Symptom Inventory (BSI)-18. Administration, scoring and procédures manual*. Minneapolis: NCS Pearson, Inc.

Ell, K., Nishimoto, R., Morway, T., Mantell, J., & Hamovitch, M. (1989). A longitudinal analysis of psychological adaptation among survivors of cancer. *Cancer, 63*, 406–413.

Favez, N. (2010). *L'examen clinique de la famille. Modèles et instruments d'évaluation*. Wavre: Mardaga.

Fichten, C. S., & Wright, J. (1983). Problem-solving skills in happy and distressed couples: Effects of videotape and verbal feedback. *Journal of Clinical Psychology, 39*, 340–352.

Gerits, P. (2000). Life events, coping and breast cancer: State of the art. *Biomedecine and Parmacotherapy, 54*, 229–233.

Giese-Davis, J., Hermanson, K., Koopman, C., Weibel, D., & Spiegel, D. (2000). Quality of couples' relationship and adjustment to metastatic breast cancer. *Journal of Family Psychology, 14*, 251–266.

Gottman, J. M. (1979). *Marital interaction: Experimental investigations*. New York: Academic.

Gottman, J. M. (1994). *What predicts divorce: The relationship between marital processes and marital outcomes*. Hillsdale: Lawrence Erlbaum Associates, Inc.

Gottman, J. M. (1998). Psychology and the study of marital processes. *Annual Review of Psychology, 49*, 169–197.

Hahlweg, K., Reisner, L., Kohli, G., Vollmer, M., Schindler, L., & Revenstorf, D. (1984). Development and validity of a new system to analyze interpersonal communication: Kategoriensystem für partnerschaftliche Interaktion KPI. In K. Hahlweg & N. S. Jacobson (Eds.), *Marital interaction: Analysis and modification* (pp. 182–198). New York: Guilford Press.

Hahlweg, K., Kaiser, A., Christensen, A., Fehm-Wolfsdorf, G., & Groth, T. (2000). Self-report and observational assessment of couples' conflict: The concordance between the communication patterns questionnaire and the KPI observation system. *Journal of Marriage and Family, 62*, 61–67.

Heavey, C. L., Larson, B. M., Zumtobel, D. C., & Christensen, A. (1996). The communication patterns questionnaire: The reliability and validity of a constructive communication subscale. *Journal of Marriage and Family, 58*, 796–800.

Helgeson, V., & Cohen, S. (1996). Social support and adjustment to cancer: Reconciling descriptive, correlational and intervention research. *Health Psychology, 15*(2), 135–148.

Hendrick, S. S. (1988). A generic measure of relationship satisfaction. *Journal of Marriage and the Family, 50*, 93–98.

Heyman, R. E. (2001). Observation of couple conflicts: Clinical assessment applications, stubborn truths and shaky foundations. *Psychological Assessment, 13*, 5–35.

Jacobson, N. S., McDonald, D. W., Follette, W. C., & Berley, R. A. (1985). Attributional processes in distressed and nondistressed married couples. *Cognitive Therapy Research, 9*, 35–50.

Kavanagh, D.J., O'Halloran, P., Manicavasagar, V., Clark, D., Piatkowska, O., Tennant, C., Rosen, A. (1997). The family attitude scale: Reliability and validity of a new scale for measuring the emotional climate of families. *Psychiatry Research, 70*, 185–195.

Kayser, K. (2005). Enhancing dyadic coping during a time of crisis: A theory-based intervention with breast cancer patients and their partners. In T. A. Revenson, K. Kayser, & G. Bodenmann (Eds.), *Couples coping with stress: Emerging perspectives on dyadic coping* (pp. 33–50). Washington, DC: American Psychological Association.

Kayser, K., & Scott, J. (2008). *Helping couples cope with women's cancers. An evidence-based approach for practitioners.* New York: Springer.

Kenny, D. A., & Acitelli, L. K. (2001). Accuracy and bias in the perception of the partner in a close relationship. *Journal of Personality and Social Psychology, 80*, 439–448.

Kornblith, A. B., Regan, M. M., Youngmee, K., Greer, G., Parker, B., Bennett, S., & Winer, E. (2006). Cancer-related communication between female patients and male partners scale: A pilot study. *Psycho-Oncology, 15*, 780–794.

Krokoff, L. J., Gottman, J. M., & Roy, A. K. (1988). Blue-collar marital interaction and a companionate philosophy of marriage. *Journal of Personal and Social Relationships, 5*, 201–222.

Kronmüller, K.-T., Backenstrass, M., Victor, D., Postelnicu, I., Schenkenbach, C., Joest, K., Fiedler, P., & Mundt, C. (2011). Quality of marital relationship and depression: Results of a 10-year prospective follow-up study. *Journal of Affective Disorders, 128*, 64–71.

Ligue Suisse contre le Cancer. (2005). *Le dépistage du cancer du sein.* Berne: Ligue suisse contre le cancer du sein.

Lister, Z. D. (2011). Diabetes and the couple dyad: Expressed emotion, diabetes control and management. *Dissertation Abstracts International, A: The Humanities and Social Sciences, 71*, 3438.

Magana, A., Goldstein, M., Karno, M., Miklowitz, D., Jenkins, J., & Falloon, I. (1986). A brief method for assessing expressed emotions in relatives of psychiatric patients. *Psychiatry Research, 17*, 203–212.

Manne, S. L., & Ostroff, J. S. (2008). *Coping with breast cancer. A couples-focused group intervention.* Oxford: University Press.

Manne, S. L., Alferi, T., Taylor, K. L., & Dougherty, J. (1999). Spousal negative responses to cancer patients: The role of social restriction, spouse mood and relationship satisfaction. *Journal of Consulting and Clinical Psychology, 67*, 352–361.

Manne, S. L., Ostroff, J., Sherman, M., Heyman, R. E., Ross, S., & Fox, K. (2004). Couples' support-related communication, psychological distress, and relationship satisfaction among women with early stage breast cancer. *Journal of Consulting and Clinical Psychology, 72*, 660–670.

Margolin, G., & Wampold, B. E. (1981). Sequential analysis of conflict and accord in distressed and nondistressed marital partners. *Journal of Consulting and Clinical Psychology, 49*, 554–567.

Möller-Leimkühler, A. M., & Jandl, M. (2011). Expressed and perceived emotion over time: Does the patients' view matter for the caregivers' burden? *European Archives of Psychiatry and Clinical Neuroscience, 261*, 349–355.

Murray, S. L., Holmes, J. G., & Griffin, D. W. (1996). The benefits of positive illusions: Idealization and construction of satisfaction in close relationships. *Journal of Personality and Social Psychology, 70*, 79–98.

Neff, L. A., & Karney, B. R. (2005). Gender differences in social support: A question of skill or responsiveness? *Journal of Personality and Social Psychology, 88*, 79–90.

Northouse, L. L. (1989). The impact of breast cancer on patients and husbands. *Cancer Nursing, 12*, 276–284.

Northouse, L. L., Mood, D., Kershaw, T., Schafenacker, A., Mellon, S., Walker, J., Galvin, E., & Decker, V. (2002). Quality of life of women with recurrent breast and their family members. *Journal of Clinical Oncology, 20*, 4050–4064.

Nye, F. (1988). Fifty years of family research 1937–1987. *Journal of Marriage and Family, 50*, 305–316.

Pistrang, N., & Barker, C. (1995). The partner relationship in psychological response to breast cancer. *Social Science and Medicine, 40*, 789–797.

Rhoades, G. K., & Stocker, C. M. (2006). Can spouses provide knowledge of each other's communication patterns? A study of self-reports, spouses' reports, and observational coding. *Family Process, 45*, 499–511.

Schulz, U., & Schwarzer, R. (2004). Long-term effects of spousal support on coping with cancer after surgery. *Journal of Social and Clinical Psychology, 23*, 716–732.

Schwarzer, R., & Leppin, A. (1989). *Sozialer Rückhalt und Gesundheit: Eine Meta-Analyse.* Göttingen: Hogrefe.

Sillars, A. L. (1985). Interpersonal perceptions in relationships. In W. Ickes (Ed.), *Compatible and incompatible relationships* (pp. 277–305). New York: Springer-Verlag.

Uchino, B. N. (2004). *Social support and physical health: Understanding the health consequences of our relationships.* New Haven: Yale University Press.

Vandeleur, C., Kavanagh, D. J., Favez, N., Castelao, E., & Preisig, M. (2013). French version of the Family Attitude Scale: Psychometric properties and relation of attitudes to the respondent's psychiatric status. *Psychiatry Research, 210*, 641–646.

Vincent, J. P., Friedman, L. C., Nugent, J., & Messerly, L. (1979). Demand characteristics in observations of marital interaction. *Journal of Consulting and Clinical Psychology, 47*, 557–566.

Weiss, R. (1974). The provisions of social relationships. In Z. Rubin (Ed.), *Doing unto other* (pp. 17–26). Englewood Cliffs: Prentice-Hall.

Weiss, R., & Heyman, R. (2004). Couples observational research: An impertinent, critical overview. In P. Kerig & D. Baucom (Eds.), *Couple observational coding systems* (pp. 11–25). Mahwah: Lawrence Erlbaum.

Wortman, C. B., & Dunkel-Schetter, C. (1987). Conceptual and methodological issues in the study of social support. In A. Baum & J. E. Singer (Eds.), *Handbook of psychology and health* (Vol. 5, pp. 63–108). Hillsdale: Lawrence Erlbaum.

Zimmermann, T., & Heinrichs, N. (2006). Psychosoziale Interventionen für Frauen mit Krebserkrankungen der Genitalorgane. *Verhaltenstherapie & Verhaltensmedizin, 27*(2), 125–141.

Zimmermann, T., & Heinrichs, N. (2008). *Seite an Seite. Eine gynäkologische Krebserkrankung in der Partnerschaft gemeinsam bewältigen: Ein Ratgeber für Paare.* Göttingen: Hogrefe-Verlag.

Zimmermann, T., Heinrichs, N., & Baucom, D. H. (2007). Does one size fit all? Moderators in psychosocial interventions for breast cancer patients. A meta-analysis. *Annals of Behavioral Medicine, 34*(3), 225–239.

Career Pathways and Professional Transitions: Preliminary Results from the First Wave of a 7-Year Longitudinal Study

Christian Maggiori, Jérôme Rossier, Franciska Krings, Claire S. Johnston, and Koorosh Massoudi

1 Introduction

Work and the professional domain represent essential aspects of adult-life and are strongly related to individuals' somatic and mental health, and potentially vulnerable situations as well (Fouad and Bynner 2008; Friedland and Price 2003). However, current career paths and professional development are challenged by increased instability and demands related to – amongst others – productivity and coping with constant uncertainty (Rudisill et al. 2010). In addition to unemployment, in the current world of work other risk-situations may contribute to the emergence of critical situations, such as frequent transitions and unstable or precarious situations (e.g., time-limited employment and positions with a high risk of lay-off and minimum wage employment). For these reasons, and considering that almost no longitudinal studies of the professional trajectories of adults from a psychological perspective are available, the need for a closer and longitudinal examination of middle-aged adults' career pathways and transitions is fundamental.

The purposes of this chapter are to present the main characteristics and implementation of our longitudinal project, the strategies used to collect data on

C. Maggiori (✉)
NCCR LIVES, University of Lausanne, Lausanne, Switzerland

School of Social Work Fribourg, University of Applied Sciences and Arts Western Switzerland, Fribourg, Switzerland
e-mail: christian.maggiori@hefr.ch

J. Rossier • K. Massoudi
Institute of Psychology, University of Lausanne, Lausanne, Switzerland

C.S. Johnston
NCCR-LIVES, University of Lausanne, Lausanne, Switzerland

F. Krings
Department of Organizational Behavior, University of Lausanne, Lausanne, Switzerland

© The Author(s) 2016
M. Oris et al. (eds.), *Surveying Human Vulnerabilities across the Life Course*,
Life Course Research and Social Policies 3, DOI 10.1007/978-3-319-24157-9_6

professional experiences using a mixed-mode approach, and to highlight initial results and indications from the first data collection wave (such as vulnerability and work stress or the predictors of the agreement to participate in the next waves). First, after introducing the general aim of the project, we present briefly some elements emerging from the current literature on workers' experience and career paths, and a definition of vulnerability to contextualize the project and position its hypothesis. Second, we introduce some methodological aspects, such as the design, the research protocol and the data collection procedure. Third, we present some of the preliminary results from the first data collection wave of our study. Finally, in the conclusion section we highlight the main findings and considerations emerging from the implementation and the first data collection wave and discuss some implications and challenges for the next waves.

1.1 Career Pathways and Professional Transitions: An Overview

Overall, adopting a broad psychological perspective including counseling, positive, work and organizational, as well as life-span psychology, this project studies the direct and indirect impacts of individual characteristics (such as personality, character strengths, or justice beliefs), individual resources (such as social support or self-regulatory skills), and socio-cultural and economic background (such as SES or acculturation) on adults' professional transitions and career pathways and their successful development (i.e., professional success, life-satisfaction, general and domain-specific well-being) (Krings and Olivares 2007; Petersen et al. 2010; Rossier et al. 2012b; Wiese and Freund 2005). A longitudinal survey design implying a yearly follow up spanning 7 years on a large sample of employed and unemployed middle-aged adults living in Switzerland was implemented. The longitudinal perspective will offer the opportunity to evaluate psychological processes, inter-individual differences and intra-individual variability across time in relation to professional experiences (including job search and unemployment) and professional transitions. Moreover we will focus on identifying the individual strengths (or resilience factors) and vulnerabilities in order to predict objective and subjective aspects of career pathways. More specifically, our study will make it possible to estimate the impact of these factors on the experienced trajectories of workers, and on employees' work conditions, such as underemployment, time-limited employment, multiple-jobs and job loss.

Another central characteristic of this study is the adoption of a mixed-mode approach for the data collection. In fact, in order to offer the opportunity to participants to choose the most convenient way to participate and to target different subgroups in our sample (Dillmann et al. 2009), we implemented several formats[1] to complete the research protocol. More precisely, participants could choose to

---

[1] That is, modes of data collection (such as, phone interview).

complete the two parts of the research protocol via a full online version, a phone interview (CATI) plus an online questionnaire or a CATI plus a paper-pencil questionnaire.

1.2 Why Study Career Pathways?

To position our study in the current labor market context, we consider some relevant literature pertaining to careers and the world of work.

Due to the changing social and economic conditions, the work context – and consequently professional pathways – has profoundly changed over the last two decades (Rudisill et al. 2010). The current labor market requires individuals to face increasing job instability and demands related to flexibility and geographical mobility, productivity and management of constant insecurity (Kanfer et al. 2001; Rudisill et al. 2010). Furthermore, current work-profiles are very heterogeneous, in terms of, for example work activity rate (part-time vs. full-time), type of contract (time-limited vs. non-time limited employment), or job security. Moreover, in the coming years individuals can expect to encounter a growing number of job transitions, and hence periods of (partial-) unemployment during their work life (Kanfer et al. 2001; Zikic and Klehe 2006). It is important to underline that individuals making these changes have to cope with different psychological (and social) challenges (e.g. cope with constant stress, adopt a new, or leave behind an old social role). This seems particularly true when these changes are not made voluntarily and are imposed by external factors (e.g. due to a layoff) (Fouad and Bynner 2008; Sapin et al. 2007). In this context, professional trajectories across adulthood are severely challenged and become more instable and less predictable (Mercure 2001; Sennett 1998; Rudisill et al. 2010). At the same time, due to societal changes, developmental tasks and personal goals have shifted across cohorts during the last five to six decades (Bangerter et al. 2001; Grob et al. 2001). Currently individuals face an increasing diversification of developmental pathways. Compared to previous cohorts, family and work-related goals have become less important for current young adults, whereas education and personal time/leisure goals (such as travelling or community involvement) have become more central concerns (Bangerter et al. 2001). This reflects a tendency towards individualism and self-fulfilment, as indicated by Grob and colleagues (2001).

In a general way, we can consider that career pathways and professional experiences are the result of the interaction between personal characteristics and socio-cultural conditions: (i) Individuals' skills, competencies, socio-economic background and/or goals; (ii) Labor market's needs and demands (for instance, in terms of adaptation skills, willingness to relocate, mastery of new technologies, or the ability to take frequent and complex decisions, and to update one's skills) (Sennett 1998; Briscoe and Hall 2006); (iii) The necessity for and competence to make several career-related choices throughout the life-span (rather than deciding once and for all upon a specific career) (Fouad and Bynner 2008). Of course, individual career choices and contextual challenges influence people's professional and personal development in terms of subjective and objective career pathways, and physical as well as psychological well-being (Klehe et al. 2011). For example, unemployment and unfavorable conditions at the workplace, such as job insecurity, underemployment and the experience of workplace incivilities have a negative impact on individuals' functioning and professional and general well-being (among others in terms of quality of life, stress, depression and work satisfaction) and can lead to vulnerability (Cortina et al. 2001; Friedland and Price 2003). Lucas et al. (2004), highlighted that the unemployment experience can also impact personal well-being in the medium- and long-term even after re-entering the labor market. In fact, even after reemployment, individuals continue to exhibit lower life satisfaction. Hence, contemporary professional trajectories occasionally induce at-risk situations, such as difficult transitions (Schlossberg et al. 1995), social and professional exclusion or discrimination (Haeberlin et al. 2004), and trajectories towards unemployment or poverty (Meyer and Stalder 2003).

For these reasons, analyzing individuals' professional experience and career paths represents an important research area. Understanding the relationship between individual characteristics, vulnerabilities and resources, and environmental aspects like job characteristics and opportunities, and their dual impact on well-being outcomes seems important in order to understand how people adapt to changing work conditions. Research on these types of topics is of prime importance for psychologists dealing with the prevention of at-risk psychosocial situations and negative health outcomes, and more generally with vulnerability processes arising within or from the domain of work (Bakker et al. 2005).

1.3 Vulnerability and the Professional Context

To understand and analyze various forms and process of vulnerability represents one of the main purposes of the NCCR-LIVES. More specifically, in our project we address aspects of vulnerability related to the work domain and professional paths (such as work stress and job loss).

According to the social cognitive theory of Lent et al. (1994), and to the life-design theoretical perspective of Savickas et al. (2009) people have to adapt to new situations in their everyday life. Thus, they need to be able to use their dispositions to respond to the environment and to maximize their capacities and resources. These models suggest that the relationship between dispositions, environment, and people's behavior (in terms of, for example, career choice, work performance or work engagement) are mediated by process variables or regulation abilities, such as self-efficacy, external expectations, career adapt-ability and emotional regulation (Rossier et al. 2012a, b). In accordance with this theoretical background, vulnerability related to entry, participation and development within the professional context is characterized by:

1. The presence of individual (e.g., disability, poor health and well-being, inadequate regulatory capacities) and/or contextual risk factors (e.g., minority, low SES, unemployment, high stress conditions);

2. The deficit or lack of individual (e.g., adaptive capacities, character strengths) and/or contextual resources (e.g., financial, social support and network, labor market situation);
3. The possible interactions between risk factors and resources.

Overall, our research design with annual measurements allows us to take a longitudinal approach to vulnerability and to deal empirically with questions such as which factors increase vulnerability in the long run and which resources mitigate these effects.

Considering the elements presented so far, the general focus for our project concerns relations between individual resources and characteristics, social support (both actual and potential support), cultural background, job conditions (e.g., job demands and job control) and, job-related (e.g. work stress and job satisfaction) and general outcomes (e.g., health and quality of life). Specifically we hypothesize that in addition to a direct impact on outcomes including professional and general well-being and career related transitions (e.g. from unemployment to employment or job-to-job transitions), individual resources and characteristics, social support, and cultural background will moderate and/or mediate the relations between job conditions and outcomes.

2   Data Collection Tools and Measures to Explore Career Paths and Professional Experiences

In this section we present some methodological characteristics of our study on career pathways and professional transitions of employed and unemployed adults and general information concerning the procedure implemented for the first data collection wave realized from January to April 2012.

2.1   Sampling

According to the Swiss State Secretariat for Economy (SECO), in the first quarter of 2011 – at the time we started the project – the number of employed individuals in Switzerland was 4.5 million which represents about 58 % of the overall Swiss resident population. Women and non-Swiss represented respectively 45.6 % and 23.3 % of the employed population. At the same period, according to the International Labour Office's (ILO) criteria, there were more than 197,000 unemployed (about 4.4 % of the active population). Women and non-Swiss represented respectively 48.2 % and 44.7 % of the unemployed population. However, only about 134,000 people were officially registered at an official regional placement office (RPO). Concerning the length of unemployment, for these registered individuals about 39 % were unemployed for 6 months or more (SECO 2012).

For the purposes of this study, a first random sampling list was realized by the Swiss Federal Statistic Office (SFSO) (N = 9000) and drawn from the national register of the inhabitants. However, it was not possible to distinguish active and non-active individuals at this step. To increase the number of unemployed participants, in order to obtain a more detailed picture and increase statistical power, a second random sample was realized by the SECO (N = 2400). This sample was drawn from the national register of unemployed. Concerning the sampling criteria, both samples included exclusively adults aged 25–55 years from the French and German speaking regions of Switzerland. It is important to note that, at the beginning of the interview, we verified additional inclusion criteria that were not possible to control at the moment of the sampling. More specifically, participants had to meet the following criteria: (a) non-Swiss citizens needed to have at least an annual work permit; (b) live in a private household (people living in an institution were not sampled); (c) have a professional activity and/or be searching for a job. For practical and economic reasons (such as the necessity to translate and validate the majority of our instruments or to have Romansh and Italian speaking interviewers) we didn't include individuals living in the Italian- and Romansh- speaking regions, that represent <8 % of the Swiss population. Moreover, women were slightly oversampled to obtain a more comparable proportion of both genders.

2.2 Design and Research Protocol

As indicated previously, the project intends to realize a 7-year longitudinal study with an annual assessment (from T1 to T7). For T1, each participant completed a research protocol, consisting of two successive steps using a mixed-mode method for the data collection. More specifically, participants could choose: (a) To fill in the two parts of the research protocol using an online self-administered form; (b) To complete the first step by CATI and the second online; (c) To complete the first part by CATI and the second with a paper-pencil questionnaire. Overall, the estimated time to complete the total research protocol (240 items) was 10–15 min for the first step and 30–40 min for the second step.

In the first step, we assessed characteristics of the professional situation (e.g. employed or unemployed, current number of jobs or different employers, work rate and main activity), and professional experience and biography (e.g., start date of first job), including factors related to unemployment (e.g., receive – or not – unemployment benefits or length of unemployment). We also evaluated job satisfaction, perceived discrimination (e.g., sexual harassment and physical violence in the current work environment and/or during the job search process) and job search characteristics for employed and unemployed individuals (e.g., external support during job search). In this first part of the research protocol we used essentially items developed specifically for the study and questions proposed in other national surveys of the SFSO. Importantly, at the beginning of this part of the research protocol inclusion criteria mentioned previously were verified. More concretely, 910 individuals did not meet the criteria, or stopped the questionnaire and were excluded from the sample.

In the second step, we evaluated professional environment (in terms of, for example, job strain, job insecurity, work stress, and perceived organizational justice) and individual characteristics and resources, such as career adapt-ability, personality, and just world beliefs. In order to evaluate the respondents' general well-being, we assessed – amongst others – health, satisfaction with life and quality of life. Finally, we collected additional personal information (such as marital status, household income and education level). In relation to the employment status, a different questionnaire was proposed to employed and unemployed people.

2.2.1 Measures

In this section we present briefly the main measures analyzed in this chapter. Regarding individuals' characteristics and personal resources, the *Career Adapt-abilities Scale* (Savickas and Porfeli 2012) was employed to assess adapt-ability resources. This questionnaire contains 24 items that yield a total score, which indicates a person's career adapt-ability. The items are divided equally into four subscales that measure the adapt-ability resources of concern, control, curiosity, and confidence as psychosocial resources to face occupational transitions and work related challenges. Career adapt-ability is conceptualized as a hierarchical construct comprised of four dimensions: (i) Concern allows one to plan, activate and prepare an adaptive response; (ii) Control allow to engage the person's subjectivity in this adaptive response; (iii) Curiosity allows one to explore and find new responses; (iv) Confidence is the perceived capacity to express an adaptive response (Savickas et al. 2009). Participants rated how strongly they have developed each ability using a five-items rating scale (1 = "Not strong", 5 = "Strongest"). Personality was evaluated using the French-version of the *NEO Five-Factor Inventory Revised* (NEO-FFI-R; McCrae and Costa 2004; Aluja et al. 2005). The NEO-FFI-R includes 60 items, with a five-point scale ranking from "Strongly disagree" to "Strongly agree". The items are equally distributed to measure five personality dimensions (i.e., neuroticism, extraversion, openness, agreeableness and conscientiousness). The *Beliefs in a Just World Questionnaire*, developed by Dalbert (1999), was used to assess general (GBJW) and personal beliefs in a just world (PBJW). GBJW concerns the belief that people generally live in a just world, while the PBJW concerns whether they are personally treated fairly or not (Dalbert 2001; Wu et al. 2011). Six items are designed to describe GBJW and seven for PBJW. The questionnaire proposes a rating scale from 1 = "Strongly disagree" to 6 = "Strongly agree". The eight-item *Functional Social Support Questionnaire* (FSSQ, Broadhead et al. 1988) is an instrument to measure the level of the perceived personal social support. The items are scored on a five-point scale (1 = "Much less than I would like", 5 = "As much as would like").

Concerning professional outcomes, to evaluate work-related stress we used the *General Work Stress Scale* (GWSS; de Bruin and Taylor 2005). Participants responded to the nine items on a five-point rating scale, where the response options were labeled from 1 = "Never" to 5 = "Always". Job satisfaction was measured by an abbreviated version of the *Inventaire JobSat* of Rolland (Massoudi 2009). The five items proposed to our participants were selected to cover different domains of the professional satisfaction (i.e., supervisor behaviors, job security, salary, working conditions and relationships with colleagues). Each item was rated on a four-point rating scale, where 1 = "Not satisfied at all" and 4 = "Very satisfied".

Regarding individual risk factors, general stress was measured with the five-item version of the *Perceived Stress Scale* (PSS; Cohen and Williamson 1988). These items assess the extent to which situations in one's life were appraised as stressful during the last month using a rating scale ranking from 1 ("Never") to 5 ("Very often"). Life satisfaction was assessed using the *Satisfaction With Life Scale* (SWLS, Diener et al. 1985). The five items were rated on a seven-point scale (1 = "Strongly disagree", 7 = "Strongly agree"). Furthermore, we introduced in the research protocol the single-items suggested by the World Health Organization Quality of Life (WHOQOL)-Group (and used for example in the WHOQOL-Bref study, Skevington et al. 2004) to assess general *quality of life* and *self-rated health*. Respondents answered on a five-point rating scale from 1 = "Very poor" to 5 = "Very good".

2.3 Data Collection Procedure

For the data collection we established a formal contract with the main Swiss polling institute in social and political sciences: Link Institut. All efforts related to the field work: CATI programming, interviewer selection, instruction and training, organizing and managing the hotline, printing and mailing initial and reminder letter (and reminder phone call) were guaranteed by the polling institute with the supervision of the research team. Concerning the interviewer instruction and training, the program was developed and realized by two PhDs of the research team in collaboration with the polling institute. In this way, we tried to guarantee a certain quality and the same information to all the interviewers (French and German speakers). Two call centers were organized, one in Lausanne for the French-speakers and one in Zürich for the German-speakers, and a free-hotline was available throughout the data collection period from Monday to Saturday. Finally, two members of the research team were available during the data collection to answer participants' questions about the content of the survey and provide additional information about its purposes.

2.3.1 Mixed-Mode Method to Collect Data in T1

First of all, an advance personalized letter was sent to all target individuals describing the purpose and importance of the study, the data collection procedure and inviting them to participate. Individuals were encouraged to visit the project's web site to fill in a complete online version of the research protocol. To do so, each individual received a personal user name and password to have immediate access to a secure server. However, in this letter we also indicated the possibility to call a free-hotline to complete the first part of the research questionnaire by phone, to schedule an appointment or just to obtain additional information. Participants choosing CATI to complete the first part, were invited at the end of the interview to answer the second part of the research protocol via a paper-pencil or an online questionnaire. To reduce the time between the two parts of the research protocol, participants choosing the online version received an invitation by e-mail immediately after the initial interview. People choosing the paper-pencil format received the questionnaire by mail within 3–4 days, with a pre-stamped envelope to return the questionnaire.

With reference to the first part of the research protocol, those who did not complete the online questionnaire or did not call the hotline received a first reminder by mail 3 weeks after the initial contact. When necessary, a second reminder took place 2 weeks later by phone (when a phone number was available) or by mail. A similar reminder procedure was implemented for participants who never sent back the questionnaire or didn't complete the second part online. Furthermore, at the end of the main data collection, a conversion-strategy was implemented and realized by specially trained interviewers. More specifically, when a phone number was available, the interviewers re-contacted individuals who initially refused participation to try and persuade them to participate. More information about rates of refusal and drop-out at the different steps, and about the completion modes are presented in section "Participation: Key Data".

2.3.2 Subsequent Data-Collection Waves

Regarding the next waves (from T2 to T7), as indicated previously data collection will be realized once a year and it will take place during the same period (i.e., from January to April) to avoid seasonal bias. It is important to note that the same data collection procedure (i.e., a research protocol consisting of two successive steps and proposing a mixed-mode method) will be implemented. However, each year – in respect to the questionnaires' rotation system–, the content of the research protocol will be adapted. In fact, some new questionnaires will be integrated to replace others and will give us the opportunity to assess additional variables such as acculturation and personal strengths and follow changes related to professional situation.

2.4 Why Use a Mixed-Mode Method?

Considering the characteristics of our sample (for example in terms of employment situation), a mixed-mode method (including a online version of the research protocol) presents several advantages compared to a single-mode survey. First, the mixed-mode method offers participants the possibility to choose the most appropriate and comfortable format to complete the research protocol. Furthermore, they had the opportunity to schedule the phone interview at a convenient time. Second, in comparison to a face-to-face or phone interview, it reduces the costs of the data collection (Herrero and Meneses 2006; McHorney et al. 1994). For our project, this reduction – estimated at 15–20 % – is essentially related to the decreased number of phone interviews. Third, if participants chose the full online version, the research protocol could be completed relatively quickly as there was no time lag between the first and second parts. Furthermore, for participants choosing to complete the first part by CATI and then to continue online, they immediately received an invitation and an Internet link to complete the second part. This short time lag helps to prevent a lack of motivation as participants did not have to wait to complete the second part (Riva et al. 2003). Furthermore, the online versions allowed participants to complete the questionnaire in more than one session, permitting the participants to choose a convenient time to complete the questionnaire. Finally, for sensitive questions, a mixed-mode format using self-administered questionnaires results in increased comfort for respondents, possibly yielding a higher response rate than other interview formats (e.g. face-to-face interview) (de Leeuw 1992, 2005). For this reason, we introduced the more sensitive questions in the second self-administered part (online or paper) of the research protocol. Overall, the different opportunities presented by this kind of mixed-mode method aims to maximize participation by reducing the annual dropout rate and to consequently obtain the largest possible sample in T7.

However, a mixed-mode method presents some disadvantages too, which could have an impact on the quality of the collected data. For instance, measurement differences may emerge because not all participants used the same response format (de Leeuw 2005). Moreover, as indicated by de Leeuw (2005), the same question proposed online or by CATI, will not necessarily offer the same stimulus to the participant. To reduce this problem, during the first step of our survey (completed by CATI or online) we essentially asked for formal and objective information. Concerning psychological constructs – such as psychological distress or personal resources and characteristics – using online or paper-pencil questionnaires, several studies show that these methods produce equivalent assessments (e.g., Aluja et al. 2007; Herrero and Meneses 2006; Riva et al. 2003; Tse 1998). Furthermore, as with other methods based on self-report, a mixed-mode solution is not immune to potential sources of common method variance (such as consistency motif, social desirability or transient mood state) (Podsakoff et al. 2003). Moreover, due to the specific data collection format and even though questions were kept as simple as possible, people needed sufficient knowledge of German or French to participate. This limitation – which is not uniquely related to the mixed-mode method – is probably more important among non-Swiss individuals and subgroups with higher levels of low skilled people (such as unemployed individuals). Nevertheless, as indicated by Laganà et al. (2011), reaching more marginal groups –for example due to language limitations – is a recurrent problem in this kind of survey. Finally, online surveys, similar to surveys based on phone interviews, are affected by coverage bias (or error) (i.e., not all the household are equipped with Internet or phone connections, and coverage could differ within groups, e.g., lower-income vs. higher-income) (de Leeuw 2005). Nevertheless, about 80 % of Swiss households have Internet access (SFSO 2012). When we consider exclusively households with individuals aged 20–50 years, Internet coverage increases to 95 %. With reference to the professional situation, about 88 % of the unemployed have Internet access at home (SFSO 2012). Moreover, mixed-mode designs permit partial compensation of the coverage bias (Parackal 2003).

2.4.1   Sample Attrition and Participant Retaining Strategies

Regarding the sample attrition, considering an annual dropout of about 20 % after the first year (from T1 to T2), and about 10–15 % for the following waves, the number of individuals at the end of the study (T7) is expected to be 800. This estimation is based on previous national longitudinal surveys conducted by polling institutes and is similar to the attrition observed for the Swiss longitudinal youth study 2001–2010 (Bergman et al. 2011). Overall, part of this attrition will partially be due to the impossibility to survey all addresses and name changes or individuals moving to other countries. However, to try and limit the problem of non-valid contact details, respondents themselves have the possibility to update personal information (via the project website or a pre-stamped card). Moreover, the polling institute guarantees a verification of the mail addresses throughout the longitudinal study.

In order to retain participants in our study, we used different strategies. First of all, each participant could choose a gift (for an amount of CHF 20, about 22 USD or 16.5€) as an incentive to participate. Gift choices included a gift card to use at a supermarket, a gift card for a department store, a book voucher or a donation to a non-profit organization for children's aid. At each wave, participants completing the research protocol will be able to choose a gift of the same amount. Second, each year they will receive a newsletter (summarizing some of the main results in an appealing and more accessible format) and a greeting card. Furthermore, participants can access non-scientific articles and general information (such as new results) on the project website. Finally, after the second wave we will definitively exclude only people not participating in two consecutive waves. This means that people who decide not to participate in T2 will be contacted again in T3.

3   First Results and Indications from the Data Collection (T1)

This section of the manuscript presents some indications and results based on T1. These results are intended to describe general tendencies and relationships using non-weighted values, knowing in particular that unemployed participants and women were oversampled.

Table 1 Participation and refusal at different stages of the data collection procedure

Contacted initially by letter	7600			
Non-valid address			439	5.77 %
Participant not at the address			100	1.31 %
Others (e.g., death, move abroad)			31	0.39 %
Valid contacts	7030			
Interviews not possible			430	6.12 %
Refusing to participate			679	9.66 %
Never responded or contacted the hotline			1376	19.57 %
Visit to Website or call the hotline without starting the RP			679	9.66 %
1st part RP:				
Start 1st part RP	3866			
(By CATI)	(1255)	(32.46 %)		
(Online)	(2611)	(67.54 %)		
Not eligible			910	23.54 %
(CATI)			(407)	(10.53 %)
(Online)			(503)	(13.01 %)
2nd part RP:				
Start 2nd part RP	2956			
(Paper after CATI)	(613)	(20.73 %)		
(Online after CATI)	(235)	(7.95 %)		
(Online after online)	(2108)	(71.31 %)		
Not returned/timed out			487	16.47 %
(Paper not returned)			(180)	(6.09 %)
(Timed out – online after CATI)			(72)	(2.43 %)
(Timed out – online after online)			(235)	(7.95 %)
Total completed RP	2469			

RP = Research protocol; Percentages (%) refer to initial value of each section

3.1 Participation: Key Data

As shown in Table 1, during the data collection procedure, with the aim to obtain a final sample of about 2400 participants, the polling institute activated a total of 7600 addresses (or target persons)[2] but 570 were not valid (e.g. participant not at the address) and for 430 individuals the interview was not possible (e.g. target person outside Switzerland for a long period, language problems, health problems or in an institution). About 670 explicitly refused to participate and more than 1370 never responded to the letters or phone calls. Regarding refusal

---

[2]Of the 7600 target persons, 6000 were from the sample drawn from the national register of the inhabitants by the SFSO, and 1600 were from the sample drawn from the national register of the unemployed by the SECO.

motivations, the majority of the individuals indicated an opposition to any form of survey, no interest in the topic or lack of time. It is important to note that interviewers registered refusal motivations during the phone contact using pre-established categories. Consequently, we do not have any information about possible motivation of individuals that never contact the hotline. Moreover, 679 people called the hotline or visited the web site (using the personal password) without starting the questionnaire.

A little <3870 individuals started to complete the first part of the research protocol, but among these more than 910 were screened-out (for example because not professional active and not searching for a job). So, 2956 participants completed the first part of the research protocol (2108 online and 848 by CATI). Of those who completed the CATI, 613 requested the paper-pencil version and 235 decided to complete the second part online. The others participants continued with the online version. At the end, of the individuals who started the second part, we obtained 2469 complete research protocols, meaning that these participants completed both parts of the protocol. So, 487 individuals didn't complete the second part or never sent back the paper questionnaire. Unfortunately, we have no information about the reasons for stopping the questionnaire. The rate of completion for the research protocol (first and second part) within the valid addresses was 35.1 %. Importantly, research protocols were considered as complete only if participants responded up until the last question. However, as suggested by McHorney and colleagues (1994), when we calculate the response rate as the ratio of completed research protocols to the eligible sample (i.e., excluding out-of-scope individuals, such as non active people), the total participation rate was estimated at 40.3 %. Concerning the choice of method to complete the protocol, to summarize, we observed that 75.9 % ($n = 1873$) of the participants choose the "full" online version (i.e., the online questionnaire both for the first and second part), 6.6 % ($n = 163$) choose the CATI and online format, and 17.5 % the CATI and paper format ($n = 433$). Although a majority of the participants chose the full online version, about one-quarter opted for another format supporting the decision to propose several ways to complete the research protocol.

3.2   Characteristics of Participants at T1

As mentioned above, the final sample for T1 was composed of 2469 participants from the French and German regions of Switzerland aged from 25 to 55 years old, with a mean age of 41.9 years ($SD = 8.6$). With reference to the age groups, 25–35, 36–45 and 46–55 years represented respectively 27.4 %, 33.5 % and 39.1 % of the total sample. About half of the participants (50.7 %) were women and 53.5 % were married. More than one third of the respondents (36.1 %) had tertiary education, 55.6 % reported a secondary education and 8.3 % a primary education. Concerning the nationality and professional situation, non-Swiss[3] and unemployed participants represented respectively 21.6 % and 23.2 %. Of the 533 non-Swiss participants, 26.1 % came from Germany, 11.6 % from France, 11.1 % from Portugal and 10.1 % from Italy. Finally, 89.1 % of the total sample gave us their consent to be contacted next year to participate in the second wave of our study.

On a descriptive level, in comparison to the active population in Switzerland, in our sample we oversampled women and unemployed. In fact, in 2012 women and unemployed aged 25–55 years represented respectively 45.5 % and 3.8 % of the active population (SFSO 2013b). The rate of non-Swiss individuals was close to the one observed in the active population (i.e., 23.8 %). Concerning non-Swiss actives individuals, about 69 % came from European Union countries and – as in our sample – the largest group was represented by German individuals (27 %) (SFSO 2013a). With reference to education, there are some notable differences in the lower levels. In fact, data from the SFSO (2011) indicated that 14.4 % of the general population had a primary education, 50.3 % a secondary education and 35.3 % a tertiary education. Regarding specific characteristics of the employed and unemployed groups, some information was presented above (see section "Sampling").

3.2.1 Employed and Unemployed Participants: Personal and Professional Characteristics

Considering the main purpose of this project, it is essential to distinguish and specify information about employed and unemployed participants.

Concerning *demographic characteristics*, among employed participants ($n = 1895$) women represented 50.8 %, and married 56.6 %. Non-Swiss individuals constituted 16.3 % (308) of this sub-sample. Within the non-Swiss group, the majority of participants were German (32.9 %). The mean age of the professionally active sub-sample was 42.0 years ($SD = 8.6$). With regard to education, 38.4 % of the employed completed a tertiary education, 55.5 % a secondary education and 6.1 % a primary education. In the group of unemployed ($n = 574$), about half (50.5 %) were women. Furthermore, 43.4 % were married, 22.6 % currently lived with their children and 39.2 % were non-Swiss. Once again, German people were the most frequently represented group (17.0 %) within the non-Swiss group. The mean age of this sub-sample was 41.7 ($SD = 8.7$). In relation to schooling, 38.3 % of the unemployed participants completed a tertiary education, 56.1 % a secondary education and 15.3 % attained a primary education.

Regarding the *professional characteristics and situation*, among *employed individuals* 66.2 % had a full-time[4] job. Caring for children (or other persons) and assumed domestic tasks (71.3 %) and the desire not to work full-time (58.9 %) were

---

[3]For these analyses, participants with double-nationality with Swiss citizenship are classified as Swiss.

[4]According to the SECO (2012), we consider an activity rate equal or >90 % as full-time rate.

the most frequently given reasons for part-time work. Furthermore, <6 % indicated that it was impossible to find a job to increase current working time. About a tenth (10.7 %) of the employed participants actively looked for a new job during the last 6 months. Concerning job insecurity 13.3 % of the employed group indicated that, in the course of the last year, they faced at least once the risk of lay-off, and 8.6 % fear losing their own job in the next 12 months. More than half (54.2 %) of the employed reported that finding a similar job would be difficult or very difficult. Furthermore, about one-third (35.2 %) of the employed participants reported being unemployed in the past. In the *unemployed subsample*, 85.4 % were registered at a RPO and 72.6 % received unemployment benefits during the last 6 months. About half of the unemployed (49.6 %) have been unemployed for 6 months or more, and three-quarters (74.0 %) were looking for a full-time job and 15.6 % for a job at an activity rate equal to or below 60 %. Similar to employed participants, the main reasons to look for a part-time job were the necessity to take care of children (or other people) and domestic responsibilities (67.1 %) and the desire to keep time for themselves (36.6 %). Among unemployed individuals, 41.8 % were forced to leave their job following restructuring or dismissal, while 11.7 % lost their job at the end of a fixed-term contract. Other frequently mentioned reasons were health problems (9.9 %) and willingness to change job or employer (11.0 %). In relation to the job search, 49.0 % reported having no-one to help and support them in their job search process, except for the person in charge of their file at the RPO. From an economic point of view, about 38.1 % indicated that it was very urgent for them to find a job, and that this should happen in the next month. To conclude, 48.3 % of the currently unemployed participants reported periods of previous unemployment.

When we asked about *unfair treatment* (e.g., sex or age-related discrimination, harassment), 20.3 % of currently employed participants reported being the target of discrimination or unfair behaviors in their current work place. Among unemployed individuals, about half (48.3 %) indicated receiving unfair treatment or discrimination at their last job. For both groups, the most frequent behaviors were mobbing and age, national origin and sex-related discrimination. Considering that the questions were not exactly the same we cannot directly compare these results. However, it is important to emphasize that jobless people reported a higher frequency of unfair treatment at the work place.

3.3 Choice of the Format to Complete the Research Protocol

To assess possible predictors of the choice of format used to answer our questions (full online, CATI and online, or CATI and paper), we conducted multinomial logistic regression with full-online format as reference category (see Table 2). To do this, we introduced in the model different personal criteria as factors (i.e., age group, professional situation, household income, nationality and education level).

The first half of Table 2 compares the *CATI and paper format against the full online format*. Analyses highlighted that both the two youngest groups (25–35,

Table 2 Choice of data collection format: Multinomial logistic regression

	β	SE β	Wald's χ^2	df	p	Odds ratio
CATI and paper						
Age (reference: 46–55 years)						
25–35 years	−1.06	0.17	38.42	1	<0.001	0.35
36–45 years	−0.61	0.14	18.33	1	<0.001	0.54
Employed	−0.25	0.15	2.95	1	>0.05	0.77
Household income (reference: >139,000)						
<60,000	1.29	0.24	30.36	1	<0.001	3.64
60–99,000	0.73	0.22	11.05	1	0.001	2.08
100–139,000	0.69	0.23	9.31	1	0.002	2.00
Swiss	−0.31	0.15	3.94	1	0.047	0.55
Level of education (reference: tertiary)						
Primary	1.18	0.23	26.78	1	<0.001	3.26
Secondary	0.71	0.16	19.35	1	<0.001	2.04
CATI and online						
Age (reference: 46–55 years)						
25–35 years	0.10	0.20	0.24	1	>0.05	1.10
36–45 years	−0.15	0.20	0.54	1	>0.05	0.86
Employed	0.08	0.21	0.13	1	>0.05	1.08
Household income (reference: >139,000)						
<60,000	0.98	0.27	13.52	1	<0.001	2.67
60–99,000	0.28	0.25	1.31	1	>0.05	1.32
100–139,000	0.12	0.26	0.20	1	>0.05	1.12
Swiss	0.46	0.24	3.68	1	>0.05	1.50
Level of education (reference: tertiary)						
Primary	−0.72	0.43	2.81	1	>0.05	0.50
Secondary	−0.15	0.18	0.68	1	>0.05	0.86

The reference category is "full online" format. Pearson and Deviance statistic tests, $p > 0.05$. Cox and Snell $R^2 = 0.09$, Nagelkerke $R^2 = 0.12$; Model χ^2 (18) = 204.83, $p < 0.001$. Household income: Evaluate in CHF; CHF 1.00 = EUR 0.82; CHF 1.00 = USD 1.06 (Exchange rate as of 31.01.2012)

36–45 years) chose the full online version more often than the oldest group (46–55 years). The model indicated also that – compared to the higher household income group (>139,000) – the others groups are more likely to choose the CATI and paper format (odd ratios varying from 2.00 for 100–139,000 CHF to 3.64 for <60,000 CHF). Concerning nationality, Swiss participants choose the CATI and paper format less often than the full online version. With reference to the level of education, results emphasized that participants with primary or secondary education opted more often for CATI and paper version than participants with a tertiary education. Finally, no differences were observed in relation to professional situation. The second half of Table 2 compares the *CATI and online format against the full online format*. Interestingly, analyses indicate that the age group, professional situation and level of education did not significantly predict whether participants chose the full online or the CATI and online format. Regarding income, the results emphasized only a significant difference between the two extreme groups. In fact, compared to the >139,000 CHF group, the lowest household income group was about 2.7 times more likely to choose the CATI and online format.

3.4 Choice of Gift

Concerning the choice of the gift, overall the most selected gifts were the supermarket card (40.9 %) and the donation (34.4 %). Concerning the other gift options, 16.8 % of the individuals chose the department store card and only 7.9 % the book voucher.

Multinomial logistic regressions were conducted to assess whether personal criteria predicted the choice of the gift (see Table 3), with donation as the reference category. When we compared *department store and donation*, results indicated that age, household income and education of the participants significantly predicted their choice. More specifically, compared to the oldest participants (46–55 years), the youngest individuals (25–35 and 36–45 years) were more likely to choose the department store card. In relation to the household income, compared to the highest income group (>139,000 CHF), others participants (i.e., <60,000 CHF and 100–139,000 CHF groups) preferred more often the department store card. Concerning education, analyses highlighted that, in comparison to the others groups, individuals with tertiary education opted more frequently for the donation. Finally, it is interesting to underline that employed participants and Swiss citizens were not more likely to make a donation compared respectively to unemployed and non-Swiss. The comparison between *supermarket card and donation* highlighted an impact of all personal criteria, except for nationality. As for the previous comparison, the younger groups (25–35 and 36–45 years) choose about two times more often the supermarket card than the oldest group (46–55 years). Employed individuals were less likely to choose the supermarket gift. With regard to household income, data highlighted that the highest income group (>139,000 CHF) opted more frequently for a donation than the other groups. Finally, the choice of the gift varied in relation to the level of education. In fact, participants with a primary or secondary education were more likely to choose the supermarket card, respectively 3.4 and 1.8 times more than participants with a tertiary education.

The last part of Table 3 compares the *book voucher with donation*. Results indicated that only the household income was a significant predictor of the choice between these two options. In fact, the highest income group chose the donation more often than the others groups, except for the 60–99,000 CHF group. However, it is important to emphasize that <8 % of the participants choose the book voucher.

Table 3 Choice of gift: multinomial logistic regression

	β	SE β	Wald's χ^2	df	p	Odds ratio
Department store						
Age (reference: 46–55 years)						
25–35 years	0.95	0.16	34.23	1	<0.001	2.59
36–45 years	0.69	0.16	29.24	1	<0.001	1.99
Employed	−0.24	0.18	20.2	1	>0.05	0.79
Household income (reference: >139,000)						
<60,000	0.60	0.22	7.64	1	0.006	1.82
60–99,000	0.29	0.19	2.37	1	>0.05	1.33
100–139,000	0.39	0.19	4.10	1	0.043	1.47
Swiss	−0.23	0.16	2.03	1	>0.05	0.79
Level of education (reference: tertiary)						
Primary	1.43	0.28	27.02	1	<0.001	4.19
Secondary	0.66	0.15	19.79	1	<0.001	1.92
Supermarket						
Age (reference: 46–55 years)						
25–35 years	0.64	0.13	24.78	1	<0.001	1.91
36–45 years	0.67	0.12	31.66	1	<0.001	1.95
Employed	−0.38	0.13	8.22	1	0.004	0.68
Household income (reference: >139,000)						
<60,000	0.74	0.17	18.21	1	<0.001	2.09
60–99,000	0.55	0.14	14.72	1	<0.001	1.73
100–139,000	0.46	0.15	9.61	1	0.002	1.58
Swiss	−0.14	0.13	0.1	1	>0.05	0.99
Level of education (reference: tertiary)						
Primary	1.22	0.24	26.76	1	<0.001	3.39
Secondary	0.61	0.11	29.73	1	<0.001	1.85
Book voucher						
Age (reference: 46–55 years)						
25–35 years	0.29	0.21	2.00	1	>0.05	1.34
36–45 years	−0.02	0.21	0.01	1	>0.05	0.98
Employed	0.32	0.23	0.02	1	>0.05	1.03
Household income (reference: >139,000)						
<60,000	0.84	0.29	8.84	1	0.003	2.31
60–99,000	0.31	0.24	1.65	1	>0.05	1.37
100–139,000	0.59	0.23	6.28	1	0.012	1.80
Swiss	−0.08	0.22	0.14	1	>0.05	0.92
Level of education (reference: Tertiary)						
Primary	−0.63	0.51	1.52	1	>0.05	0.59
Secondary	−0.19	0.18	1.06	1	>0.05	0.83

The reference category is "donation". Pearson and Deviance statistic tests, $p > 0.05$. Cox and Snell $R^2 = 0.10$, Nagelkerke $R^2 = 0.11$; Model χ^2 (18) = 227.51, $p < 0.001$. Household income: Evaluate in CHF; CHF 1.00 = EUR 0.82; CHF 1.00 = USD 1.06 (Exchange rate as of 31.01.2012)

Table 4 Intention to participate in the future waves: binary logistic regression (final model)

	β	SE β	Wald's χ^2	df	p	Odds ratio
Age (reference: 46–55 years)						
25–35	0.42	0.19	4.98	1	0.026	1.52
36–45	0.04	0.16	0.07	1	>0.05	1.04
Employed	−0.14	0.19	0.56	1	>0.05	0.87
Household income (reference: >139,000)						
<60,000	−0.89	0.25	12.51	1	<0.001	0.41
60–99,000	−0.55	0.23	5.81	1	0.016	0.58
100–139,000	−0.53	0.23	5.36	1	0.021	0.59
Swiss	0.26	0.17	2.33	1	>0.05	1.30
Level of education (reference: tertiary)						
Primary	−0.12	0.27	0.22	1	>0.05	0.88
Secondary	0.02	0.17	0.01	1	>0.05	1.02
Neuroticism	−0.34	0.16	4.47	1	0.035	0.70
Extraversion	0.01	0.17	0.01	1	>0.05	1.01
Openness	0.82	0.16	26.57	1	<0.001	2.27
Agreeableness	0.19	0.16	1.37	1	>0.05	1.21
Conscientiousness	0.08	0.16	0.26	1	>0.05	1.09
Self-rated health	−0.02	0.10	0.03	1	>0.05	0.98
General stress	0.33	0.14	5.38	1	0.020	1.20

Cox and Snell $R^2 = 0.10$, Nagelkerke $R^2 = 0.11$; Model χ^2 (18) = 227.51, $p < 0.001$. Hosmer & Lemeshow χ^2 (8) = 14.36, $p > 0.05$

3.5 Intention to Participate in the Next Wave

We also conducted a binary logistic regression to assess possible predictors of the initial agreement to participate in the next wave of the study (0 = No, reference category; 1 = Yes, predicted category). More specifically, after controlling for personal criteria (i.e., age group, professional situation, household income, nationality and education), we introduced in the model personality dimensions in the second step. Moreover, we decided to also enter self-rated health and perceived general stress in the second step as independent variables. We expected that these two variables could contribute to explain the variance in the intention to participate (Etter and Perneger 1997).

The final model (see Table 4) highlighted that age group, household income, neuroticism, openness and general stress were important variables in predicting the agreement for the second wave. In fact, compared to the oldest group of participants, the youngest group (25–35 years) was more likely to agree to be contacted again the next year. Regarding household income, participants in the highest income group (CHF >139,000) gave from 1.5 to 2.5 times more frequently the agreement to continue to participate compared to those with a lower household income. Moreover, analyses highlighted that participants with higher scores on openness and stress and lower scores on neuroticism indicated agreement to participate in the next wave more frequently.

It is important to underline that – in terms of odd ratio – income and openness were the most important predictors of the intention to participate in the future waves. With regard to stress, although higher levels of stress seemed to predict agreement to participate, actually participants in our study reported very low levels of stress. Alternatively, individuals who feel stress may appreciate the opportunity to share their personal situation and concerns by participating in the survey. Finally, the intention to continue in the survey was not predicted by nationality, professional situation, level of education, health and the other dimensions of personality. Concerning the health state, as emphasized by the main reasons relating to non-participation, it is possible that individuals with poorer health were not integrated in the first wave of this survey.

3.6 Vulnerability and Resources Promoting Well-Being

To conclude the results section, we present some results concerning several characteristics and resources related to vulnerability, such as adapt-ability, quality of life, health and social support.

3.6.1 Quality of Life as an Indicator of Vulnerability

Overall, the *participants in this study* ($N = 2468$) indicated a more than satisfactory quality of life ($M = 4.10$, $SD = 0.74$). However, a series of ANOVAs revealed that Swiss ($M_{Swiss} = 4.15$, $M_{Non-Swiss} = 3.92$, $F(1, 2450) = 40.92$, $p < 0.001$), women ($M_{Men} = 4.06$, $M_{Women} = 4.14$, $F(1, 2452) = 7.82$, $p = 0.005$) and employed ($M_{Employed} = 4.22$, $M_{Unemployed} = 3.71$, $F(1, 2452) = 4224.90$, $p < 0.001$) reported a higher quality of life. Moreover, results highlighted significant differences between the three levels of education for all possible comparisons ($M_{Primary} = 3.62$, $M_{Secondary} = 4.03$, $M_{Tertiary} = 4.31$). Subsequently we repeated the analyses independently for both employed and unemployed subgroups. Among *employed*, consistent with the previous results, Swiss ($M_{Swiss} = 4.25$, $M_{Non-Swiss} = 4.08$, $F(1, 1884) = 16.84$, $p < 0.001$), and participants with higher education level ($M_{Primary} = 3.89$, $M_{Secondary} = 4.14$, $M_{Tertiary} = 4.38$) indicated a higher quality of life score. Interestingly, data showed no difference in relation to gender, work activity rate and type of contract (fixed-term contract and permanent contract). Quite a different picture emerged among *unemployed individuals*. In fact, women reported a greater perceived quality of life ($M_{Men} = 3.60$, $M_{Women} = 3.83$, $F(1, 565) = 10.53$, $p = 0.001$), while no differences emerged concerning nationality. Once again, individuals with a higher education level ($M_{Primary} = 3.26$, $M_{Secondary} = 3.66$, $M_{Tertiary} = 4.00$) indicated a greater quality of life. Finally, all these effects were verified using ANCOVAs to control for possible effects of the format choice used to

Table 5 Quality of life and personal resources – correlation coefficients

	Quality of life	
	Employed ($n = 1895$)	Unemployed ($n = 574$)
Career adapt-abilities (CAAS)		
Concern	0.21***	0.28***
Control	0.26***	0.23***
Curiosity	0.18***	0.15***
Confidence	0.19***	0.16***
Social support (FSSQ)	0.39***	0.45***
Beliefs in a just world (BJW)		
General	0.03	0.10*
Personal	0.42***	0.48***

$*p < .05, **p < .01, ***p < .001$

complete the research protocol. Overall, the patterns of results were similar to those indicated here.

3.6.2 Personal Resources as Protective Factors Against Vulnerability

Regarding personal resources, overall the participants of our entire sample reported more than satisfactory perceived social support ($M = 4.13, SD = 0.83$) and adequate adapt-ability resources. In fact, adapt-ability dimensions' scores varied from 3.55 for concern ($SD = 0.67$) to 3.94 for control ($SD = 0.63$). Furthermore, they indicated a higher belief in a personal just world ($M = 4.19, SD = 0.88$) than in a general just world ($M = 3.13, SD = 0.90$).

When we analyzed the association between perceived quality of life and personal resources, analyses pointed out a similar pattern of results for employed and unemployed (see Table 5). In fact, except for the general beliefs in a just world, both for employed and unemployed individuals the perceived quality of life is positively correlated with all adapt-ability dimensions (i.e., concern, confidence, control and curiosity), functional social support and personal justice beliefs. Finally, partial correlations (controlling for the mixed-mode format) confirmed these patterns of association.

3.6.3 Career Adapt-Ability, Professional Context and Vulnerability for Employed Respondents

Concerning the employed participants in T1 ($n = 1884$), the impact of job insecurity (past and future) on career adapt-ability and, general and professional well-being (i.e., life satisfaction, general health, job satisfaction and work stress) were tested with ANCOVAs (Maggiori et al. 2013). Regarding perceived past job insecurity (i.e., the risk of being dismissed during the last year), those employed with higher insecurity indicated lower scores on the concern and control dimensions of the CAAS. Furthermore, compared to employees with lower job insecurity, they also reported a poorer health status, lower life and professional satisfaction and a higher level of work-related stress (Maggiori et al. 2013). Moreover, when we considered future job insecurity (i.e., the fear of losing one's job in the coming year), the results highlighted the same pattern of trends concerning adapt-ability resources and well-being. In other words, people in a more insecure professional situation (past and/or future) were more vulnerable and seemed to possess fewer career resources to face and cope with professional challenges and career paths. Once again, analyses showed no impact of the chosen research protocol format. Finally, structural equation modeling highlighted that career adapt-ability resources partly mediated the impact of work conditions (in terms of job strain and both past and future professional insecurity) on employees' professional and general well-being (Maggiori et al. 2013).

4   Conclusions

In this chapter we presented the main purposes, an overview of some method-ological aspects and initial results from the first wave of our 7-year longitudinal study on professional trajectories. However, unlike other research focused mainly on economic and sociopolitical aspects of the current labor market and the different professional realities (e.g., professional security and unemployment), this project adopts several psychological perspectives to address the role and impact of personal characteristics and resources (such as, adapt-ability resources, justice beliefs and functional social support) on career paths and professional experiences. To do this, we analyzed a large sample of middle-aged employed and unemployed adults living in Switzerland.

Concerning the data collection, a mixed-mode method combining CATI, online and paper-pencil questionnaires was implemented to offer the participants a more flexible and adaptable format to complete the research protocol, and as a way to reduce the costs (de Leeuw 2005; Herrero and Meneses 2006). Even if a large major-ity of the participants chose the full online version to answer to the questions, some differences related to age, household income, level of education and nationality in the preference for the format were observed. These indications support the decision to offer different options to match the sample characteristics and preferences thus maximizing the participation. However, the implemented procedure is not without some limitations. For example, in such studies some less well-integrated subgroups (such as individuals with poorer health or low language skills) could be more difficult to contact and convince to participate (Laganà et al. 2011). Consistent with previous studies (e.g., Aluja et al. 2007; Riva et al. 2003), the first analyses indicated no differences in the evaluation of psychological processes related to survey format. Nevertheless, it would be important to assess more in detail and in a longitudinal perspective the possible impact of the way information is transmitted on participants' evaluations and answers (cf. de Leeuw 2005). Regarding the choice of the gift – which is an important element for the retention of the participants – data highlighted different preferences related, amongst others, to the age group, the household income and professional situation. So, giving multiple gift choices rather than one appears to match more with individuals' preferences. However, it would be interesting, to compare these results with those that emerge from studies proposing for example a gift of a different value (or simply cash) or a unique gift (so, the same present for all the participants) in terms of participation rates. Moreover, personality dimensions (notably in terms of openness and agreeableness) and income represented an important factor in determining this choice.

Further to some demographic and economic variables (such as household income), personality dimensions predicted initial agreement to participate in the next wave of our study. In fact, openness and neuroticism seem to influence the intention to participate in the next wave. In our point of view, personality, which was probably under emphasized until now in this kind of study, plays an important role in the conduct of a study and represents an aspect to take into consideration in future research, for example at the time of data analysis. However, it is important to stress that initial agreement to participate in future waves was not determined by personal characteristics such as health, nationality, professional situation or level of education (and only partly by age).

With reference to vulnerability criteria, although the participants overall reported a more than satisfactory quality of life, some differences existed in relation to level of education, nationality, gender or professional situation for example. Moreover, independent of the professional situation, quality of life was positively associated with several personal characteristics and resources (such as just-world beliefs and career adaptability resources). However, it would be interesting to repeat analyses with weighted data (for example, for professional situation and age) to confirm the observed pattern of results. Concerning employed participants, previous analyses highlighted a negative impact of job insecurity on individuals' general and professional well-being, in terms of work-related stress, job satisfaction or general health (Maggiori et al. 2013). Moreover, employees' with a more insecure professional situation reported lower adapt-ability resources to face work-related everyday challenges and demands. On a practical level, this pattern of preliminary results seem to support the importance of developing interventions based on strengths and resources, with the goal of ameliorating work-related outcomes (e.g. job satisfaction and work engagement) and decreasing the impact of precarious professional situations, such as underemployment and unemployment, on people's well-being.

To conclude, the data collected in the next waves will permit us to study more in depth the personal characteristics and resources involved in the professional experience and transitions – such as becoming unemployed or reentering the work force – in a changing career context. Furthermore, new data will give us the opportunity to verify and assess more intricately the pattern of results presented in this chapter, for instance concerning the real impact of the personality dimensions on actual participation and not just on the intention to participate in the successive waves of the study.

References

Aluja, A., García, O., Rossier, J., & García, L. F. (2005). Comparison of the NEO-FFI, the NEO-FFI-R and an alternative short version of the NEO-PI-R (NEO-60) in Swiss and Spanish samples. *Personality and Individual Differences, 38*, 591–604. doi:10.1016/j.paid.2004.05.014.

Aluja, A., Rossier, J., & Zuckerman, M. (2007). Equivalence of paper and pencil vs internet forms of the ZKPQ-50-CC in Spanish and French samples. *Personality and Individual Differences, 43*, 2022–2032. doi:10.1016/j.paid.2007.06.007.

Bakker, A. B., Demerouti, E., & Euwema, M. C. (2005). Job resources buffer the impact of job demands on burnout. *Journal of Occupational Health Psychology, 10*, 170–180. doi:10.1037/1076-8998.10.2.170.

Bangerter, A., Grob, A., & Krings, F. (2001). Personal goals at age 25 in three generation of the twentieth century: Young adulthood in historical context. *Swiss Journal of Psychology/Schweizerische Zeitschrift für Psychologie/Revue Suisse de Psychologie, 60*, 59–64. doi:10.1024//1421-0185.60.2.59.

Bergman, M., Hupka-Brunner, S., Keller, A., Meyer, T., & Stalder, B. E. (2011). *Youth transitions in Switzerland: Results from the TREE panel study.* Zürich: Seismo.

Briscoe, J. P., & Hall, D. T. (2006). The interplay of boundaryless and protean careers: Combinations and implications. *Journal of Vocational Behavior, 69*, 4–18. doi:10.1016/j.jvb.2005.09.002.

Broadhead, W. E., Gehlbach, S. H., de Gruy, F. V., & Kaplan, B. H. (1988). The duke-UNC functional social support questionnaire: Measurement of social support in family medicine patients. *Medical Care, 26*, 709–723. doi:10.2307/3765493.

Cohen, S., & Williamson, G. M. (1988). Perceived stress in a probability sample of the United States. In S. Spacapan & S. Oskamp (Eds.), *The social psychology of health* (pp. 31–67). Newbury Park: Sage.

Cortina, L. M., Magley, V. J., Williams, J. H., & Langhout, R. D. (2001). Incivility in the workplace: Incidence and impact. *Journal of Occupational Health Psychology, 6*, 64–80. doi:10.1037/1076-8998.6.1.64.

Dalbert, C. (1999). The world is more just for me than generally: About the personal belief in a just world scale's validity. *Social Justice Research, 12*, 79–98. doi:10.1023/A:1022091609047.

Dalbert, C. (2001). *The justice motive as a personal resource: Dealing with challenges and critical life events.* New York: Springer.

De Bruin, G. P., & Taylor, N. (2005). Development of the sources of work stress inventory. *South African Journal of Psychology, 35*(4), 748–765.

de Leeuw, E. D. (1992). *Data quality in mail, telephone, and face-to-face surveys.* Amsterdam: TT-Publicaties.

de Leeuw, E. D. (2005). To mix or not to mix data collection modes in survey. *Journal of Official Statistics, 21*(2), 233–255.

Diener, E., Emmons, R. A., Larsen, R. J., & Griffin, S. (1985). The satisfaction with life scale. *Journal of Personality Assessment, 49*(71), 75. doi:10.1207/s15327752jpa4901_13.

Dillman, D. A., Smyth, J. D., & Melani, L. C. (2009). *Internet, mail, and mixed-mode surveys: The tailored design method.* Hoboken: Wiley & Son.

Etter, J.-F., & Perneger, T. V. (1997). Analysis of non-response bias in a mailed health survey. *Journal of Clinical Epidemiology, 50*, 1123–1128. doi:10.1016/S0895-4356(97)00166-2.

Fouad, N. A., & Bynner, J. (2008). Work transitions. *American Psychologist, 63*, 241–251. doi:10.1037/0003-066X.63.4.241.

Friedland, D. S., & Price, R. H. (2003). Underemployment: Consequences for the health and well-being of workers. *American Journal of Community Psychology, 32*, 33–45. doi:10.1023/A:1025638705649.

Grob, A., Krings, F., & Bangerter, A. (2001). Life markers in biographical narratives of people from three cohorts: A life span perspective in its historical context. *Human Development, 44*, 171–190. doi:10.1159/000057057.

Haeberlin, U., Imdorf, Ch., & Kronig, W. (2004). *Von der Schule in die Berufslehre. Untersuchungen zur Benachteiligung von ausländischen und von weiblichen Jugendlichen bei der Lehrstellensuche.* [From school to apprenticeship. Investigations of the disadvantage of foreign and female adolescents during the search for an apprenticeship]. Bern: Haupt.

Herrero, J., & Meneses, J. (2006). Short web-based versions of the perceived stress (PSS) and center for epidemiological studies-depression (CESD) scales: A comparison to pencil and paper responses among internet users. *Computers in Human Behavior, 22*, 830–846. doi:10.1016/j.chb.2004.03.007.

Kanfer, R., Wanberg, C. R., & Kantrowitz, T. M. (2001). Job search and employment: A personality–motivational analysis and meta-analytic review. *Journal of Applied Psychology, 86*(5), 837–855. doi:10.1037/0021-9010.86.5.837.

Klehe, U.-C., Zikic, J., Van Vianen, A. E. M., & De Pater, I. E. (2011). Career adaptability, turnover and loyalty during organizational downsizing. *Journal of Vocational Behavior, 79*, 217–229. doi:10.1016/j.jvb.2011.01.004.

Krings, F., & Olivares, J. (2007). At the doorstep to employment: Discrimination against immigrants as a function of applicant ethnicity, job type and raters' prejudice. *International Journal of Psychology, 42*, 406–417. doi:10.1080/00207590701251721.

Laganà, F., Elcheroth, G., Penic, S., Kleiner, B., & Fasel, R. (2011). National minorities and their representation in Swiss surveys (II): Which practices make a difference? *Quality and Quantity, 47*, 1287–1314. doi:10.1007/s11135-011-9591-1.

Lent, R. W., Brown, S. D., & Hackett, G. (1994). Toward a unifying social cognitive theory of career and academic interest, choice, and performance. *Journal of Vocational Behavior, 45*, 79–122. doi:10.1006/jvbe.1994.1027.

Lucas, R. E., Clark, A. E., Georgellis, Y., & Diener, E. (2004). Unemployment alters the set point for life satisfaction. *Psychological Science, 15*, 8–13. doi:10.1111/j.0963-7214.2004.01501002.x.

Maggiori, C., Johnston, C., Krings, F., Massoudi, K., & Rossier, J. (2013). The role of career adaptability and work conditions on general and professional well-being. *Journal of Vocational Behavior.* Advance online publication. doi:10.1016/j.jvb.2013.07.001

Massoudi, K. (2009). *Le stress Professionnel: Une analyse des vulnérabilités individuelles et des facteurs de risque Environnementaux.* Bern: Peter Lang.

McCrae, R. R., & Costa, P. T., Jr. (2004). A contemplated revision of the NEO five-factor inventory. *Personality and Individual Differences, 36*, 587–596. doi:10.1016/S0191-8869(03)00118-1.

McHorney, C. A., Kosinski, M., & Ware, J. E. (1994). Comparisons of the costs and quality of norms for the SF-36 health survey collected by mail versus telephone interview: Results from a national survey. *Medical Care, 32*(6), 551–567.

Mercure, D. (2001). *Une Société-monde? Les dynamiques sociales de la mondialisation [A world-society? Social dynamics of globalization].* Québec: Presses de l'Université Laval – De Boeck Université.

Meyer, T., & Stalder, B. E. (2003). *Ungebildet in die Wissengesellschaft? Ein Blick auf die VerlierInnen im Transitionsprozess* [Uneducated into the knowledge society? A look at the losers in the transition process]. Communication présentée à la conférence internationale "Übergänge/Transitions". Aarau (Suisse).

Parackal, M. (2003). Internet-based and mail survey: A hybrid probabilistic survey approach. In A. Treloar & A. Ellis (Eds.), *Proceedings of AusWeb03, the ninth Australian world wide web conference: Changing the way we work* (pp. 1–12). Lismore: Southern Cross University.

Peterson, C., Stephens, J. P., Park, N., Lee, F., & Seligman, M. E. P. (2010). Strengths of character and work. In P. A. Linley, S. Harrington, & N. Page (Eds.), *Oxford handbook of positive psychology and work* (pp. 221–233). New York: Oxford University Press.

Podsakoff, P. M., MacKenzie, S. B., Lee, J.-Y., & Podsakoff, N. P. (2003). Common method biases in behavioral research: A critical review of the literature and recommended remedies. *Journal of Applied Psychology, 88*, 879–903. doi:10.1037/0021-9010.88.5.879.

Riva, G., Teruzzi, T., & Anolli, L. (2003). The use of the internet in psychological research: Comparison of online and offline questionnaires. *CyberPsychology & Behavior, 6*, 73–80. doi:10.1089/109493103321167983.

Rossier, J., Verardi, S., Genoud, P. A., & Zimmermann, G. (2012a). Ouverture émotionnelle et personnalité [Emotional openness and personality]. In M. Reicherts, P. A. Genoud, & G. Zimmermann (Eds.), *L'ouverture émotionnelle: Une nouvelle approche du vécu et du traitement des émotionnels* (pp. 69–84). Wavre: Mardaga.

Rossier, J., Zecca, G., Stauffer, S., Maggiori, C., & Dauwalder, J.-P. (2012b). Career adaptabilities scale in a French-speaking Swiss sample: Psychometric properties and relationships to personality and work engagement. *Journal of Vocational Behavior, 80*, 734–743. doi:10.1016/j.jvb.2012.01.004.

Rudisill, J. R., Edwards, J. M., Hershberger, P. J., Jadwin, J. E., & McKee, J. M. (2010). Coping with job transitions over the work life. In T. W. Miller (Ed.), *Handbook of stressful transitions across the lifespan* (pp. 111–131). New York: Springer.

Sapin, M., Spini, D., & Widmer, E. (2007). *Les parcours de vie. De l'adolescence au grand âge [Life course. From adolescent to old age]*. Lausanne: Presses polytechniques et universitaires romands.

Savickas, M. L., & Porfeli, E. J. (2012). Career adapt-abilities scale: Construction, reliability, and measurement equivalence across 13 countries. *Journal of Vocational Behavior, 80*, 661–673. doi:10.1016/j.jvb.2012.01.011.

Savickas, M. L., Nota, L., Rossier, J., Dauwalder, J. P., Duarte, M. E., Guichard, J., Soresi, S., van Esbroeck, R., & van Vianen, A. E. M. (2009). Life designing: A paradigm for career construction in the 21st century. *Journal of Vocational Behavior, 75*, 239–250. doi:10.1016/j.jvb.2009.04.004.

Schlossberg, N. K., Waters, E. B., & Goodman, J. (1995). *Counseling adults in transition: Linking practice with theory* (2nd ed.). New York: Springer.

Sennett, R. (1998). *The corrosion of character: The personal consequences of work in the New capitalism*. New York: W. W. Norton.

Skevington, S. M., Lotfy, M., & O'Connell, K. A. (2004). The World Health Organization's WHOQOL-BREF quality of life assessment: Psychometric properties and results of the international field trial. A report from the WHOQOL group. *Quality of Life Research, 13*, 299–310. doi:10.1023/B:QURE.0000018486.91360.00.

Swiss Federal Statistic Office. (2011). *Niveau de formation de la population résidante selon l'âge et le sexe.(je-f-15.03.01.01)* [Excel file] [Education level of the resident population by age and sex]. Retrieved from http://www.bfs.admin.ch/bfs/portal/fr/index/themen/15/01/new.html

Swiss Federal Statistic Office (SFSO). (2012). *Internet dans les ménages en Suisse – Résultats de l'enquête Omnibus TIC 2010* [Internet in Swiss households – Results of the Omnibus TIC 2010 survey]. Retrieved from http://www.bfs.admin.ch/bfs/portal/fr/index/news/02/03/04.html

Swiss Federal Statitstic Office. (2013a). *Vie active et rémunération du travail* [Working life and remuneration of work]. Neuchâtel: Office Fédéral de Statistique.

Swiss Federal Statistic Office. (2013b). *Statut sur le marché du travail selon le sexe, la nationalité, les groupes d'âges, le type de famille* [Status in the labor market by sex, nationality, age and type of family]. Retrieved from http://www.bfs.admin.ch/bfs/portal/fr/index/infothek/erhebungen__quellen/blank/blank/enquete_suisse_sur/08.html

Swiss State Secretariat for Economy. (2012). *La situation sur le marché du travail en avril 2012* [Labor market situation in April 2012]. Retrieved from http://www.seco.admin.ch/themen/00385/00387/index.html

Tse, A. C. B. (1998). Comparing the response rate, response speed, and response quality of two methods of sending questionnaires: E-mail vs. mail. *Journal of the Market Research Society, 40*(4), 353–361.

Wiese, S. B., & Freund, A. (2005). Goal progress makes one happy, or does it? Longitudinal findings from the work domain. *Journal of Occupational and Organizational Psychology, 78,* 287–304. doi:10.1348/096317905X26714.

Wu, M. S., Yan, X., Zhou, C., Chen, Y., Li, J., Zhu, Z., Shen, X., Han, B. (2011). General belief in a just world and resilience: Evidence from a collectivistic culture. *European Journal of Personality, 25,* 431–442. doi:10.1002/per.807

Zikic, J., & Klehe, U.-C. (2006). Job loss as a blessing in disguise: The role of career exploration and career planning in predicting reemployment quality. *Journal of Vocational Behavior, 69,* 391–409. doi:10.1016/j.jvb.2006.05.007.

How to Survey Displaced Workers in Switzerland: Ways of Addressing Sources of Bias

Isabel Baumann, Oliver Lipps, Daniel Oesch, and Caroline Vandenplas

1 Introduction

Involuntary job loss often comes as a shock for the affected individuals. Dismissal not only hampers individuals' health (Kuhn et al. 2009) and life satisfaction (Oesch and Lipps 2013), but may also negatively affect their occupational trajectory. Displaced workers are deprived of the positive components of work – they lost not only a source of income but also their social contacts, an important determinant of their social status, and the time structure implied by an economic activity (Andersen 2008). Threatened by the risks of financial deprivation and social exclusion, displaced workers are in a state of heightened vulnerability. Yet not all individuals are exposed to these threats to the same extent: some are more disadvantaged than others.

When trying to determine workers' occupational trajectories after job dismissal, researchers face a number of methodological problems. The fact that workers displaced individually are probably a self-selected group of people makes the causal analysis of the impact of job loss on the ensuing work career tricky: the same factor causing the workers to lose their jobs such as poor health or lack of motivation may also reduce their re-employment prospects (Brand 2015).

I. Baumann (✉) • D. Oesch
NCCR LIVES, Lausanne, Switzerland

Center for Health Sciences, Zurich University of Applied Sciences (ZHAW), Winterthur, Switzerland
e-mail: isabel.baumann@zhaw.ch

O. Lipps
FORS (Swiss Centre of Expertise in the Social Sciences), Lausanne, Switzerland

C. Vandenplas
FORS (Swiss Centre of Expertise in the Social Sciences), Lausanne, Switzerland

Centre for Sociological Research, Catholic University of Leuven, Leuven, Belgium

© The Author(s) 2016
M. Oris et al. (eds.), *Surveying Human Vulnerabilities across the Life Course*,
Life Course Research and Social Policies 3, DOI 10.1007/978-3-319-24157-9_7

This chapter discusses some of the problems afflicting the survey-based analysis of how displaced workers overcome the critical event of a job loss and then tries to present a few empirical solutions. A way out is to use plant closure – a reason beyond people's control – as an exogenous instrument for job displacement to tackle the endogeneity problem (Schwerdt et al. 2010).

Since the Swiss Labour Force Survey does not distinguish between different reasons for involuntary job loss, we ran our own survey on workers who lost their job 2 years earlier. The achieved sample consists of around 1200 people – the entire workforce of five Swiss manufacturing plants that had closed down completely after the financial crisis of 2008. The research objective was to identify the workers' re-employment prospects.

The chapter is structured as follows. The first section discusses two types of survey bias: selection bias and nonresponse bias. The second section describes the nuts and bolts of our survey on displaced workers and presents the data. The third section shows the empirical analysis of nonresponse bias in our sample. The fourth section then presents the re-employment rates of displaced workers based on different data subsets. The conclusion sums up the main findings and discusses some challenges faced in the survey process.

2   Selection and Nonresponse Bias in Survey Studies

When conducting a survey, researchers must be aware of a set of error sources – an approach summarized in the concept of the total survey error approach – and, more specifically, survey bias (Groves and Lyberg 2010:850). Bias occurs at the variable level when the factors that drive the bias are correlated with the relevant variables (Groves and Peytcheva 2008:169). In the following sections we discuss two types of bias that we consider particularly relevant for our study and briefly address a third one.

2.1   Selection Bias

Selection bias emanates from a non-random attribution of individuals into a sample and implies that the selected individuals are not representative of the population. Part of the problem is that one does not know whether such a selection has taken place and if so, which characteristics drove the process (Antonakis et al. 2010). Selection bias implies that the independent variables are endogenous, making causal inference on the basis of these data impossible (Hamilton and Nickerson 2003).

The ideal solution to avoid selection bias would be to run an experiment. Since in the social sciences experiments are often difficult for ethical and practical reasons, other methods for causal inference must be adopted (for an overview, see Angrist and Pischke 2008). A way around experiments is to choose natural experiments – events that occur without the contribution of the researcher, where an exogenous source of variation in the social phenomenon of interest randomly determines individuals' assignment to a *treatment* (Meyer 1995:151).

Plant closure comes close to such a setting: at the individual level, the assignment to the treatment is random because the workers are dismissed independently of their health or work performance. The fact that the entire workforce of a company loses their job suggests that selection into displacement is limited (Eliason and Storrie 2009:1397; Gibbons and Katz 1991:353). Moreover, reverse causality is unlikely in the case of plant closure: if displaced workers are in poor health, it is unlikely that their sickness has caused the plant to close, but rather that plant closure and job loss have negatively affected their health (Kuhn et al. 2009:1099). The advantage of plant closure as an analytical instrument for unemployment thus is that displaced people were not primarily selected into unemployment – that is, dismissed – on the basis of other characteristics such as lack of motivation, poor health or an insubordinate personality. It is thus possible to identify the causal effect of redundancy on workers' ensuing trajectories (Schwerdt et al. 2010:137).

At the same time, this instrument is not immune to two types of selection bias. First, there may be some extent of self-selection of workers into industries and plants that are more vulnerable to economic and structural problems (Cha and Morgan 2010:1141). Evidence from Germany suggests that older workers and workers without technical training or university education are more likely to be made redundant (Burda and Mertens 2001:22–24). Thus, belonging to the workforce of a non-profitable plant is not completely random – confronted with a choice, much sought-after specialists may think twice before seeking employment in a plant that shows evidence of economic difficulties. The same study additionally shows that workers employed in small firms have a higher propensity to be dismissed.

A second selection bias arises from the fact that some workers anticipate the closure of their plant and leave it before the closure is officially announced. If more ambitious or motivated workers select themselves out of the sample, the remaining sample is not representative for the total population. In an Austrian study, Schwerdt (2011:100) shows that early plant leavers tend to have higher re-employment rates and lower earning losses than workers displaced at the very end. According to the author the outcome is due to compositional differences between the two groups in terms of productivity-related characteristics. Turnover before plant closure thus seems to be selective.

2.2 Nonresponse Bias

Despite the use of plant closure as a methodological instrument to limit selection bias in the sample to be surveyed, individual differences in survey participation behaviour may still result in a selective sample. If the group of nonrespondents were missing completely at random, this would only reduce the statistical power of results without inducing systematic bias. Unfortunately, nonresponse most often is biased:

Individuals who are not participating in a survey are likely to be less interested in the topic or to have lower literacy in the questionnaire's language (Groves and Couper 1998; Stoop 2005). It is thus important to understand the mechanism behind nonresponse and, if possible, to correct for it.

Some subgroups may be particularly difficult to observe. For example, it has been shown for Switzerland that individuals with an immigration background from a country where none of the survey languages is spoken are heavily underrepresented in surveys such as the Swiss Household Panel or the Swiss Labour Force Survey (Lipps et al. 2013:248–251; Laganà et al. 2011:2). The participation rate is particularly low among Turks, Ex-Yugoslavians and Albanians. In contrast, Italian, French and German nationals have participation rates similar to that of Swiss nationals.

Conventional efforts to increase the overall response rate such as repeated contact attempts or government survey sponsoring tend to lead to the inclusion of more respondents of the same type instead of accessing subgroups that are traditionally less likely to participate (Laganà et al. 2011:22; Groves and Peytcheva 2008:176). These methods thus seem to increase the under-representation of minorities with immigrant backgrounds. While a high participation rate leads to more robust estimates, the increase in the response rate does not guarantee the sample's representativeness (Groves and Peytcheva 2008:168). Therefore, the objective of increasing the response rate should always be coupled with an effort to reduce bias by obtaining answers from under-represented subgroups (Luiten and Schouten 2013). In order to reach individuals belonging to subgroups with traditionally low participation rates, a more effective solution is to alter the survey protocol, for instance through a shorter questionnaire – a practice often applied in nonrespondent follow-up surveys (Peytchev et al. 2009:786; Lynn 2003).

A second possibility to reduce nonresponse bias is to use financial incentives. Incentives have proven successful at pulling in those respondents who otherwise would not answer the questionnaire (Dillman et al. 2009:249). They encourage respondents to reciprocate by completing the survey (Dillman et al. 2009:238). According to the economic exchange theory, the amount of the incentive should compensate the respondents for the opportunity costs of the time invested to partic-ipate in the survey (Citro 2010:73). Research in survey methodology indicates that unconditional and cash incentives are more effective than incentives contingent on completing a survey (Harrison 2010:519; Lipps 2010:84). Incentives are particularly important in written or online surveys where there is no interviewer to motivate and support the participants (Mehlkop and Becker 2007:8).

A third possible solution for addressing nonresponse bias consists in mixing sur-vey modes. Mixed-mode approaches using combinations of face-to-face, telephone, internet and paper-pencil questionnaires tend to be more effective at enhancing rep-resentativeness than single-mode surveys: different modes usually help to activate different subgroups of the surveyed sample (Dillman et al. 2009; Hayashi 2007). However, taken on their own, every single survey mode has its downside: internet coverage is still limited, notably among older people; landline telephone coverage has decreased in recent years; mail surveys are known to have a comparably high nonresponse rate; and face-to-face interviews are resource intensive (Schräpler 2001:13; Kempf and Remington 2007; Ernst Stähli 2012; Lipps and Kissau 2012). While the combination of different modes may help to increase representativeness, its drawback is an incomparable measurement error across modes (Dillman and Messer 2010:551–553; Vannieuwenhuyze and Loosveldt 2013).

A last possibility to deal with nonresponse bias is to adopt postsurvey adjustments by means of weighting. The idea is to give underrepresented groups a higher weight than overrepresented groups (Little and Vartivarian 2005). The quality of the weights depends on the available data: if the socio-demographic variables used to construct the weights do not affect the phenomenon of interest, the adjustments weights will not correct for nonresponse bias (Groves and Peytcheva 2008).

Finally, a third source of bias needs to be briefly discussed: measurement error. This source of bias typically arises if the questionnaire is poorly designed: ambiguous questions, confusing instructions, and easily misunderstood terms are examples of questionnaire problems that lead to measurement error (Biemer 2010:32). A technique to reduce measurement error is to validate survey answers by means of external data sources. For instance, the combination of survey data with register data allows controlling for the accuracy of the survey data (Sakshaug et al. 2012:536). Yet obtaining register data is often challenging because of data protection legislation, matching problems, and the need of informed consent by the concerned individuals.

3   Survey Procedure and Data

3.1   Sampling Strategy

In autumn 2011, we conducted our survey on the workforce of five companies in Switzerland's manufacturing sector that closed down in 2009 or 2010. The objective was to examine the re-employment prospects of displaced industrial workers about 2 years after their dismissal. In this section, we briefly present the nuts and bolts of our survey.

To begin with, the selection of companies was based on the following four criteria. First, we limited our sample to workers from production sites that closed down completely. As discussed earlier, this is relevant because plants that dismiss only parts of their workforce are likely to hold on to their most valuable workers, while making those with lower work performance redundant – which would result in a selective sample of workers. Second, we chose plants that closed down about 2 years before the survey. We thus try to capture long-term unemployment and, more specifically, the crucial moment when the unemployed exhaust their right to draw unemployment benefits. This happens in Switzerland – depending on the workers' age and duration of contribution – after 1–2 years of entitlement. Third, we selected plants that employed, at the moment of closure, no less than 150 employees. In order to limit time costs, we focused on mid-sized and large plants. Fourth, we focused

Table 1 Information on the five manufacturing plants included in the survey

Plant	Sector	Workers displaced	Displacement dates
Plant A	Metal and plastic products	204	September 2009 to March 2010
Plant B	Metal products	169	January 2010
Plant C	Printing	262	December 2009
Plant D	Chemicals	430	January 2009
Plant E	Machinery	324	October 2009 to August 2010
Total workers displaced		1389	
Refusal and invalid addresses		186	
Eligible sample		1203	

on manufacturing – the sector most strongly affected by job displacement. These criteria helped us to reach a critical mass of workers with a small number of plants.

Through media screening and contact with the cantonal employment offices, we made an inventory of plants that corresponded to these four criteria and identified ten plants. This inventory constitutes our sampling frame. We then contacted all these plants by mail and telephone, succeeding in convincing five plants to participate in the survey. The five missing plants are similar to the participating firms in terms of size, sector, displacement date and geographic location. Table 1 gives an overview over the surveyed plants and shows that they had been active in the sectors of metal and plastic production, printing, chemicals or machinery, employed between 169 and 430 workers at the moment of closure and closed down between January 2009 and August 2010.

For two plants we accessed the workers through the company's management, for one plant through the works council and for two plants through the cantonal employment offices. For data protection reasons, we had to obtain the workers' consent to use their addresses. Workers thus received a letter informing them about our study and the intention of the address providers – company management, work council, or employment office – to give us access to their postal addresses. For practical reasons, the workers only had to react in case of refusal.

Table 1 shows that 186 or 15 % of all displaced workers either had invalid addresses (because they moved or – in a few cases – were deceased) or refused access. The main reasons for refusals were (a) that workers did not feel concerned by our study, (b) that workers did not speak the survey languages (French and German), and (c) that some individuals were frustrated by their occupational situation. After all, a non-negligible share of our original sample dropped out and the surveyed sample resulted in 1203 individuals.

Since we selected those units easiest to be surveyed (that is, those companies agreeing to participate), our sampling strategy at the level of companies provides us with a *convenience sample* (Lohr 1999:5). Convenience sampling implies that the data are not generated by a known probability mechanism such as random sampling – and hence does not allow for inferring from the sample to the whole population (Western and Jackman 1994:412; Berk 2004:51). A conservative interpretation would thus be that our findings need to be read as the results of a case study.

3.2 Data Collection

Our data collection instrument was a questionnaire with about 60 mainly closed-ended questions. Many of the questions were adopted from established surveys such as the Swiss Household Panel or the Swiss Labour Force Survey. Since the target group consists in individuals living in both, the German- and French-speaking regions of Switzerland, the questionnaire was fielded in two languages. It was first cross-examined by survey experts and then completed by and discussed with four workers of the survey population. The questionnaire was both printed on paper and provided online. Furthermore some workers answered by telephone; they had the possibility to answer only to a sub-selection of the questions. We hence conducted a mixed-mode survey where questionnaires were mainly self-administered.

We started the survey at the end of September 2011 by sending out an advance letter. The aim of this letter was to describe the purpose of our study and to announce the arrival of the questionnaire. The letter contained the URL to the online questionnaire that allowed workers to start participating right away. A recommendation letter by the Swiss State Secretariat of Economic Affairs (SECO) – whose purpose was to enhance the survey's legitimacy by showing governmental support – accompanied the advance letter. One week later, at the beginning of October, workers received the paper and pencil version of the questionnaire for the first time, including a pre-stamped return envelope. This mailing was accompanied by an unconditional financial incentive in the form of a voucher worth ten Swiss Francs for Switzerland's biggest retail trade company. About 1 month later, at the beginning of November, workers who had not yet participated received the paper and pencil questionnaire for a second time.

A crude analysis of response rates by a national origin proxy suggested that immigrants tended to be under-represented in our study. Since we did not have information for all workers about their nationality, the proxy for national origin was created on the basis of workers' family names. Thereby, we distinguished four groups: (1) Switzerland, France and Germany, (2) Spain and Portugal, (3) Italy, and (4) other countries, notably Ex-Yugoslavia and Turkey. Group (1) represents 71 % of the workers, group (2) 3 %, group (3) 8 % and group (4) 17 %. When checking the response rates across these four proxy groups – an admittedly rough indicator for immigration background – we found the expected differences: group (1) had a response rate of 66 %, group (2) of 56 %, group (3) of 55 % and group (4) of 40 %. To increase the response rate of group (4), we drew a random sample of nonrespondents in this group and succeeded, in December, to conduct 15 telephone interviews with workers with an Ex-Yugoslavian or Turkish origin. This measure led to a final response rate of group (4) of 52 % – a response rate similar to that of the proxy groups (2) and (3).

The overall response rate for the survey was 62 % and the responding sample included 748 workers. The properties of our responding sample are shown in Table 5 in the appendix. 83 % of the workers in our survey were male, the mean age was 47.3 years, 57 % had an upper secondary education (apprenticeship) and 55 % were employed as craft workers, machine operators or workers in elementary jobs (henceforth: production workers).

3.3 Combining Survey Data with Plant and Register Data

A potential problem of our mixed-mode survey is differential measurement error. We tried to address this bias by linking our survey data with data from the firms and with administrative data from the unemployment register. The advantage of the data from the companies is that it is available for all workers. This allows us to examine whether respondents are representative for the surveyed sample. However, the same variables were not available for all plants: while we received important information such as occupation or age for workers in some plants, we only obtained information on the displacement date for other plants.

The administrative data stems from the AVAM/PLASTA[1] database of the public unemployment insurance. Access was subject to two conditions: first, we could only obtain information on those displaced workers who did not refuse access.[2] This implies that both, survey respondents who did not refuse access and all survey nonrespondents (who, by definition, did not refuse since refusing implied to tick a box in the questionnaire) were covered by this data source. Second, workers needed to be identifiable in the unemployment insurance database on the basis of their name and address – which was not possible for everybody, because not all the displaced workers were enrolled in the unemployment insurance: some had found a job right away, others went into early retirement, and a third group may have preferred to avoid the stigma of living from unemployment benefits. Moreover, some workers' address could not be tracked since it had changed.

At the end, it was possible to identify 355 workers in the database of the unemployment insurance, 165 of whom did not participate in the survey. Combining survey and register data we thus have information on 913 workers or 76 % of the total surveyed sample. For the post-displacement occupational situation – our central dependent variable – we have employment status for 884 workers (74 % of the total surveyed sample).

---

[1] Informationssystem für die Arbeitsvermittlung und Arbeitsmarktstatistik/Système d'information en matière de placement et de statistique du marché du travail.

[2] In order to receive the worker's agreement we included a question in the questionnaire which was formulated in a way that the respondents had to inform us if they did not wish us to access their data. Only 144 workers – corresponding to 19 % of the respondents and 12 % of the survey population – refused access.

4 Survey Participation

As mentioned, the overall response rate in our survey was 62 %. This comparatively high response rate is probably due to the features of our survey design: multiple contact attempts, mixing modes, unconditional financial incentives and an official recommendation letter by the SECO. In addition, the focus on specific populations may also result in higher response rates because respondents feel concerned by the survey topic and are interested in the goals of the study (Sweet and Moen 2011:9). Comments that we received with the questionnaires suggest that the displaced workers were happy to be able to communicate about their experiences after plant closure.

However, the crucial question is not whether the response rate is high or low, but whether different worker subgroups had a similar propensity to participate in the survey. First, we examine this question by analysing the response rate for different worker subgroups, relying on *firm data* that is available for both respondents and nonrespondents. Second, we analyse whether the groups of respondents and nonrespondents are different in terms of socio-demographic characteristics by relying on *register and survey data*.

Table 2 presents the response rates by plant, sex and occupation in the predisplacement job. Since the latter two variables are available only for three firms, the number of observations for former occupation and sex is smaller than for the survey population (N = 1203). The response rates do not vary much across plants, ranging from 55 to 66 %. Large response rate differences according to company could be problematic if the firms had very different characteristics and would differ in the labour market prospects of their workforces. Yet since we are not confronted with large differences, this issue is not relevant here. What we know is that there does not seem to be a relationship between the number of months since plant closure and

Table 2 Response rate according to plant, former occupation and sex

	Characteristics	Response rate (%)	N
By plant	Plant A (19–24 months since closure)	55	183
	Plant B (21 months since closure)	61	147
	Plant C (22 months since closure)	62	228
	Plant D (33 months since closure)	63	357
	Plant E (13–24 months since closure)	66	288
By former occupation	Machine operators and elementary occupations	60	185
	Clerks	62	29
	Craft and trade workers	66	145
	Technicians and associate professionals	69	126
	Managers	75	62
	Professionals	81	32
By sex	Men	59	630
	Women	69	130

the response rate: the response rate in plant D, having closed 33 months prior to the survey, is very similar to that of plant B and plant C, which closed 21 or 22 months prior to the survey (63 % as compared to 61 and 62 %).

Table 2 shows greater differences in response rates with respect to the former occupation. Not surprisingly, we find that machine operators and workers in elementary occupations have the lowest response rate, whereas professionals and managers have the highest. While four out of five professionals participated in our survey, only three out of five machine operators did so. We expected clerks to stand out in comparison with production workers since the former are more used to filling in forms than their colleagues in manual occupations. Contrary to our expectations, however, we found that the response rates between clerks on the one hand and craft workers and machine operators on the other hand do not vary much, ranging between 60 and 66 %. Finally, the response rates with respect to sex confirm prior findings in survey research that women are more likely to participate in surveys than men (Voorpostel 2010:367). We find that only 59% of the men, but 69 % of the women responded to our questionnaire.

In the next section we compare a series of socio-demographic characteristics between *respondents* and *nonrespondents* (Table 3). While for the respondents register and survey data is available, for the nonrespondents we only rely on register data. If we compare the respondents (all) and the nonrespondents (UEI register) we can see that the respondents are on average substantially older, more highly educated and were less often employed as production workers.

By comparing the profile of respondents for each survey mode in terms of age, education and occupation, we get an idea about how different modes affect the socio-demographic composition of our sample. Twenty-one percent of all respondents completed the questionnaire online, 76 % used the paper and pencil questionnaire, and 3 % answered by telephone. It is not surprising that paper and

Table 3 Respondents characteristics by survey mode and unemployment insurance register status

Response and mode	N	Mean age at displacement (in years)	Share of less educated (in %)	Share of production workers (in %)
Respondents – all	748	47.3	14	55
Internet	157	45.5	8	40
Paper and pencil, 1st mailing	398	47.7	15	57
Paper and pencil, 2nd mailing	165	48.3	13	62
Telephone interviews	22	43.4	38	85
Respondents – UEI register	190	48.5	13	59
Respondents – not in UEI register	558	46.8	14	54
Nonrespondents – all	455	–	–	–
Nonrespondents – UEI register	165	41.6	36	69

UEI stands for unemployment insurance. The less-educated include individuals with less than upper secondary education. Production workers include individuals who were employed before displacement in the International Standard Classification of Occupations (ISCO) groups 7, 8 or 9 pencil was clearly the most frequently used mode since we had workers' postal address, but not their e-mail address. Participants who answered on Internet are somewhat younger, more likely to be better educated and less likely to have worked in a production job compared with participants having answered the questionnaire on paper. Furthermore workers who responded by the paper and pencil questionnaire after the first mailing are similar to those who answered by means of the same mode after the second mailing. Differences between respondents using Internet as compared to paper and pencil are somewhat larger, but still not very substantial. In contrast, differences are noteworthy with respect to respondents who had answered the questionnaire by telephone: this specifically targeted group is younger, more likely to be lower educated and to have worked in a production job as compared to respondents who answered the survey by other means.

The strategy of mixing modes and multiple contact attempts seems to have paid off in terms of a higher response rate. The modes partially coincided with different moments of contact. The first contact gave participants access to the online questionnaire. The first survey participants therefore responded by Internet; yet the online questionnaire was open throughout the entire survey. The second and third contact allowed workers to fill in the paper and pencil questionnaire. The fourth contact by telephone concerned exclusively a small subsample. However, some additional workers who did not belong to this subsample contacted us via telephone and answered the survey by this means. Our results reveal that the second mailing of the paper questionnaire to nonrespondents brought in more people who are much like those respondents who already answered by paper and pencil after the first mailing. By reminding people to participate, the second mailing was effective in increasing the response rate by 14 percentage points. However, unlike the telephone interview, it does not seem to have done much to improve the sample's representativeness.

Participants who responded by telephone seem to be much more similar to nonrespondents than respondents using the two dominant modes (paper and pencil and Internet). The difference is particularly marked with respect to education: while 36 % of the nonrespondents have not obtained upper secondary education, this is the case for only 8 % of Internet respondents and for 14 % of paper and pencil respondents. Among the telephone respondents in contrast, the share of workers with a lower level of education is even higher than among nonrespondents (38 %). This finding suggests that telephone interviews were effective in motivating workers who, otherwise, would not have participated in the survey.

Table 3 also shows us that, overall, participants who registered in the unemployment insurance are similar to those who did not register: while the former are somewhat older and more likely to have worked as production workers, the share of low-educated workers is almost identical. In contrast, the small group of workers who registered in the unemployment insurance and who did not respond to our survey present a very different profile than respondents: on average, they are much younger and those with a lower level of education, as well as production workers, make up a much larger share. Clearly, having access to register data provides us with observations for potentially more disadvantaged workers.

Table 4 Variables taken from plant register data to construct nonresponse adjustment weights

	Displacement date	Sex	Occupation	Age	Nationality	Country of residence
Plant A	x					x
Plant B		x				
Plant C		x	x	x		
Plant D			x		x	
Plant E		x				

The difference in the subgroups' characteristics suggests that we are possibly still confronted with nonresponse bias. A relatively simple method to correct for this problem is unit nonresponse adjustment weighting. Accordingly, we use a technique that is based on a missing at random (MAR) assumption. This means that subgroups based on variables available for respondents *and* nonrespondents are created, with the assumption that non-participation happened at random within these subgroups. This method is often used in nonresponse adjustment (Little 1986) and consists in adjusting each subgroup separately for nonresponse.

Since for every plant in our sample, other variables are available, we used different variables for each plant when constructing the individual-level weights. The variables used for nonresponse adjustment depending on the plant are shown in Table 4. This type of nonresponse adjustment is most effective when the available variables used to construct the subgroups (sex, occupation, age, nationality) correlate with the variable of interest in the study (re-employment). The literature suggests that this is the case: sex, occupation, age, and nationality affect re-employment chances (e.g. Fallick 1996; Kletzer 2001; Jolkkonen et al. 2012). However, it might be problematic to construct adjustment weights on the basis of different variables. Yet since no variable is available for all firms, we assume that our construction is still better than no weighting at all. How these weights change our results in terms of reemployment rates will be shown in the next section.

5 Re-employment Rates of Different Subsets

The crucial question is whether nonresponse, different survey modes and weighting lead us to draw different conclusions as to the re-employment prospects of displaced workers. Figure 1 answers this question by showing workers' occupational status about 2 years after displacement for different data subsets. If we use the *survey data for all workers* (1) we find that 67.9 % of the workers are re-employed. 15.9 % are still unemployed, 13.1 % are retired and the remaining 3.1 % exited the labour market for training, childcare or due to disability. If we consider the *weighted survey data* (2), the re-employment rate is 68.7 % – slightly higher than for the unweighted survey data. The nonresponse adjustment weight thus does not

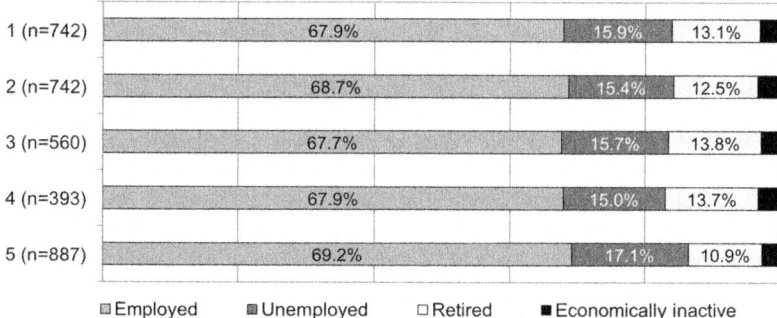

Fig. 1 Employment status of workers about 2 years after displacement by different data subsets. Note: *1* Survey data (for all workers), *2* Survey data (for all workers) – weighted, *3* Survey data for workers responding by paper and pencil questionnaire, *4* Survey data for workers responding before second mailing of the questionnaire, *5* Survey data (for all workers) combined with register data

seem to have a substantial effect on the result. We would have expected a lower reemployment rate for the weighted than the unweighted data as the characteristics of nonrespondents typically do not favour re-employment. This implies that – with respect to the weighting variables – the group of respondents is similar to the group of non-respondents in terms of re-employment. Yet the weighting induces a slightly lower rate of retired workers. This suggests that the retired are slightly overrepresented among the survey respondents. As a matter of fact, Table 3 above suggests that respondents are on average several years older than nonrespondents.

If we use *survey data for workers who responded by paper and pencil* (3), the reemployment rate amounts to 67.7 %. If we use *survey data of workers who responded before the second mailing of the questionnaire* (4), the re-employment rate is 67.9 %. These results are basically the same as those for *survey data for all workers* (1) and suggest that the re-employment prospects of those workers who responded to the survey through the paper and pencil questionnaire or before the second mailing are very similar to the whole group of survey respondents.

Finally, if we *combine the survey data with register data* (5), the share of workers who have found a new job increases to 69.2 %. Similarly, the unemployment rate is higher if we base our analysis on this subset of data. This is not surprising since our unemployment register data does not include workers who went into (early) retirement or exited the labour market for other reasons. In contrast, it is remarkable that the unemployment rate is not higher than 17.1 %: the socio-demographic characteristics of the nonrespondents (see Table 3) might have suggested that they are substantially more likely to be unemployed than the respondents.

If we compare our results for re-employment rates after plant closure with other studies, the outcomes are similar. In a recent study focusing on six industrial Swiss companies, the author finds re-employment rates of between 72 and 92 % and unemployment rates between 8 and 28 % (Wyss 2009:27). Yet this result does not consider the share of workers who quit the labour market because of retirement or training. If we adopt the same approach as Wyss (2009), we find a re-employment rate of 80 % and an unemployment rate of 20 %.

Likewise, a study on plant closure in Finland highlights that 1 year after displacement 62 % of the workers were re-employed, 14 % were unemployed, 19 % were in education or training and 5 % had dropped out of the labour force (Jolkkonen et al. 2012:88). While the re-employment and unemployment rate in the Finnish study are slightly lower than in our case, a much higher share of workers was in education or training, probably organized within the unemployment institution. Similarly, a thorough analysis of the American Displaced Worker Surveys 1984–2000 finds the reemployment rate for displaced mid-age, mid-educated male manufacturing workers in the United States to be 62 % in the early 1990s (Kletzer 2001:45). These comparisons provide some evidence that the findings from our survey also apply to other countries. Yet since the reported studies are set at different moments in the business cycles and in countries with a different labour market structure, we should not make too much of the similarities between these studies and our results.

6 Conclusion

Our survey on displaced manufacturing workers in Switzerland strives at understanding occupational trajectories after job loss. Based on a mixed-mode questionnaire, we surveyed about 1200 workers who lost their job after a financial crisis. The collected data were matched with firm data and register data from the unemployment insurance in order to obtain information about nonrespondents. When conducting this survey, we were confronted with two main problems likely to threaten the quality of the collected data: selection bias, referring to the problem that individuals are non-randomly selected into the sample, and nonresponse bias, referring to the problem that survey respondents and nonrespondents differ in characteristics (e.g. age or education) that are relevant for the outcome.

In this chapter, we have presented possible solutions to deal with survey bias and have evaluated whether these techniques were successful. Selection bias was addressed by using plant closure as an instrument. If a production site closes down completely, it is likely that workers did not lose their job because of poor performance and thus did not self-select into job displacement. Selection of workers into closing firms may not be a major problem in our case since we studied workers from mid-sized and large plants that are less likely to close down. The experiment-like setting of plant closure allows us to study the net effect of workers' socio-demographic characteristics on their re-employment prospects. We dealt with the problem of nonresponse bias by using financial incentives, mixed-mode, telephone interviews with national minorities, the inclusion of unemployment register data and weighting.

Although we cannot completely exclude selection and nonresponse bias, our adjustments seem to have reduced them. Our analyses suggest that some methods such as repeated contact attempts to reach the surveyed sample increased the response rate but did not reduce nonresponse bias. In contrast, telephone interviews helped to substantially improve the participation of typically underrepresented subgroups. Still, the survey respondents differ from nonrespondents in terms of age, education and occupation: the nonrespondents are on average substantially younger, more often with a lower level of education, and more likely to have worked in production jobs than the respondents. But interestingly these differences have no significant impact on the substantial conclusion about displaced workers' re-employment prospects. When we compare the re-employment rate based on weighted data with the re-employment rate based on data that combine survey and register data, the differences are marginal. One reason might be that the weights did not include variables that are relevant for the substantive variable. Another reason could probably be that those characteristics favouring participation in our survey – age and education – have contradictory effects on re-employment chances. While higher levels of education lead to both higher survey participation and reemployment rates, the opposite mechanism is true for age. Age increases survey participation, but strongly hampers job prospects – notably for workers aged 55 and more (Oesch and Baumann 2015).

Finally, we conclude by highlighting three challenges we faced when conducting the survey. The first challenge was the difficulty to convince companies and plants to participate in the survey since mass displacement implies negative publicity for a company, particularly if workers who were made redundant have not found new employment. A second challenge was the time-consuming construction of the questionnaire, made worse by the need to translate questions and to check its validity in both languages. A third challenge was the, ultimately unsuccessful, attempt to use an optical reading program to automatically input the responses of the questionnaires into a data file.

In contrast, particularly helpful for the survey process was the support provided by the Swiss State Secretariat of Economic Affairs. A first recommendation letter facilitated the contact with companies and employment offices. Once we had access to addresses, the external funding enabled us to provide financial incentives to respondents. The effect of a second recommendation letter that we added to the questionnaire is open: we do not know whether this letter incited – because of the official appearance of the survey – or discouraged – because of potentially negative resentment towards governmental actors – workers to participate in the survey. Our only indicator is the high participation rate, which rather points to a positive effect of the letter. Finally, collaboration with the government facilitated access to the unemployment register data, which proved to be extremely useful in the analyses of nonresponse bias presented here.

Appendix

Table A.1 Descriptive statistics of the responding sample

Variable		Share in %
Sex	Men	83
	Women	17
Education	Less than upper secondary education	14
	Upper secondary education	57
	Tertiary education	29
Mean age (in years)		47.3
Age (in categories)	16–29 years	10
	30–39 years	14
	40–49 years	28
	50–59 years	28
	60–65 years	19
Occupation	Managers (1-digit ISCO 1)	9
	Professionals (1-digit ISCO 2)	6
	Technicians (1-digit ISCO 3)	20
	Clerks (1-digit ISCO 4)	9
	Craft workers (1-digit ISCO 7)	27
	Machine operators (1-digit ISCO 8)	25
	Elementary jobs (1-digit ISCO 9)	3
Plant	A (Bern-Mittelland)	15
	B (Geneva)	12
	C (Bern-Mittelland)	19
	D (Bern-Mittelland)	30
	E (Bern-Mittelland)	24

Each subgroup sums up to 100 %. As an example, 83 % of the workers are men and 17 % are women

References

Andersen, S. H. (2008). The short- and long-term effects of government training on subjective well-being. *European Sociological Review, 24*(4), 451–462. doi:10.1093/esr/jcn005.

Angrist, J. D., & Pischke, J.-S. (2008). *Mostly harmless econometrics. An empiricist's companion.* Princeton: University Press.

Antonakis, J., Bendahan, S., Jacquart, P., & Lalive, R. (2010). On making causal claims: A review and recommendations. *The Leadership Quarterly, 21*(6), 1086–1120. doi:10.1016/j.leaqua.2010.10.010.

Berk, R. A. (2004). *Regression analysis. A constructive critique*. London: Sage Publications.

Biemer, P. P. (2010). Overview of design issues: Total survey error. In P. V. Marsden & J. D. Wright (Eds.), *Handbook of survey research* (pp. 83–137). Bingeley: Emerald.

Brand, J. E. (2015, forthcoming). The far-reaching impact of job loss and unemployment. *The Annual Review of Sociology, 41*, 1–36.

Burda, M. C., & Mertens, A. (2001). Estimating wage losses of displaced workers in Germany. *Labour Economics, 8*(1), 15–41. doi:10.1016/S0927-5371(00)00022-1.

Cha, Y., & Morgan, S. L. (2010). Structural earnings losses and between-industry mobility of displaced workers, 2003–2008. *Social Science Research, 39*(6), 1137–1152. doi:10.1016/j.ssresearch.2010.08.002.

Citro, C. F. (2010). Legal and human subjects consideration in surveys. In P. V. Marsden & J. D. Wright (Eds.), *Handbook of survey research* (pp. 59–79). Bingeley: Emerald.

Dillman, D. A., & Messer, B. L. (2010). Mixed-mode surveys. In P. V. Marsden & J. D. Wright (Eds.), *Handbook of survey research* (pp. 551–574). Bingeley: Emerald.

Dillman, D., Smyth, L., & Leani, C. (2009). *Internet, mail, and mixed-mode surveys: The tailored design method*. Bingeley: Emerald.

Eliason, M., & Storrie, D. (2009). Job loss is bad for your health – Swedish evidence on cause-specific hospitalization following involuntary job loss. *Social Science & Medicine, 68*(8), 1396–1406. doi:10.1016/j.socscimed.2009.01.021.

Ernst Stähli, M. (2012). Switzerland. In S. Häder, M. Häder, & M. Kühne (Eds.), *Telephone surveys in Europe. Research and practice* (pp. 25–36). Berlin: Springer.

Fallick, B. C. (1996). A review of the recent empirical literature on displaced workers. *Industrial and Labor Relations Review, 50*(1), 5–16. doi:10.2307/2524386.

Gibbons, R., & Katz, L. F. (1991). Layoffs and lemons. *Journal of Labor Economics, 9*(4), 351–380.

Groves, R. M., & Couper, M. (1998). *Nonresponse in household interview survey*. New York: Wiley.

Groves, R. M., & Lyberg, L. (2010). Total survey error: Past, present, and future. *Public Opinion Quarterly, 74*(5), 849–879. doi:10.1093/poq/nfq065.

Groves, R. M., & Peytcheva, E. (2008). The impact of nonresponse rates on nonresponse bias: A meta-analysis. *Public Opinion Quarterly, 72*(2), 167–189. doi:10.1093/poq/nfn011.

Hamilton, B. H., & Nickerson, J. A. (2003). Correcting for endogeneity in strategic manamagement research. *Strategic Organization, 1*(1), 51–78.

Harrison, C. H. (2010). Mail survey and paper questionnaires. In P. V. Marsden & J. D. Wright (Eds.), *Handbook of survey research* (pp. 499–526). Bingeley: Emerald.

Hayashi, T. (2007). The possibility of mixed-mode surveys in sociological studies. *International Journal of Japanese Sociology, 16*, 51–63.

Jolkkonen, A., Koistinen, P., & Kurvinen, A. (2012). Reemployment of displaced workers – The case of a plant closing on a remote region in Finland. *Nordic Journal of Working Life Studies, 2*(1), 81–100.

Kempf, A. M., & Remington, P. L. (2007). New challenges for telephone survey research in the twenty-first century. *Annual Review of Public Health, 28*, 113–126. doi:10.1146/annurev.publhealth.28.021406.144059.

Kletzer, L. (2001). *Job loss from imports: Measuring the costs*. Washington, DC: Institute for International Economics.

Kuhn, A., Lalive, R., & Zweimüller, J. (2009). The public health costs of job loss. *Journal of Health Economics, 28*, 1099–1115. doi:10.1016/j.jhealeco.2009.09.004.

Laganà, F., Elcheroth, G., Penic, S., Kleiner, B., & Fasel, N. (2011). National minorities and their representation in social surveys: Which practices make a difference? *Quality and Quantity*. doi:10.1007/s11135-011-9591-1.

Lipps, O. (2010). Effects of different incentives on attrition and fieldwork effort in telephone household panel surveys. *Survey Research Methods, 4*(2), 81–90.

Lipps, O., & Kissau, K. (2012). Nonresponse in an individual register sample telephone survey in Lucerne (Switzerland). In S. Häder, M. Häder, & M. Kühne (Eds.), *Telephone surveys in Europe. Research and practice* (pp. 187–208). Berlin: Springer.

Lipps, O., Laganà, F., Pollien, A., & Gianettoni, L. (2013). Under-representation of foreign minorities in cross-sectional and longitudinal surveys in Switzerland. In J. Font & M. Méndez (Eds.), *Surveying ethnic minorities and immigrant populations: Methodological challenges and research strategies* (pp. 241–267). Amsterdam: University Press.

Little, R. J. (1986). Survey nonresponse adjustments for estimates of means. *International Statistical Review, 54*(2), 139–157.

Little, R. J., & Vartivarian, S. L. (2005). Does weighting for nonresponse increase the variance of survey means? *Survey Methodology, 31*(2), 161–168.

Lohr, S. L. (1999). *Sampling: Design and analysis.* Pacific Grove: Duxbury Press.

Luiten, A., & Schouten, B. (2013). Tailored fieldwork design to increase representative household survey response rate: An experiment in the Survey of Consumer Satisfaction. *Journal of the Royal Statistical Society A, 176*(1), 169–189.

Lynn, P. (2003). PEDASKI: Methodology for collection about survey non-respondents. *Quality & Quantity, 37,* 239–261.

Mehlkop, G., & Becker, R. (2007). The effects of monetary incentives on the response rate in mail surveys on selfreported criminal behavior. *Methoden – Daten – Analysen, 1*(1), 5–24.

Meyer, B. D. (1995). Natural and quasi-experiments in economics. *Journal of Business & Economic Statistics, 13*(2), 151–161.

Oesch, D., & Baumann, I. (2015). Smooth transition or permanent exit? Evidence on job prospects of displaced industrial workers. *Socio-Economic Review, 13*(1), 101–123. doi:10.1093/ser/mwu023.

Oesch, D., & Lipps, O. (2013). Does unemployment hurt less if there is more of it around? A panel analysis of life satisfaction in Germany and Switzerland. *European Sociological Review, 29*(5), 955–967. doi:10.1093/esr/jcs071.

Peytchev, A., Baxter, R. K., & Carley-Baxter, L. R. (2009). Not all survey effort is equal: Reduction of nonresponse bias and nonresponse error. *Public Opinion Quarterly, 73*(4), 785–806. doi:10.1093/poq/nfp037.

Sakshaug, J. W., Couper, M. P., Ofstedal, M. B., & Weir, D. R. (2012). Linking survey and administrative records: Mechanisms of consent. *Sociological Methods & Research, 41*(4), 535–569. doi:10.1177/0049124112460381.

Schräpler, J.-P. (2001). Respondent behaviour in panel studies. A case study of the German Socio-Economic Panel (GSOEP). *DIW-Discussion Paper* 244. Berlin: DIW.

Schwerdt, G. (2011). Labor turnover before plant closure: "Leaving the sinking ship" vs. "Captain throwing ballast overboard". *Labour Economics, 18*(1), 93–101. doi:10.1016/j.labeco.2010.08.003.

Schwerdt, G., Ichino, A., Ruf, O., Winter-Ebmer, R., & Zweimüller, J. (2010). Does the color of the collar matter? Employment and earnings after plant closure. *Economics Letters*, 137–140. doi:10.1016/j.econlet.2010.04.014

Stoop, I. (2005). *The hunt for the last respondent: Nonresponse in sample survey.* Hague: Sociall en Cultureel Planbu.

Sweet, S., & Moen, P. (2011). Dual earners preparing for job loss: Agency, linked lives, and resilience. *Work and Occupations, 39*(1), 35–70. Retrieved from http://wox.sagepub.com/cgi/doi/10.1177/0730888411415601.

Vannieuwenhuyze, J., & Loosveldt, G. (2013). Evaluating relative mode effects in mixed-mode surveys: Three methods to disentangle selection and measurement effect. *Sociological Methods and Research, 42*(1), 82–104.

Voorpostel, M. (2010). Attrition patterns in the Swiss household panel by demographic characteristics and social involvement. *Swiss Journal of Sociology, 36*(2), 359–377.

Western, B., & Jackman, S. (1994). Bayesian inference for comparative research. *The American Political Science Review, 88*(2), 412–423.

Wyss, S. (2009). Stellenverlust und Lohneinbusse durch die Globalisierung? University of Basel: Eine Fallstudie. *WWZ Studie* 05/09 (B-100).

Using Life History Calendars to Survey Vulnerability

Davide Morselli, Nora Dasoki, Rainer Gabriel, Jacques-Antoine Gauthier, Julia Henke, and Jean-Marie Le Goff

1 Vulnerability: The Ordinary Facet of Life

European post-industrial societies are characterized by a high level of instability and fluctuation at economic, political and social levels (Crouch 1999). Hence at the turn of the twenty first century European countries are less stable than in previous historical periods (Sennett 2011). Confidence in the ability to keep social risks under control has been replaced by the idea that risks are not fully predictable or controllable. The side effect of such a change is a consequently greater exposure to risk factors that could force individuals to experience negative social and economical outcomes such as falling below the poverty threshold (Beck 1992).

The picture becomes more complicated than in previous (industrial) societies because new social risks emerge as the consequence of interactions between labour markets families and welfare systems producing a broad spectrum of negative outcomes (Ranci 2010). For instance the compensations for losses such as reintegration in the labour market after losing a job are not always effective in reducing social and psychological vulnerability and they perform differently for different segments

D. Morselli (✉) • J.-A. Gauthier • J.-M. Le Goff
NCCR LIVES, IP 201, Chavannes-près-Renens, Switzerland

Social Sciences Institute, University of Lausanne, Lausanne, Switzerland
e-mail: davide.morselli@unil.ch

N. Dasoki
NCCR LIVES, IP 213, Chavannes-près-Renens, Switzerland

Social Sciences Institute, University of Lausanne, Lausanne, Switzerland

R. Gabriel • J. Henke
NCCR LIVES, IP 213, Geneva, Switzerland

Centre for the Interdisciplinary Study of Gerontology and Vulnerability,
University of Geneva, Geneva, Switzerland

© The Author(s) 2016
M. Oris et al. (eds.), *Surveying Human Vulnerabilities across the Life Course*,
Life Course Research and Social Policies 3, DOI 10.1007/978-3-319-24157-9_8

of society. Negative outcomes must be framed in an analytical strategy that includes individual interpretations of the events in relation to their social and historical context on the one side and the personal and family history on the other. The interaction between the social context and individual life courses defines to a great extent the meaning and expectations individuals attach to life events.

In a context of uncertainty stability of the life course marked by a constant exposure to multidimensional risk factors, vulnerability is not only the possibility for an individual to experience a negative outcome or significant damage as a consequence of exposure to specific risk factors but also the lack of possibilities for individuals or social groups to activate protective and compensatory factors at different levels—material social and psychological. In other words vulnerability is not a state but a dynamic condition and can be defined as the time needed to recover from a negative outcome. Vulnerability is also multidimensional as it concerns simultaneously different aspects and dimensions of life their interactions in time and the interpretations given to them (Ranci and Magliavacca 2010).

Thus we can define social and psychological vulnerability as the difficulty to access resources to exit a particular negative and undesired state. This definition explains why the same risk factor may have different effects on different individuals (Ranci 2010). For this reason the study of vulnerability benefits from the adoption of a life course approach that accounts for multidimensional aspects of life and their interpretation. In this chapter we will focus on the life history calendar as a powerful tool for the study of multidimensional vulnerability.

2 Life History Calendars: A Pragmatic Approach

Researchers may use either prospective or retrospective methods to study life-histories (Scott and Alwin 1998; Levy et al. 2005). Both methods have advantages and disadvantages. Researchers should therefore evaluate the method in relation to the research questions.

In prospective studies such as panels cohort studies and other longitudinal designs researchers maintain contact with participants over time and repeatedly interview them on their current conditions. The analyst reconstructs the respondents' life courses by looking at the answers given at the different observation points. The drawbacks of prospective studies would make the study of vulnerability across the whole life extremely difficult if not in some cases impossible.

By contrast in retrospective designs respondents are interviewed once to collect data on their past life courses. Retrospective methods are sometimes less efficient than longitudinal panels in which data are collected at precise intervals during the life course (Bidard 2010) because retrospective methods have to rely on the respondents' willingness and capability to disclose their past to the researcher; several factors may influence memory possibly leading to omission or misreporting of life events (Auriat 1996; Reimer 2001).

Surveying a population requires some prior information to be able to design the sample. In the case of surveying vulnerability this would mean knowing beforehand who might potentially be in a vulnerable condition. Such priors are drawn from previous results and surveys that indicate which population strata are more at risk of being vulnerable and need particular attention.

For instance it is a common practice in birth cohort studies to oversample children from immigrant or low-income families. This approach produces high-quality data to investigate important issues concerning for instance inter-generational transmission of vulnerability. However it focuses on the life trajectories that have a vulnerable condition as their starting point but may fall short of capturing transitions into vulnerability. In addition while birth cohort studies can easily survey second-generation immigrants they provide poor information on the first generation. Collecting the same type of data on this population would require starting the study in a foreign country and monitoring the migration to the country of interest. Given these drawbacks it appears retrospective methods may be necessary to investigate certain research questions.

Starting from these considerations researchers have used different methods to minimize memory errors in surveys including decomposition (e.g. breaking a class of events into subclasses) the use of reversed chronological order the use of landmarks (e.g. transition points) and incrementing the time to answer survey questions (see Tourangeau 2000). Among these methods life history calendars (LHCs) seem to perform particularly well because they enhance several aspects of memory retrieval (Caspi et al. 1996; Freedman et al. 1988). The LHC is typically a two-way grid with the temporal dimension on one side and different life domains (e.g. residence family employment) on the other. Respondents report events for each life domain relating them to what happened in other life domains or to other time markers. With LHCs respondents can visualize their life trajectory linking what happened to when where it happened and for how long it lasted. Thus the calendar tools facilitate respondents' ability to place events into a temporal context by relating them to other synchronic (parallel) or diachronic (hierarchical) events and episodes that occurred in the life span (Belli 1998).

Researchers have produced a large corpus of evidence in the last 30 years comparing the quality of data obtained with LHCs and conventional question-naires. For instance Becker and Sosa (1992) showed the LHC resulted in more consistent reports (i.e. less superposition of mutually exclusive behaviours) than the conventional questionnaire. Goldman et al. (1989) and Yoshihama et al. (2005) argued that the calendar was more effective in enhancing the recall and reporting of specific events (e.g. contraceptive use domestic violence victimization). Engel et al. (2001a) suggested that the LHC performed better than the traditional question-list in terms of completeness. The visual nature of the calendar makes it easier for the interviewee and the interviewer to spot incongruous answers in the data reducing the unaccounted for amount of time in the respondent's life course. Test-retest reliability studies showed very high agreement for reported life events such as marriages and migrations (Engel et al. 2001b).

In addition to these indirect evaluations some experimental comparisons between calendar instruments and conventional questionnaires showed that adding a timeline to the questionnaire enhanced data quality in comparison to the regular questionnaire procedure (Van der Vaart 2004). Similarly Belli et al. (2001) showed that the calendar produced lower levels of reporting error than conventional question lists concerning the number of residential moves income weeks unemployed and illness but it over-reported history of cohabitation and number of jobs.

Why do LHCs help to report retrospective data? According to Conway (1992, 1996) autobiographical memory is a non-linear process that works through different association mechanisms. Events can be recalled through their hierarchy (e.g. from more important to least important) through their sequence (e.g. in chronological order) or in relation to other events and episodes. In addition different individuals may be more comfortable or used to recollecting events in different ways. Thus Belli (1998) argued that the calendar facilitates the use of all three memory retrieval mechanisms as well as facilitating a flexible interaction between the respondent and the interviewer to clarify intended meanings and to reconstruct the past.

In line with these assumptions Glasner (2011) compared the number of edits (i.e. corrections) by respondents who answered the same questions in an online conventional biographical questionnaire as compared to an online LHC. Congruently with Belli's rationale but without the interviewer/respondent interaction Glasner found the number of edits in the calendar mode were twice as high as those in the conventional questionnaire. In other words respondents were more likely to correct and improve the quality of biographical calendar data by respondents than conventional questionnaire data.

Consistent with this results from cognitive interviews conducted at the Swiss National Centre of Competence in Research LIVES with respondents aged 35–66 with medium to low levels of education showed that in seven out of ten interviews the calendar structure encouraged respondents to re-edit their answers concerning several life domains (residence cohabitation couple relationships family work and education health other unexpected events). During the cognitive interviews the sequence through which respondents completed a self-administered calendar was recorded by an external observer.

Table 1 reports the sequence used by the respondents to fill in the different columns of the calendar (ordered from A = *residence* to G = *other unexpected events*). In the most linear sequence (Type 1) three out of ten respondents filled the columns of the calendar in order starting from the first one on the left (*residence*) then passing to the second (*cohabitation*) and so on until they reached the last one on the right (column 7 *other unexpected events*).

Type 2 respondents (three out of ten) completed the calendar in sequential order except for the first two columns (*residence* and *cohabitation*). They used residence and cohabitation as anchors for recollecting the changes in both domains. Once these two columns were properly completed respondents went through the rest of the calendar in an almost linear manner from columns 3 to 7. Type 3 respondents (four out of ten) completed the task in a less sequential order using the information of certain columns to step back and make changes in the previous data.

Table 1 Sequence of the edits for each column during the LIVES cognitive interviews

Type of respondents by editing style	Editing sequence													
Type 1 respondents	A	B	C	D	E	F	G							
	A	B	C	D	E	F	G							
	A	B	C	D	E	F	G							
Type 2 respondents	A	B	C	B	A	C	D	E	F	G	F	G	F	
	A	B	C	B	A	B	A	B	A	B	C	D	E	F	G
	A	B	C	B	A	B	C	D	E	F	G			
Type 3 respondents	A	B	C	D	E	F	E	G						
	A	B	C	D	A	B	D	E	F	G				
	A	B	C	D	E	F	G	E	F	B	G			
	A	B	C	G	D	E	E	B	C	E	F	D	E	

A = residence B = cohabitation C = couple relationships D = family E = work and education F = health G = other unexpected events

While the Type 1 respondents did not re-edit the information they had reported the graphical and conceptual structure of the calendar helped Type 2 and 3 respondents to retrieve and report autobiographical memories. Without the calendar Type 2 respondents may have had more difficulties in accurately recalling their residence and cohabitation history and Type 3 respondents may not have gone back and corrected the information they had reported previously.

Auriat (1993) argued that when people are asked to remember episodes in a sequential order misdating a certain point of the sequence is likely to produce errors in reporting the subsequent events. Thus the calendar methods may decrease distortion by forcing respondents to visualize the sequence and anchor it to surrounding events (as with the Type 2 respondents). Cross-referencing between life events becomes then a resource that can be used by the respondent but also by the interviewer. The calendar format facilitates the interaction between interviewer and respondent in face-to-face interviews leading to a more precise check of the reported information (Belli et al. 2001; Sutton et al. 2011). Engel and colleagues (2001b) compared the calendar method to a self-reporting questionnaire and concluded that people are more willing to provide correct information and are more cooperative during the administration of LHCs.

3 Memory Bias as a Hidden Resource for Understanding Life Histories

So far we have discussed how LHCs help to reduce the probability of memory biases and misreporting of dates. A provocative alternative approach is not to consider errors as a problem for data analysis but as an important source of information in their own right. According to Couppié and Demazière (1995) memory errors are not distributed at random but depend on specific social variables that may be connected to the phenomenon under investigation. From a sociological perspective memory is not a simple restoration or reproduction of the past but a reconstruction of the life trajectory; this partly depends on the situation respondents are in when asked to recollect information on their experiences (Halbwachs 1994[1925]).

For Halbwachs the recollection of events is the result of two interrelated thinking strategies. The first consists of "locating" an event in its social context in terms of time and space. Like some sort of time travel people progressively place themselves in a frame that facilitates the recollection of personal events. In the second mnemonic process people transfer their focus from one single event to another focusing on its nature and its meaning (Halbwachs 1994 p. 201).

The meaning of what is recollected has a social frame that depends at the same time on the different social groups the participant was a member of when a particular event occurred and on the social groups the participant belongs to at present. Coenen-Huther (1994) mentioned for instance that reports of past events differ according to the respondents' gender age or social class. In the case of gender she argued that women tend to structure their memory according to family events while men structure their memory in relation to the professional domain.

In Halbwachs' perspective some events and objects fade from memory because they are no longer meaningful if related to a social frame that no longer exists. For example when a specific social group to which the respondent belonged no longer exists at the moment of the interview the respondent is more likely to omit events experienced in relation to that group or situation. Such omissions are therefore not due to the fact that the events were not important in the past but because they are no longer relevant at the time of the interview.

A comparison of two life events calendars completed by the same respondents the first completed 5 years after they left school and the second one completed 9 years later showed some time differences in the job history (Couppié and Demazière 1995). For example respondents were more likely to omit precarious jobs and short spells of unemployment in the second wave if the respondents had been employed in a permanent position between the two waves. Memory is therefore a dynamic process which generates information reconstructs life events and attributes meaning according to both current and past conditions.

Answering retrospective biographical questionnaires as with any autobiographical process is thus not only a means to provide information on social phenomena but also represents processes of social construction that attach meanings to questions and answers. When respondents use biographical memory to communicate life events and experiences to others (e.g. an interviewer) they organize their memory in an ordered and coherent way in which casual and unexpected events may take on a coherent (and sometimes causal) structure (Bertaux 1981; Ricoeur 1985). The respondent becomes the author of a narrative in which he or she is the main character attributing a sense of coherence to his or her life. In other words in the autobiographical narrative respondents order their life events into a matrix that is culturally and socially constructed and gives sense and meaning to what happened (Bruner and Weisser 1991).

The structure of a LHC in particular serves as a standardized grid that helps respondents report their life trajectories and assists researchers in framing the data. However the choice of standardization and the type of information requested are bound to interact with the respondents' reconstruction of their lives. They obligate respondents to re-organize their lives in a certain way; the reported information is therefore shaped by this constraint. The biographical questionnaire forces respondents to elaborate a socially-constructed theory of their lives. Respondents have to select the events to report among the wide range of their life events. They do so in relation to the type of events requested and the way the questions are formulated. In this process they sort the events giving them different importance and different priorities. They then order the events following the logic of the questionnaire (e.g. chronological). Thus responding to a biographical questionnaire such as the LHC is a social action. Respondents use life events to tell a story (with all its meanings and implications) to someone: the interviewer, the research project, the scientific world or the social and political environment (Bruner 1990; Eco 1984).

Taking these aspects into account to analyze social events and survey data can open the door to new and multi-faceted insights and the analysis of LHC data is particularly interesting in this respect. Embarking in this direction a scientific paradigm that considers autobiographical narratives in terms of self-construction is needed (Bruner 1990; Ricoeur 1985). This type of approach is not new to the hermeneutic and phenomenological traditions which are commonly based on a relatively small sample or single case analysis. In contrast LHCs are the junction between autobiographical narrative and quantitative data and they can be used in large-scale surveys. LHCs produce biographical data that are at the same time narrative and quantitative and for this reason they are useful for analysis using either qualitative or quantitative paradigms. Introducing LHCs into survey designs can therefore extend the hermeneutic approach to investigate large populations superimposing constructivist and positivist paradigms.

For example Couppié and Demazière (1995) showed that the absence of reported unemployment episodes is strongly influenced by the way the category "unemployment" is defined in the calendar and by the current occupational status (employed or unemployed) of the respondents at the time of the interview. Instead of considering discrepancies in the data or misreporting as errors the authors analysed the missing information as a dependent variable. In other words they treated non-response as a way of answering the question that indicates a specific process of social integration (Bourdieu 1979). Researchers can estimate the size of non-response by comparison with other studies or subsamples with lower missing values and cross that information with other socio-demographic indicators to estimate whether the missing data are random. However the risk of this approach is to link results to a particular context and setting undermining the generalisation of the results. Using a similar approach Couppié and Demazière proposed replacing the notion of memory error (or memory bias) which implies a fault in the data with the notion of *memory deviation* stressing the process of social construction of the reported information. This research approach is intriguing in many ways but largely unexplored in survey research.

In summary LHC methods not only perform better than conventional questionnaires in collecting retrospective data but also serve as a tool for different scientific paradigms. Researchers can use LHCs to investigate how people interpret and define the social world and their self-positioning within it. LHCs allow researchers to account for the interaction between events (objective/factual data) and their interpretation (subjective/perceived factors) in different life domains.

As noted earlier this approach is close to the phenomenological perspective in which the interactions between people the social world and cognitive processes are the objects of investigation (Gadamer 1975; Fisher 2004). How people interpret facts and why they formulate certain interpretations instead of others is central in the phenomenological approach. According to Schutz (1962) people structure their lives in socially defined life spheres that are interconnected and interact with each other. The life spheres are structured in a hierarchy in which some are more important than others for both individual and social reasons. The interaction between the life spheres shapes the meaning attributed to life events. When things happen which specific life spheres are involved and the way the life spheres are interconnected with each other are all elements that structure individuals' interpretation of their lives and different reactions to the same life events.

4   Using a Life History Calendar to Survey Vulnerability

We defined vulnerability as a dynamic and pervasive process embedded within social life. In this chapter we focus on three interrelated processes of vulnerability: diffusion accumulation and interpretation. The process of diffusion is based on Schutz's (1962) definition of life spheres according to which an individual life is categorized into different domains—e.g. family work social relations political life and so on. The definition of each sphere is socially constructed and as we discussed the way researchers define each sphere in designing questionnaires or LHCs is charged with meanings.

Nevertheless each sphere can be the object of specific disciplinary investigations given that the notion of a sphere itself presumes that life spheres are independent of each other to some extent. However they are not completely independent; both positive and negative spill-overs may occur. For instance events that happen within the family life can influence the work sphere or social relations. Experiencing a divorce can strongly affect the network of interpersonal relations of the two ex-partners (Widmer 2010). Accounting simultaneously for different life domains allows researchers to study spill-over effects with LHCs.

In addition as life spheres are framed as interdependent interdisciplinary research is needed. The LHC tool is particularly suitable for multi-disciplinary research because it produces a relatively large amount of data suitable for analysis from different perspectives (demography sociology psychology social-psychology and more).

Besides diffusion processes the interaction among events that happen within each life-sphere is also fundamental for understanding vulnerability. The accumulation of disadvantages including the temporal distance between negative and positive outcomes as well their sequence can put people in a severe condition of risk affecting the reconstruction of resources needed to exit from vulnerability (Dannefer 2003, 2009). The temporal structure of LHC data is particularly suitable for accounting for these aspects and can be used for performing sequence analysis event-history analysis or other longitudinal models (Axinn and Barber 2001; Axinn et al. 1999).

Last but not least the interpretation of events is at the same time a dependent and an independent variable in the study of vulnerability. The same event can assume very different meanings and affect peoples' lives in very different ways. For instance members of different social classes or members of the same class may not experience losing a job or being fired in the same way. Thus an event that for one person can start a dangerous domino effect may be a minor problem for another person.

In addition the meaning attached to events is culturally and socially embedded. Losing a job in a period of economic crisis may be a different experience compared to losing it in a period of economic growth. On the other hand in a period of crisis the loss of the job becomes sadly common while in other historical periods it could represent a less likely and for this reason more stigmatizing experience (Oesch and Lipps 2012). The interpretation of events and their relationships with the social-historical contexts are tightly related and researchers can address them both easily in two ways with LHCs.

Data in LHCs are both connected to temporal—i.e. the year in which events occurred—and spatial dimension—i.e. where the respondent was located at the time the event occurred. This makes it possible to relate events to places and consequently to social and historical contexts. In addition LHCs can allow a retrospective evaluation of events providing information on individual interpretations of life trajectories. This is probably one of the less developed uses of LHCs although it is central to the study of vulnerability. In the next section we present some experiences with using LHCs to tap the three processes of diffusion accumulation and interpretation as examples of the use of LHCs to survey vulnerability.

5 Designing Live History Calendars for Research on Vulnerability

5.1 The 'Devenir Parent' Survey

The *Devenir Parent*[1] [Becoming a Parent] survey was conducted between November 2005 and May 2009 by an interdisciplinary team from the universities of Lausanne and Geneva. The aim was to investigate the factors of differentiation in professional trajectories between men and women during the transition to parenthood in contemporary Switzerland (Le Goff and Levy 2011). The Swiss welfare system

[1] Swiss National Science Foundation grants no 100012-109692/1 100012-113598/1 100012-115928/1 and 100017_130233/1.

lacks adequate childcare infrastructures (OFS 2008) and women risk being forced
to abruptly change their professional careers because of the impossibility of leaving
their child in day care (e.g. Le Goff 2005). Thus after the birth of the first child one
partner—often the woman—may be forced to diminish working hours or to resign
from her job with evident repercussions for the household economy and equality
between partners.

The *Devenir Parent* survey was a three-wave panel: 235 Swiss-French couples
volunteered for three interviews, the first during the second half of the pregnancy,
the second 4–6 months after childbirth and the third a year later. Researchers
asked questions on the redefinition of personal identity social roles everyday life
professional activities family and friendship networks in face-to-face interviews
conducted separately with both partners. The researchers also conducted in-depth
qualitative interviews.

In the third wave the participants filled out two LHCs. The first retraced events
in different life domains from the age of 15; the second focused on the professional
trajectory from the moment of conception to the year after childbirth. This short
calendar tapped periods of non-activity due to maternity leaves as well as from
unemployment and other possible reasons. In the case of women the calendar also
traced childcare trajectories with details about the type of care and the average
duration per week. Although this calendar focused on factual data it allowed
researchers to connect events to subjective expectations and intentions as formulated
in the first and second waves and eventually in qualitative interviews.

Figure 1 displays the story of a woman "Annette" (a fictitious name) in the
months following the conception of her first child. In the first wave Annette
mentioned she was working full-time but she had intended to convert her contract to
a half-time job after the maternity leave. She also declared that her employer did not
agree to restructuring the contract and she expressed her intention to change jobs.
During the first interview Annette mentioned an intention of leaving the child at a
nursery five half-days a week which corresponded to a 50 % part-time job. At the
time of this first wave she was still waiting for an answer from the nursery.

The LHC questionnaire showed the uncertainties related to these two intentions
and more deeply some vulnerable dimensions linked to the transition to parenthood.
At the end of her maternity leave which in the Swiss canton of Geneva where
Annette lived was a maximum of 4 months the lack of an available place at
the day nursery made it impossible for Annette to register at the unemployment
office because an administrative Swiss rule stated that a person can be considered
unemployed only if he or she is immediately available to take a job. Because the
child could not be left unsupervised Annette could not be considered available and
therefore "unemployed." She was forced to take unpaid leave until a place in the
nursery became available 4 months later.

Eventually the nursery accepted the child for five half-days a week. Annette could
then look for new employment. After three more months she began a 50 % part-
time job. During all this period her husband worked full-time as a manager of an
administrative department in a corporation. The story had a happy ending with the
situation fulfilling the initial intentions about work and childcare.

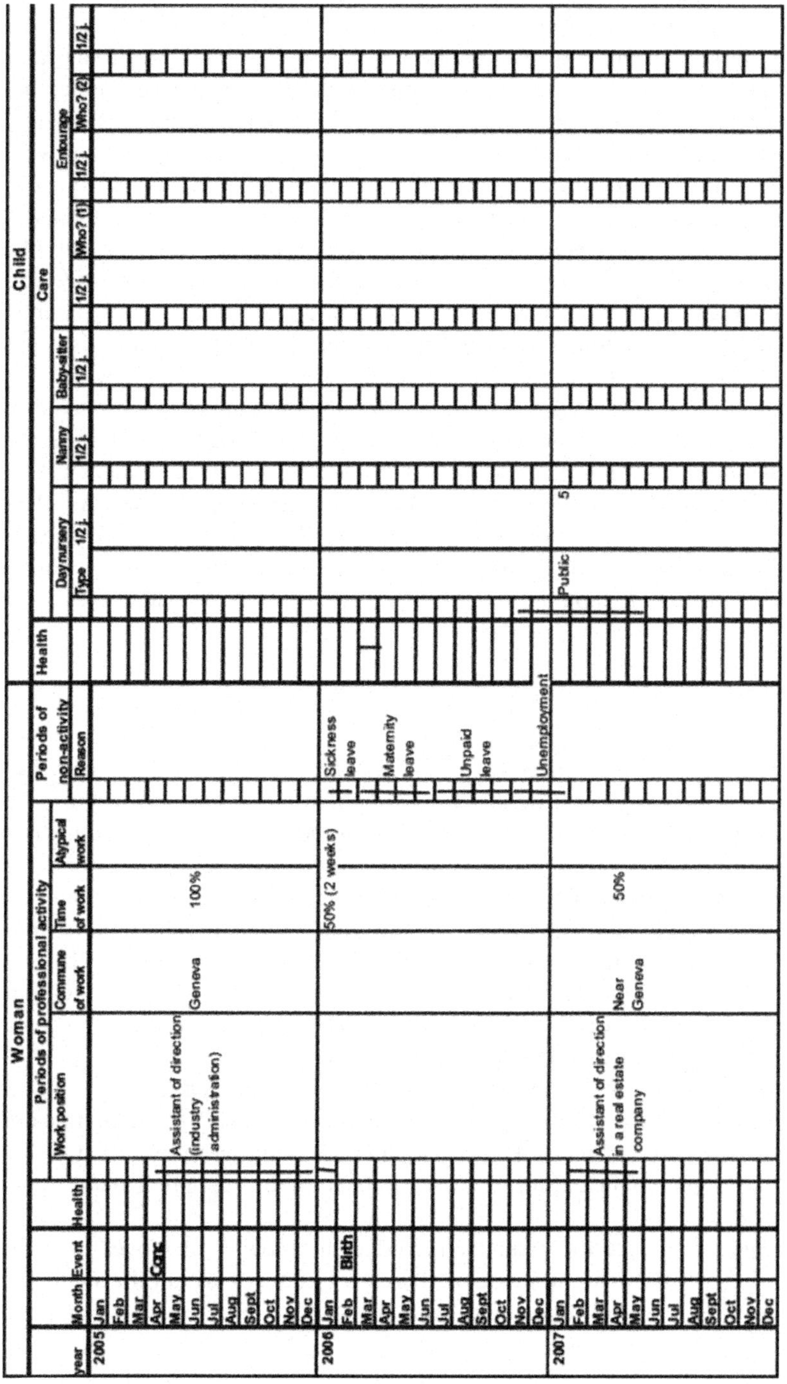

Fig. 1 Annette's "short" calendar in the *Devenir Parent* survey

However Annette was exposed to social risk in two regards: the first related to the necessity to end her first job; the second related to the non-availability of a place in the day nursery at the end of the maternity leave. If she had not found a new job or if the unavailability of childcare would have been longer the vulnerability of her situation would have been more serious. The initial expectations would not have been fulfilled creating a potential situation of psychological distress as well as a redefinition of the household economy and family roles. In the months preceding the important social transition of becoming a parent the partners project themselves in the future with baggage full of personal and social norms. We thus speak of the birth of the first child as a normative event that generates a series of expectations and plans. When these expectations are not fulfilled the potential for parents to experience negative outcomes and remain constrained by the situation is greater. Unexpected events may have significant consequences.

The *Devenir Parent* LHC constrained individuals' life trajectories into sequences of events concerning two life domains: employment and childcare. Thus the analysis of the LHC alone does not indicate what happened outside these parameters. The LHC in the *Devenir Parent* was only one part of a more complex survey. A different approach would be to use the LHC to directly collect data on unexpected or unwanted events in each of the life domains. The next example shows how life calendars can be used to tap non-normative (i.e. unexpected) critical events.

5.2   Family tiMes

Two cohorts of 400 individuals born in 1950–1955 and 1970–1975 and drawn from a representative sample of the Swiss population participated in the *Family tiMes*[2] survey. Like *Devenir Parent* but not concerned with the specific transition to parenthood this survey was also aimed at capturing from a life course perspective the changing web of constraints and opportunities in which family and occupational trajectories of individuals unfold. Besides questions on values and opinions and an instrument measuring the personal networks of relationships (Widmer 2010) that were recorded with computer-assisted personal interview (CAPI) mode the *Family tiMes* survey included a LHC (Fig. 2) designed to be hetero-administered by means of a paper questionnaire in a face-to-face interview setting.

The calendar brought together six life domains (cohabitation residence intimate relationships occupational activities and critical life events) with 6-month time units. On this basis the researchers asked respondents to mention information on what happened in each domain and for how long indicating the beginning and the end of each episode.

Concerning residence the calendar recorded the number of moves as well as the corresponding destination area code (even for changes within the same area). For intimate relationships longer than 3 months respondents identified each partner

[2]Swiss National Science Foundation grants no 100017_130343/1.

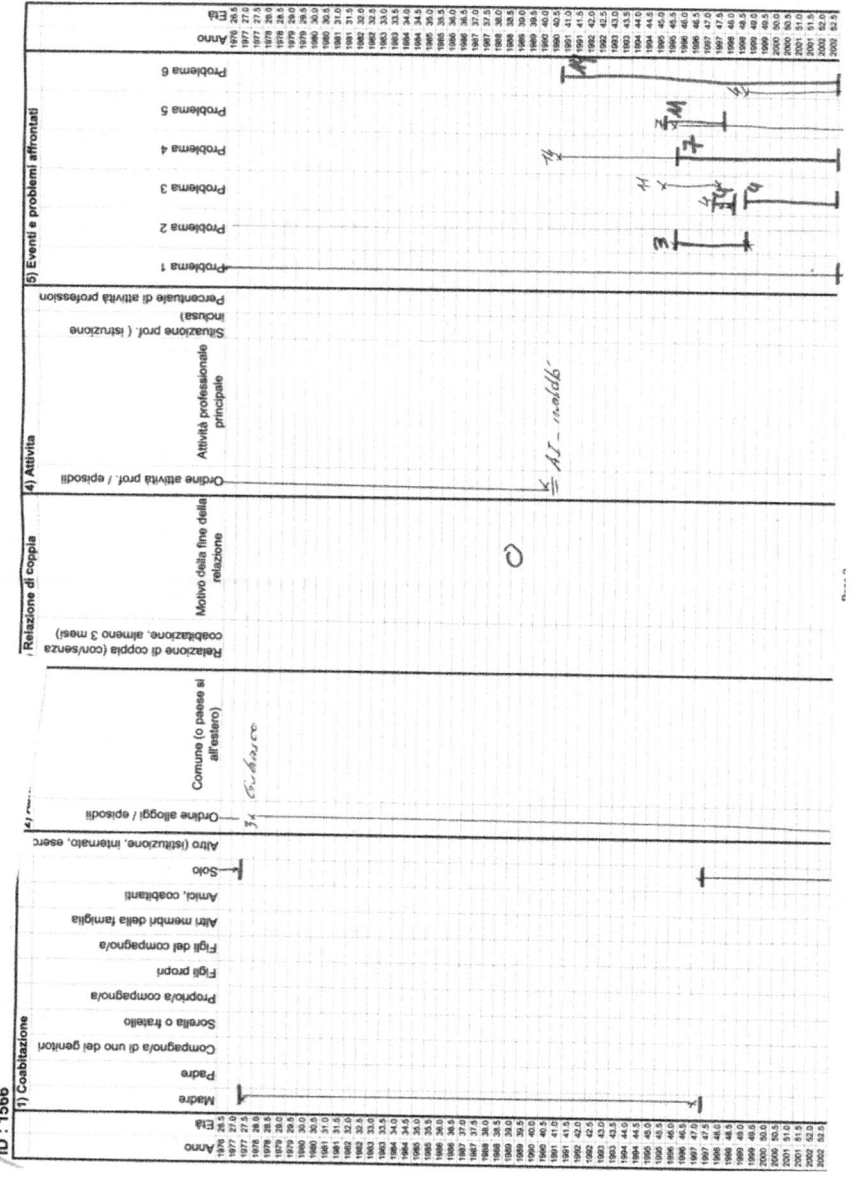

Fig. 2 Example of a completed Family TiMes calendar. The last column refers to critical events

and recorded the reasons for separation. The LHC also included inquiries into the number of jobs type status and activity rates to tap occupational careers.

In addition to these events the last part of the calendar was dedicated to non-normative and unexpected critical events. The survey asked respondents to indicate up to a maximum of six simultaneous critical events (e.g. serious accident or illness depression severe conflict long unemployment period) relative to themselves or one of their close relatives. Non-normative events have cumulative properties and are systemically associated—as dependent independent or intervening variables—with dysfunctions in other life domains (e.g. Hill 1958). On the other hand these types of events may be more susceptible to being misreported in conventional retrospective interviews.

In conventional questionnaires the interviewing sequence may affect the likelihood of reporting non-normative events with respondents' recollections of more recent events impairing their ability to remember earlier occurrences (Belli et al. 1997). By contrast in LHCs the iterative structure of the interview and the use of temporal landmarks help the respondents access and report memories on unexpected events (Yoshihama et al. 2005). Thus LHCs seem particularly useful in collecting data on vulnerability factors and their cumulation.

Inspired by the French Ageven tradition (Vivier 2006; Antoine and Lelievre 2009) and in line with the life course paradigm (e.g. Mortimer and Shanahan 2003) the *Family tiMes* calendar focused on individual trajectories as produced by an events-related logic rather than by an underlying generative process. It aimed at explaining a trajectory through the chronological order of events and the social statuses linked to it. This process is supposed to be multidimensional. In this sense it is the result of a double interaction: one synchronic (level of normativity/compatibility between various statuses at a given time point) the other diachronic (the kind of path dependencies resulting from antecedent configurations). In this holistic perspective researchers can display and eventually explain patterns of linked trajectories.

The face value of the filled calendars confirms the above statements as relational features (absence or multiplicity of partners divorce and separation) are associated with the occurrence of problems. Sometimes residential mobility solo living and unstable intimate relationships are characteristic of a trajectory. Parental separation childbirth and chronic illness often appear synchronically or diachronically together. Such interrelated mechanisms are visible in the example (Fig. 2). In this case the respondent suffered from chronic conditions: at age 20 his father and sister died in an accident reducing his social resources to his mother. After a period of relative stability the death of his mother associated with his unemployability left him completely isolated facing financial difficulties and depression.

The combination between the four life domains (cohabitation residence intimate relationships and occupational activities) and the non-normative critical events returns a complex—not simplistic—and holistic picture of individual life courses. In *Family tiMes* the critical life events were unexpected problems that respondents had to face during their life histories. As discussed above the weight for the personal trajectory derives from the (synchronic) interaction of life domains and by the (diachronic) accumulation of negative critical events. However this approach assumes that certain types of events may be generally understood as advantages or disadvantages. This may not always be the case and some events that can be disruptive for certain individuals or social categories may have a different weight for others. Thus the subjective interpretation of events assumes an important role in understanding the incidence of events on life histories. The next two examples illustrate the use of LHCs to assess subjective evaluations of trajectories.

5.3   Vivre/Leben/Vivere and the Swiss Panel LIVES Calendar

The *Vivre/Leben/Vivere* (VLV) survey[3] on the health and living conditions of the elderly population in Switzerland implemented another LHC. The aim of this choice was to collect retrospective data on the respondents' life trajectories but also to help the target population of individuals aged 65 and older with memory recall through the graphical visualization of their life histories. In addition the VLV calendar aimed to collect retrospective evaluations of respondents' life trajectories.

The VLV calendar was self-administered and later checked by an interviewer by means of a CAPI protocol to correct or complete information if necessary when unclear or incoherent. It included five life domains: residence family and relationships job health and nationality. Because the calendar was self-administered it also provided general guidelines on the type of events to consider and two examples of correctly filled-out calendars. To assess the subjective interpretation the interviewer asked respondents to indicate with an orange marker directly on the calendar sheet the periods during which they felt most vulnerable (also defined as fragile or difficult periods) and with a yellow marker the periods they considered the happiest. This procedure collected important data about respondents' perceptions of their vulnerability.

Figure 3 shows the year count of vulnerable periods by age groups. It reveals some interesting patterns. Two distinct profiles emerge.

Respondents aged 85 and older frequently indicated vulnerable periods during their childhoods and early adulthoods which coincided with the Second World War. That period represented a peak of vulnerability with 12 % of the 85-and-older respondents reporting experiences of vulnerability. Their vulnerability curve drastically decreased after the war and stayed more or less constant until an increment in reported vulnerability in the most recent 10 years which in this subsample corresponded to their entry into older age—i.e. 60–70 years.

The second group consisting of people younger than 85 years had a less marked profile of vulnerable periods. For all four subgroups the percentage of respondents

---

[3]VLV is the third of a set of transversal studies on conditions of the elderly population in Switzerland. The first one was conducted in 1979, and the second in 1994 (Lalive d'Epinay et al. 1999).

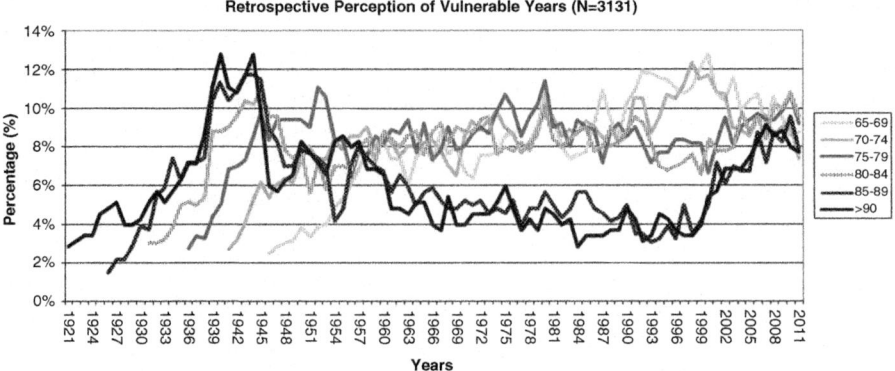

Fig. 3 Percentages of respondents by age groups marking vulnerable years in the VLV survey

reporting vulnerability during childhood was low and especially lower for those 65–69 years old born after the end of the war. However all the groups converged in reporting experienced vulnerability in the 1950s. Therefore while vulnerability was less frequent than in the 85+ group in the following years it held constant at about 8–9 % in the younger group. All groups converged again in the most recent years.

The data also showed multiple response patterns reflecting different ways respondents understood or perceived vulnerability. Approximately 46 % of the respondents indicated only one period during which they felt particularly vulnerable followed by 20 % with two and 11 % with three periods. Long periods of vulnerability running through a major part of life were the exceptions: the periods tended to be short (less than 10 years) and got shorter when participants mentioned multiple periods.

The data showed multiple styles of reporting vulnerability. For instance some respondents reported vulnerability as a single enduring experience which covered several years. Some others reported instead recurring vulnerability experiences of shorter length. Similarly the correlation between vulnerability and happy periods was not monotonic. Some reported happiness as opposed to vulnerability while some others superposed periods of happiness and vulnerability to some extent. The combination of these different reporting styles returned a detailed picture of individual interpretations of life trajectories *vis-à-vis* normative expectations and social contexts. Two examples from the VLV survey may better illustrate these aspects.

The first is the story of "Felicja" (fictional name) a 78-year-old Polish woman living in Geneva. She marked only one period of vulnerability which started at her birth in 1933 and continued until the age of 19. In the calendar she linked no specific event to this long negative period; however it was likely connected to the historical context and possibly the death of her two brothers in 1945 and 1947. Given the absence of objective information an analytic approach based only on factual data would have most likely skipped or undervalued the link between Felicja's experience and the context. But the story is not finished and it has a happy

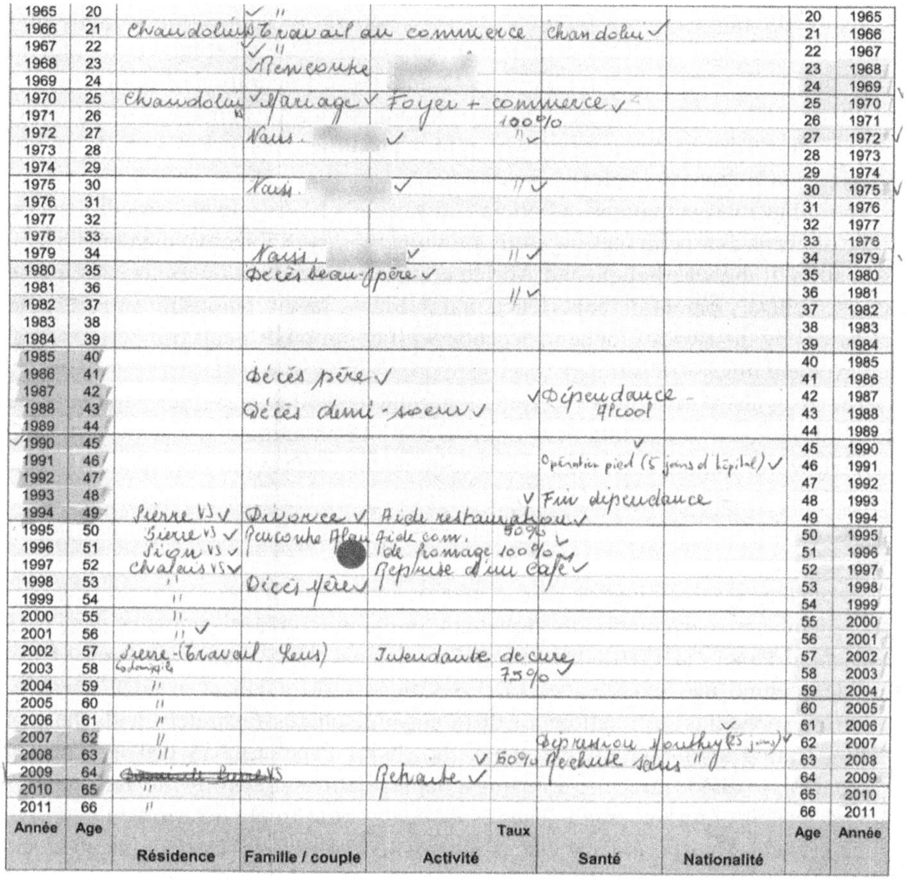

Fig. 4 Adrian's completed *Vivre/Leben/Vivere* calendar. The *orange* marks on the *left* indicate the most vulnerable periods; the *yellow* marks on the *right* the happiest ones

ending. Besides this single vulnerable period Felicja indicated one single happy period that started at the age of 30 in 1963 and persisted to the time of the interview when she was 78 years old. In contrast to the blurred edges of the vulnerable period the happy one started with the birth of her daughter in 1963. What is also interesting is that neither the loss of her father in 1979, her divorce in 1981, or the death of her mother in 1982 affected her positive evaluation of life since her daughter's birth.

In contrast with Felicja's style of experiencing and reporting vulnerability Adrian (fictional name) a 66-year-old man from the Valais Canton marked multiple episodes of vulnerability and happiness which seemed to be linked to specific events (Fig. 4). Adrian's most vulnerable period of life started in 1985 1 year before the loss of his father and continued with the loss of his half-sister in 1989 until his divorce in 1994. In addition the loss of his father had very likely triggered a phase of alcoholism indicated in the health section of the calendar. Before this 10-year period of great difficulties Adrian reported positive periods in connection to particular events such as the completion of his education in 1963 meeting his partner in 1968 and the birth of his children in 1972 and 1975. In addition after his divorce in 1994 Adrian marked the beginning of a long period of happiness which was ongoing at the time of the interview despite other difficulties including sinking into a depression a few years before his retirement.

The subjective evaluations in Felicja and Adrian's LHCs add an extra dimension to the analysis that is pivotal for studying vulnerability. Subjective data enables an estimation of the way Felicja and Adrian counterbalanced hard periods or negative events. Felicja's parenting experience and Adrian's new relationship were used *a posteriori* by the two respondents to cope with common difficult life periods (e.g. bereavement illness transitions).

The assessment of subjective evaluation implemented in VLV thus augments the study of vulnerability adding new value to the interpretation and analyses of LHC data. However the questionnaire asked respondents to provide judgments on their general life conditions (in terms of happiness and vulnerability). In some cases people could feel particularly vulnerable in one specific life domain but not in others.

To overcome this limitation researchers designed a different tool for the assessment of subjective evaluation to implement in the third cohort sample of the Swiss Household Panel (SHP-III). Instead of focusing on the overall evaluation of life the idea behind the Swiss Panel LIVES Calendar (Morselli et al. 2012) was to capture respondents' evaluations of different life spheres separately with the aim of pinpointing spill-over effects. Thus the Swiss Panel LIVES Calendar asked respondents to divide three life domains (couple relationship family life and activity) into periods of different length. The respondents could freely determine the length of the periods. Thus period and events did not necessarily overlap. For instance one may get married once (event) but the marriage can have different phases (periods) with ups and downs. Once respondents had completed the task of sub-setting the three life domains into periods the researchers asked them to express a present-state evaluation for each period on a 5-point bipolar scale ranging from very negative to very positive.

In addition to the considerations drawn from Felicja's and Adrian's LHC this method makes it possible to capture with more precision the counterbalancing between evaluations of one life sphere (e.g. family) and what respondents experienced or perceived in the others (e.g. health job and so on). Moreover by asking respondents to divide the whole trajectory into periods that might not be linked to the specific events asked in the calendar (e.g. residential moves jobs births) this method is particularly suitable for tapping extra information that would otherwise be lost especially when researchers use LHCs to collect highly standardized data.

For instance young respondents' calendars on cohabitation and family events risk having little information compared to older respondents given their shorter life histories. Youths are likely to live with their parents not to have experienced changes in civil-status not to have had children and are not yet inserted into the labour market. The division of life domains into periods makes it possible to detect easily and quickly if and when things got better or worse within each life domain even in the absence of specific events. For instance the respondents may report little factual data in the family trajectory but researchers or respondents could divide the family history into periods of relative happiness and periods of conflict.

A limitation of this approach is that it shows that something happened within the trajectory and has changed the evaluation but it is not always possible to explain what happened and why the evaluation changed. All of the examples reported in this chapter proposed complementary tools for the use of LHC in surveying vulnerability. The best solution would be to implement all the specificities of each example into a single tool. Unfortunately this is not always possible in surveys and research requires compromises regarding costs administration times and questionnaire length. Nevertheless the use of one or more of these tools may produce rich data for understanding vulnerability dynamics and processes.

6   Is It Gold or Just Glittering?

So far we have made the case for implementing LHCs in research on vulnerability. However all that glitters is not gold and the LHC method has also a number of drawbacks that researchers must consider. Time and costs are problems of the LHC technique (Belli 1998) especially when the calendar has open answers that must be manually entered into a database and eventually coded. However the use of new technologies like tablets may overcome part of these problems and drastically reduce the costs (e.g. Glasner 2011).

More problematic are the administration time and the relative difficulty of the task. Both can easily increase for complex and atypical trajectories but vulnerable populations are the most likely to have complex atypical trajectories that do not follow normative transitions. Thus difficulties in filling LHCs could add to other problematic aspects of surveying vulnerable populations in particular those with low personal resources such as low socio-economic status or low cultural capital. Though the concept of life history calendars is becoming more popular thanks to its implantation on recreational platforms (e.g. Facebook Timelines) filling a calendar-based questionnaire is a cognitively demanding operation.

On the one side we showed that LHCs are suitable to study vulnerability processes from different perspectives considering vulnerability as the interrelation between diffusion accumulation and interpretation processes. By allowing for integrated analytical approaches the LHC can stimulate researchers towards complex and multifaceted understandings of vulnerability interconnecting subjective evaluations with factual episodes. On the other side specific segments of the society especially those at the margin that may be more at risk of experiencing prolonged vulnerability may encounter more difficulties in filling calendar-based questionnaires. Thus researchers should take extreme care in designing questionnaires for potentially vulnerable populations.

The visual potential of LHCs is still underexplored. LHCs are particularly useful for visualizing and structuring an individual's life trajectory. The graphical layout helps respondents access different types of memory allowing them to change correct and fill gaps during the interview. We showed that the cognitive testing confirmed that certain individuals (but not all) use the calendar in a synchronic way. The calendar's format allows those people to correct the reported information and enhance the reliability of data. Capitalizing on these considerations researchers could enhance the graphical layout of LHCs exploring for instance whether different graphical solutions could help respondents understand and more easily report events in LHCs. If it is not possible to lighten the cognitive task of memory recollection it could be at least made easier by means of graphical and multimedia tricks. Similarly the use of web-based LHCs still needs exhaustive experimentation and may be able to help some categories of respondents as well as making the task more pleasant and less tiring.

Aside from these aspects another point researchers on vulnerability must consider is the non-linearity and non-normativity of life trajectories under vulnerable conditions. As pre-constructed grids LHCs ask respondents to define their trajectories in standardized ways specifying family connections work activity and inactivity and residential history. Even if researchers could control for the social desirability of their questions, the fact that the LHC asks only some information and not others may return to the respondents an unwanted normative message indicating the "important" aspects of life. Thus, the construction of LHCs for surveying vulnerability should allow accounting for unexpected non-normative events and non-typical trajectories. Researchers should seek the right balance between standardization and unexpected types of transition. Recording non-normative events in the *Family tiMes* LHC as well as the assessments of subjective interpretations in VLV and the Swiss Panel LIVES Calendar were attempts to address this delicate point.

Another aspect worth considering is the role of interviewers *vis-à-vis* the high variability of how respondents fill in the calendar. Research so far has been inconclusive on the size and likelihood of interviewer effects in LHCs with general population respondents. Belli et al. (2007) did not find any difference in the interviewer variance between LHCs and conventional questionnaires while Sayles et al. (2010) reported a small increase in the interviewer variance for life calendar methods when compared to standardized questionnaires. Morselli et al. (2012) found the interviewer effect was not negligible in face-to-face interviews but was reduced when respondents filled out the LHCs themselves and the interviewer followed a standardized protocol to help them with the task.

Careful training of interviewers should be part of research plans for studies using LHCs. Aside from the interaction with the respondent during the interview, interviewers should also learn how to check the calendar once the respondents have filled them out and to verify with the respondent the exactness of the information.

Despite these aspects that require consideration especially in the design of large-scale surveys, the richness and complexity of data produced by LHCs may be worth the drawbacks. LHCs are able to capture essential dimensions of vulnerability accounting for the complex multidimensional time-related processes of individual lives.

References

Antoine, P., & Lelievre, E. (2009). *Fuzzy states and complex trajectories: Observation, modelization and interpretation of life histories*. Paris: Institut national d'études démographiques.

Auriat, N. (1993). "My Wife Knows Best": A comparison of event dating accuracy between the wife, the husband, the couple, and the Belgium population register. *Public Opinion Quarterly, 57*(2), 165–190.

Auriat, N. (1996). *Les défaillances de la mémoire humaine*. Paris: Presses Universitaires de France, INED.

Axinn, W. G., Pearce, L. D., & Ghimire, D. (1999). Innovations in life history calendar applications. *Social Science Research, 28*(3), 243–264.

Axinn, W. G., & Barber, J. S. (2001). Mass education and fertility transition. *American Sociological Review*, 481–505.

Beck, U. (1992). *Risk society: Towards a new modernity*. London: Sage Publications.

Becker, S., & Sosa, D. (1992). An experiment using a month-by-month calendar in a family planning survey in Costa Rica. *Studies in Family Planning, 23*, 386–391.

Belli, R. F. (1998). The structure of autobiographical memory and the event history calendar: Potential improvements in the quality of retrospective reports in surveys. *Memory, 6*(4), 383–406.

Belli, R. F., Schuman, H., & Jackson, B. (1997). Autobiographical misremembering: John Dean is not alone. *Applied Cognitive Psychology, 11*, 187–209.

Belli, R. F., Shay, W., & Stafford, F. (2001). Event history calendars and question-list surveys: A direct comparison of interviewing methods. *Public Opinion Quarterly, 65*, 45–74.

Belli, R. F., Smith, L. M., Andreski, P. M., & Agrawal, S. (2007). Methodological comparisons between CATI event history calendar and standardized conventional questionnaire instruments. *Public Opinion Quarterly, 71*(4), 603–622.

Bertaux, D. (Ed.). (1981). *Biography and society: The life history approach in the social sciences*. London: Sage.

Bidard, C. (2010). Bifurcations biographiques et ingrédients de l'action. In M. Bessin, C. Bidard, & M. Grossetti (Eds.), *Bifurcations: Les sciences sociales face aux ruptures et à l'événement* (pp. 224–238). Paris: La Découverte.

Bourdieu, P. (1979). *La distinction. Critique social du jugement*. Paris: Editions de Minuit.

Bruner, J. S. (1990). *Acts of meaning*. Cambridge: Harvard University Press.

Bruner, J., & Weisser, S. (1991). The invention of self: Autobiography and its forms. *Literacy and Orality, 129*–148.

Caspi, A., Moffitt, T. E., Thornton, A., Freedman, D., Amell, J. W., Harrington, H., Smeijers, J., & Silva, P. A. (1996). The LHC: A research and clinical assessment method for collecting retrospective event-history data. *International Journal of Methods in Psychiatric Research, 6*, 101–114.

Coenen-Huther, J. (1994). *La mémoire familiale: un travail de reconstruction du passé*. Paris: Editions L'Harmattan.

Conway, M. A. (1992). A structural model of autobiographical memory. In M. A. Conway, D. Rubin, H. Spinnler, & W. A. Wagenaar (Eds.), *Theoretical perspectives on autobiographical memory.* Dordrecht: Kluwer Academic Publishers.

Conway, M. A. (1996). Autobiographical knowledge and autobiographical memories. In D. Rubin (Ed.), *Remembering our past: Studies in autobiographical memory.* Cambridge: Cambridge University Press.

Couppié, T., & Demaziere, D. (1995). Se souvenir de son passé professionnel: Appel à la mémoire dans les enquêtes rétrospectives et construction sociale des données. *Bulletin de Méthodologie Sociologique, 49,* 23–57.

Crouch, C. (1999). *Social change in western Europe.* Oxford: Oxford University Press.

Dannefer, D. (2003). Cumulative advantage/disadvantage and the life course: Cross-fertilizing age and social science theory. *Journal of Gerontology, 58,* 327–337.

Dannefer, D. (2009). Stability, homogeneity, agency: Cumulative dis/advantage and problems of theory. *Swiss Journal of Sociology, 35,* 193–210.

Eco, U. (1984). *The role of the reader: Explorations in the semiotics of texts.* Bloomington: Indiana University Press.

Engel, L. S., Keifer, M. C., & Zahm, S. H. (2001a). Comparison of a traditional questionnaire with an icon/calendar based questionnaire to assess occupational history. *American Journal of Industrial Medicine, 40,* 502–511.

Engel, L., Keifer, M., Thompson, M. L., & Zahm, S. (2001b). Test-retest reliability of an icon/calendar-based questionnaire used to assess occupational history. *American Journal of Industrial Medicine, 40,* 512–522.

Fisher, W. P. (2004). Meaning and method in the social sciences. *Human Studies, 27,* 429–454.

Freedman, D., Thornton, A., Camburn, D., Alwin, D., & Young-DeMarcco, L. (1988). The LHC: A technique for collecting retrospective data. *Sociological Methodology, 18,* 37–68.

Gadamer, H.-G. (1975). *Truth and method.* New York: Seabury Press.

Glasner, T.J. (2011). *Reconstructing event histories in standardized survey research: Cognitive mechanisms and aided recall techniques.* Unpublished doctoral dissertation, Vrije Universiteit, Amsterdam.

Goldman, N., Moreno, L., & Westoff, C. F. (1989). Collection of survey data on contraception: An evaluation of an experiment in Peru. *Studies in Family Planning, 20,* 147–157.

Halbwachs, M. (1994[1925]). *Les cadres sociaux de la mémoire.* Paris: Albin Michel.

Hill, R. (1958). Generic features of families under stress. *Social Casework, 39,* 139–150.

Lalive d'Epinay, L., Bickel, J.-F., Maystre, C., & Vollenwyer, N. (1999). *Vieillesses au fil du temps, 1979–1994: Une révolution tranquille: Santé, situations de vie, formes de participation et visions du monde des personnes âgées en Suisse.* Lausanne: Réalités sociales.

Le Goff, J.-M. (2005). Articulation entre la vie familiale et la vie professionnelle. In J.-M. Le Goff, C. Sauvain-Dugerdil, C. Rossier, & J. Coenen-Huther (Eds.), *Maternité et parcours de vie. L'enfant a-t-il toujours une place dans les projets des femmes en Suisse ?* (pp. 239–277). Berne: Peter Lang.

Le Goff, J.-M. & Levy, R. (2011). *Enquête Devenir parent.* Rapport technique. Pavie Working Paper, 11.2.

Levy, R., Ghisletta, P., Le Goff, J.-M., Spini, D., & Widmer, E. (2005). Incitations for interdisciplinarity in life course research. In R. Levy, P. Ghisletta, J.-M. Le Goff, D. Spini, & E. Widmer (Eds.), *Towards an interdisciplinary perspective on the life course* (pp. 361–391). Amsterdam-Boston: Elsevier.

Morselli, D., Roberts, C., Brändle, K., Dasoki, N., Mugnari, E., & Spini, D. (2012). *Self- and interviewer-administered life history calendars.* Paper presented at the Eucconet/Society for Longitudinal and Life Course Studies International Conference, 29–31 Oct 2012.

Mortimer, J. T., & Shanahan, M. J. (2003). *Handbook of the life course.* New York: Springer.

OFS. (2008). *Les familles en Suisse. Rapport statistique 2008.* Neuchâtel.

Oesch, D., & Lipps, O. (2012). *Does unemployment hurt less if there is more of it around? A panel analysis of life satisfaction in Germany and Switzerland.* European Sociological Review.

Ranci, C. (2010). Social vulnerability in Europe. In C. Ranci (Ed.), *Social vulnerability in Europe: The new configuration of social risks* (pp. 3–24). Basingstoke: Palgrave Macmillan.

Ranci, C., & Magliavacca, M. (2010). Social vulnerability: A multidimensional analysis. In C. Ranci (Ed.), *Social vulnerability in Europe: The new configuration of social risks* (pp. 219–249). Basingstoke: Palgrave Macmillan.

Reimer, M. (2001). *Die Zuverlässigkeit des autobiographischen Gedächtnisses und die Validität retrospektiv erhobener Lebensverlaufsdaten.* Berlin: Max-Planck-Insitut für Bildungsforschung.

Ricoeur, P. (1985). *Temps et récit. Tome: Le temps raconté.* Paris: Le Seuil.

Sayles, H., Belli, R. F., & Serrano, E. (2010). Interviewer variance between event history calendar and conventional questionnaire interviews. *Public Opinion Quarterly, 74*(1), 140–153.

Schutz, A. (1962). *Collected papers.* The Hague: Martinus Nijhoff.

Scott, J., & Alwyn, D. F. (1998). Retrospective vs prospective measurement of life histories in longitudinal research. In J. Z. Giele & G. H. Elder (Eds.), *Methods in life course research. Qualitative and quantitative approaches* (pp. 98–127). Thousand Oaks: Sage.

Sennett, R. (2011). *The corrosion of character: The personal consequences of work in the new capitalism.* New York: WW Norton & Company.

Sutton, J. E., Bellair, P. E., Kowalski, B. R., Hutcherson, D. T., & Hutcherson, D. T. (2011). Reliability and validity of prisoner self-reports gathered using the life event calendar method. *Journal of Quantitative Criminology, 27*, 151–171.

Tourangeau, R., Rips, L. J., & Rasinski, K. (2000). *The psychology of survey response.* Cambridge: Cambridge University Press.

Van der Vaart, W. (2004). The timeline as a device to enhance recall in standardized research interviews: A split ballot study. *Journal of Official Statistics, 20*(2), 301–317.

Vivier, G. (2006). Comment collecter des biographies? De la fiche Ageven aux grilles biographiques, Principes de collecte et Innovations recentes. *Population et travail Dynamique et Travail*, 119–131.

Widmer, E. (2010). *Family configurations: A structural approach to family diversity.* Ashgate Publishing, Ltd.

Yoshihama, M., Gillespie, B., Hammock, A. C., Belli, R. F., & Tolman, R. M. (2005). Does the LHC method facilitate the recall of intimate partner violence? Comparison of two methods of data collection. *Social Work Research, 29*, 151.

Studying Youth Transitions Through a Social Network: First Impressions

Véronique Eicher, Mouna Bakouri, Christian Staerklé, Marlene Carvalhosa Barbosa, and Alain Clémence

1 The Study of Youth Transitions

Young adulthood is a period during which many important life transitions in the professional and educational domain occur, for example choosing an educational track, passing selection procedures into higher education, selecting an occupation, finding a job (e.g., Fleeson and Cantor 1995; Pimentel 1996). It has been shown that successful or unsuccessful regulation of these transitions influences future transitional choices and actions (Heckhausen and Schulz 1995; Nurmi 1993). The transitional choices, as well as the way young individuals deal with developmental tasks and challenges, are influenced by various factors, ranging from the available choices and perceived opportunities to specific regulation strategies of failures to differential levels of vulnerability (e.g., Salmela-Aro 2009). The present study focuses on the relationship between different types of vulnerability (internal and external), regulation strategies, and life transitions in young adults aged 15–30 years. We specifically investigate how young people manage professional and educational transitions, in particular transitions from school to higher education and from school or vocational training to first employment. We assume these transitions to be influenced by different levels of internal and external vulnerability, as well as by different types of regulation strategies. External vulnerability refers to factual aspects like material (e.g., low income) or categorical (e.g., member of

V. Eicher (✉)
Social Work, Zurich University of Applied Sciences, Zurich, Switzerland

NCCR LIVES, IP 9, Chavannes-près-Renens, Switzerland
e-mail: eicr@zhaw.ch

M. Bakouri • C. Staerklé • M.C. Barbosa • A. Clémence
NCCR LIVES, IP 9, Chavannes-près-Renens, Switzerland

Institute of Psychology, University of Lausanne, Lausanne, Switzerland

© The Author(s) 2016
M. Oris et al. (eds.), *Surveying Human Vulnerabilities across the Life Course*,
Life Course Research and Social Policies 3, DOI 10.1007/978-3-319-24157-9_9

lower status group) vulnerability that increase the likelihood of negative events and decrease the number of opportunities (e.g., Eccles 1994; Pascoe and Richman 2009). Internal vulnerability, in turn, refers to the internalization of factual vulnerabilities affecting people's sense of agency, efficacy and motivation that can be expressed as psychological (e.g., perceived lack of control) or relational (e.g., perceived lack of social support) forms of vulnerability (Eccles and Wigfield 2002; Salmela-Aro 2009). Different types of regulation strategies include the attribution of success and goal selection and adjustment (e.g., Brandstädter 2009; Heckhausen 1999) (i.e., cognitive-motivational strategies), in-group identification and endorsement of collective norms (e.g., Turner et al. 1994) (i.e., group-based strategies), as well as ideological beliefs and political activism (e.g., Staerklé 2009) (i.e., political-institutional strategies).

The online network to be described in this chapter was intended to provide the opportunity to investigate two research questions understood as instances of *group-based* regulation of developmental tasks and life transitions (i.e., exchange with others, identification with significant others). In order to be as close to participants' everyday life and their preferred communication tools as possible, we designed an *online social network*, which would allow participants to communicate with each other on topics of their own choosing. In the following, we first give the theoretical background of the two research questions before presenting the *methodology* with which we planned to investigate these group-based regulatory strategies.

1.1 Research Questions Related to the Online Social Network

In line with developmental research demonstrating the importance of co-regulation in dealing with life course transitions (Salmela-Aro 2009), we expected *exchange of experiences* with individuals facing similar challenges to be a central regulatory strategy. Sharing the struggles and fears, but also successes of life course transitions may indeed be beneficial for both sides. 'Talking' about one's experience may help to better understand and cope with it. 'Hearing' about other people's experiences can procure a sense of sharedness, knowing that other people face similar difficulties.

Prior research has analysed whether online social networks are associated with social capital and exchange with friends in general. For instance, it has been shown that people who use Facebook often have more *bridging* capital (i.e., weak ties with dissimilar others that may provide information but no emotional support; Putnam 2000) independent of their level of self-esteem or life satisfaction, while less intensive Facebook users with lower self-esteem or satisfaction indicate less bridging capital (Ellison et al. 2007). In an extension of this study, Steinfield et al. (2008) showed that Facebook use led to more bridging social capital 1 year later, rather than the other way around.

Bonding capital, in contrast, refers to social connectedness with similar others, typically in-group members. This "feeling of belonging to a social group" (Köbler et al. 2010, p. 2) has been studied in association with Facebook use where it was shown that the more people post information on social networks, the more connected they feel to others (Köbler et al. 2010). When asked why they are on Facebook, users indicated mostly social motives like connecting with others and meeting like-minded people (only a small group of people indicated using Facebook mainly for playing games). Additionally, they liked to tell others about what happened to them and to look at what others were doing (Joinson 2008). Online social networks are thus used as a facilitator for social relationships. Introverted individuals and those with lower self-esteem for example indicate using the network mainly to build new relationships and considering online communication as more effective for developing in-depth communication than face-to-face interactions (Valkenburg and Peter 2007; Valkenburg et al. 2005).

Beyond the beneficial aspect of enlarging the social network and sharing experiences, Valenzuela et al. (2009) investigated the association between Facebook use and different well-being outcomes. They showed that, although these effects were not large, Facebook use was positively associated with social trust, life satisfaction, political participation, and civic engagement. These findings suggest that use of social networks does not lead to social isolation – as is often proclaimed by "cyberpessimists" (Valenzuela et al. 2009, p. 893) – but can even have beneficial effects on real-life interactions. Overall, these studies point to the usefulness of online networks to strengthen and widen the social network and the perceived importance of social interactions. We thus assumed that participants may want to share their transition experiences with others and extend their network to similar others. As a first research question, we are therefore *interested in the role of exchange of experiences with other individuals facing similar transitions in life course regulation and its implications for well-being*.

A second major research question concerns the role of *identification with significant others* as a way to cope with difficult transitional demands. Social-psychological theories concerned with the psychological manifestations of group membership (i.e., Social Identity Theory, Self-Categorization Theory) analyse how individuals shift between personal and social identities as a function of their memberships in social groups (e.g., Tajfel 1978; Turner et al. 1987). Identifying oneself with a group can provide social support such that difficult or negative experiences may be better regulated when one feels like a member of a group (e.g., Outten et al. 2009).

One of the first social psychological studies of computer-mediated communication (CMC) analysed communication patterns in computer-mediated vs. face-to-face settings (Kiesler et al. 1984). The authors showed that participants interacted more equally (there were fewer dominant individuals) in CMC and suggested that, because dominance and group information are less visible over computer, computer-mediated interactions may be more equal and less influenced by existing group differences. This quite optimistic view of CMC – of breaking down social barriers and norms – has been questioned by the Social Identity model of Deindividuation

Effects (SIDE; Reicher et al. 1995). Here, anonymity and deindividuation make the social identity more salient and thus provoke strong reliance on the norms of the in-group and a rejection of the out-group rather than a breakdown of social barriers (Postmes et al. 1998). Thus, it appears that the anonymity of CMC, and thus of social networks, does not eliminate existing group boundaries. Rather, it leads to an emphasis of social identity that transforms an interpersonal interaction into an intergroup interaction, thus re-establishing the group boundaries found in real life. Such a view is supported by a study on the formation of group norms in CMC carried out over several months in the context of a computerized statistics course (Postmes et al. 2006). In this study, groups of students differed from each other with regard to length of messages, time frame of messages or the number of references to oneself, for instance. Analysing the messages over time, the authors found that they tended to get more prototypical for each group over time, but only for communication among group members: When participants sent messages to an out-group, their messages were not prototypical for their group. All of these studies point to the salience of group identities in CMC and suggest similar group effects in online social networks. We therefore examine *the role of group identification in the context of online social networks and analyse whether this identification helps individuals to cope with the demands of life transitions.*

1.2   Outline of the Study Methodology

The present study on youth transitions follows a longitudinal mixed-methods design over a period of at least 4 years during which participants are contacted once a year. All participants first complete a *questionnaire*, assessing a broad range of different types of vulnerability and regulation strategies as well as transitional projects and life course goals. In this questionnaire, they are asked for their email address and a username for their registration to the online social network. For all participants who indicate an email address a user account is created in the *online social network* of the study. Besides the analysis of the role of communicational exchange and social identification in life course regulation, the social network is also used as a way to stay in contact with the participants for the duration of the study. Finally, a small subgroup of participants is selected for in-depth *interviews* about their use of specific regulation strategies.

We use these different methods of data collection to answer different types of research questions, but also to adapt our methodology as much as possible to commonly-used communication channels of participants. They are young adults aged 15–30 years who are in a more or less vulnerable position regarding their professional trajectory (i.e., some already have stable employment, while others have trouble even finding an apprenticeship place) and their level of education (ranging from compulsory schooling to university diploma). The network may thus help to encourage participation by young adults who may not be used to completing questionnaires and writing texts.

2 Online Social Networks

Online social networks have become increasingly popular among young adults as a method of connecting with peers. The first online social networks were created in the 1990s and became a mass phenomenon during the 2000s with the creation of MySpace, Facebook, Google+, etc. Today, the most widely used online social network, Facebook, has more than 900 million users (ranging from 5 % of the total population in Africa to 45 % of the total population in North America), half of which log in every day (Socialbakers 2012). In Switzerland, where our study was conducted, approximately 40 % of the population has a Facebook account, a percentage that rises to more than 75 % among young adults (16–34 years old) (Socialbakers 2012). These statistics suggest at the very least a widespread use of computer-mediated communications tools among young adults.

2.1 Reasons for Using an Online Social Network in a Study on Youth Transitions

The assumption that a *majority of young adults in Switzerland uses online social networks* was one of the key reasons why we decided to use this method. In contrast to standardized questionnaires, an online network would give participants the opportunity to express themselves via a media they are supposedly comfortable with and used to. And as we are particularly interested in more vulnerable populations, this option seemed even more important: Instead of frightening off (or boring) participants with standardized questions, we wanted to give them the possibility to participate in the study with the method they often use to communicate with others.

A second major reason to use an online social network was its *flexibility as a method of data collection*. Participants can use the network whenever they want for as long as they want. This permits a completely flexible time schedule both for participants and for researchers. Participants could 'talk' about their experiences as soon as they happen instead of several weeks or months later (when researchers happen to collect data). This immediacy might minimize recall effects, which are often particularly strong for emotional experiences (Thomas and Diener 1990). The same way that participants can choose freely when to use the network, researchers can use the network flexibly to ask questions and stimulate discussions at different time points. The flexibility of networks is not limited to the temporal aspect, but also extends to the format of the data collection. Researchers can post closed and open-ended questions, invite participants for one-item-polls, invite discussions on specific topics and so on. The network thus offers a more flexible way to study different topics than questionnaires and interviews typically allow.

A third advantage of the online social network is the ease of contacting *the participants*. Our participants are young adults who experience many life transitions, like starting a new school or job, moving out of the parental home or moving in with a partner or friends. This period in life is thus marked by many changes, which can make it more difficult to stay in contact with participants. By using participants' email address to create an account on an online social network, participants could be contacted independently of employment changes or moving house. If participants change their email address, they can adapt this in their user account, making the continuity of the account potentially independent of changes in people's lives.

Another reason that led to the decision of the creation of an online social network was to increase the *fidelity of participants* over the course of the study. Through an online social network we hoped to be able to stay in contact with them, so they would not have forgotten about the study by the time they were next contacted. Additionally, we wanted to increase identification with our study through direct interaction with participants, a strategy also intended to decrease attrition rates.

2.2   Reasons for Creating a New Online Social Network

In order to build a strong study identity for our study, we wanted to create a new online social network for which we were able to decide the layout and the functions and connect it with a public website for the study. The new network would be closely linked to our study and by using the network, participants would also identify with the study itself, thus ensuring continuous participation.

The second major reason for creating a new network was to have a network that is exclusive to the participants in our study. All participants enter the network without previous and outside contacts and can focus solely on other participants of the study. In existing networks, people are already connected with other people and often have already developed a specific behavioural pattern on how to use the network. By creating a new network, we would be able to give all participants the same 'starting point' and could also analyse relevant behaviours of co-regulation that would have been difficult to study in an existing network (e.g., newly formed connections between individuals, creation of groups around specific topics).

A final reason for not relying on an existing network relates to data privacy. If we had integrated the study within an existing network, it would not have been possible to guarantee participants the privacy of their data, as it would be owned by the specific network. By creating our own network, we are able to ensure that participants' data is not used for commercial purposes and is solely used for research purposes within the research group.

3   The Online Social Network "Projet Expériences"

In this section, we present the online social network created for the purposes of the present study, named "Projet Expériences". First, we describe the concrete decisions and steps we took in the creation of the network. Then, we give an overview over some of the functions of the network and indicate how they relate to our research questions. In a third subsection, we show first results based on 365 participants. Finally, we conclude with the difficulties faced in the creation and maintenance of the network.

3.1   Building the Network: Steps, Choices, and Difficulties

Various functional goals determined the planning and the construction of the network. We wanted to be able to post closed and open-ended questions and short polls (i.e., flexibility of data collection), contact participants easily through a website and newsletters (i.e., ease of access to participants) and control access to the network (data privacy). Access control was also intended to link the network closely to the study and thus strengthen identification with it. Additionally, to study our research questions, we needed to create a platform, where participants could post texts and media contents (e.g., pictures, videos, music) to everyone or just the research team, as well as interact with other users online through friendship connections and exchange private and public messages. Finally, we wanted the network to be similar to existing networks so that participants would feel comfortable and experienced in using it.

We started exploring the different possibilities for creating a social networking platform, inspired by the features of the most popular existing ones (Facebook and Twitter). Giving the current success of online communities, many Content Management Systems (CMS) are freely available on the internet. CMS are applications providing tools for creating, editing, and publishing web content for non-expert users (among the most used CMSs are Drupal, Joomla, and Wordpress). The main difficulty was to compare and choose between the different options, as there are many different applications and plug-ins (software components that add specific functions) and it thus takes time to explore the advantages, compatibility and performance of each one. Together with the IT team of the university of Lausanne, we decided to use Wordpress, as the IT centre already had experience with the must-have plug-ins for this CMS and was ready to collaborate in the construction of the network.

3.2   Building Our Online Social Network Using Wordpress

Wordpress is a free and open-source software allowing the creation of blogs and websites. With the multitude of plug-ins available, Wordpress is also able to transform a website into a real network. We made sure that all the features we wanted were possible with this CMS and checked with the IT team that we had the necessary system requirements to use it. Before installing WordPress, we had to define our domain name and register it on a domain registration website (e.g., GoDaddy). The domain name should reflect the content of the website, be easy to remember and of course be available. As our project was interested in young people's life experiences, we chose "ProjetExperiences.ch" (i.e., project experiences).

As we wanted to include social networking features in addition to simple blogs, we installed Buddypress, a powerful plug-in for Wordpress that enables participants to interact with each other and transforms Wordpress into a social network platform. Before we customized our website and social network, we chose a theme that handles the layout of the site and its content and determines the features available on the platform. We chose "Buddypress social" as it allows us to display different pages to users who are signed in versus others who are not. This way, we were able to make the description and results of our project public to all visitors, while restraining the social network part (e.g., profiles and activities of participants) to logged users. This theme allows additional interaction features like displaying the most commented posts and the most popular groups, improving the interactive experience of the network. The only disadvantage of this theme is that it is not free (around $100 per year). After installing the theme, we created the different pages of our public website, which is visible to everyone without registration. On this public website, we describe our project, present the research team and give regular updates on the results of the project. We also present the social network and shortly describe its main functions and uses. On this public website, we also suggest a calendar with regional events that could be of interest to our participants. Finally, we offer them "Useful links", a list of relevant websites (associative, informative, pedagogical or preventive) that may be useful for education, hobbies or health. After this public, and more classic, part of the platform, we customized the network using Buddypress plug-ins.

3.2.1 Functions (and Related Plug-Ins)

Buddypress is an elaborate plug-in with many features that can be individually activated. We outline the different functions and describe the features of Buddypress required for each function.

Participants can *update their profile* using a variety of categories, like favourite films and books, and they can also give a brief description of themselves. The profile can give interesting information on how the participants define themselves and if they identify with specific groups (e.g., describing themselves as an apprentice or employee at a specific company). This function is possible with the feature "Extended Profiles".

The users can *make friend connections* by asking other users to be their friends. These connections are especially important for our research question on group identification as we can investigate if people make connections solely within their group (e.g., employees at a company) or if they try to enlarge their network by connecting with participants from other groups. This function is enabled by the feature "Friends".

The users can *post texts, links, pictures or videos* they want to share with other members of the network and their activities are then displayed on the network for other members to see. This function is central to our research as it allows participants to express themselves on their day-to-day-life, but also on specific experiences. Additionally, they can choose to comment on posts of other participants, which is interesting in the context of shared experiences: Do participants comment by sharing similar experiences, offer advice, give feedback, or do not respond at all? The feature "Activity stream" allows the display of recent activities of each member, while an additional plug-in "Buddypress Activity Plus" allows sharing links, pictures, and videos. In addition to posting public texts, participants can *send personal messages* to other users directly, which only they can see (like emails). This function is possible with the feature "Private messaging".

Finally, participants can *create and join groups* based on specific topics that may interest them. This function is also central for our research as participants can write or discuss about topics that may be of specific concern to them at that time (e.g., their apprenticeship, their boss, their relationships). We are interested to see if people will discuss about their experiences regarding specific topics and if so, how this discussion will develop: Will people actively encourage each other or give advice or will they passively tell their own experiences while not engaging in a discussion with others. Additionally, it will be interesting to see if the language used in such groups (e.g., positive vs. negative "atmosphere", abbreviations, longer vs. shorter texts) will be different from group to group (similarly to the emergence of norms in the statistics course by Postmes et al. 2006). Next to these public groups, participants can also create private groups, which are only visible to the participant and the research team. Here, participants can talk about private experiences or use it as a diary to document their everyday life and events. This final function is enabled through the feature "Groups".

These plug-ins and features are integrated in the Buddypress package and are mostly designed to enrich the interpersonal and intergroup interactions, which was one of our priorities. To facilitate the management of our network we installed the following additional plug-ins, tested them and checked their compatibility with our BuddyPress theme: "Add New Users" (facilitates the addition of new users and attribution of different roles, e.g., subscriber for participants, administrator for research team), "Contact Form 7" (allows the creation of contact forms so participants and people interested on our project can easily contact us), "WP-polls" (enables the creation of quick polls on specific topics), "BP Redirect to profile for Buddypress" (redirects users to their profile and activity-page when they log in), and "Wysija Newsletters" (allows the design and creation of newsletters and makes it possible to import and manage our list of participants). Finally, we included "Connection attempts limit" to increase the security of our network: With this plug-in, we prevent individuals or a robot from making unlimited login attempts, making the network more secure against attacks from outsiders.

3.2.2 Network Preparation and Maintenance

Before registering the first users on our network, we *created several groups* on topics which we thought might be relevant to participants and would be interesting for us to collect data (e.g., my apprenticeship, my boss, my worries, my projects, feeling lonely). We wanted participants to join these groups, talk about their experiences in these different domains and discuss them with each other. We were interested to see how participants would talk about their experiences, how they would interpret them, but also how other users would react (e.g., by sharing their own experiences or offering their advice). Next to these research-relevant topics, we also created several groups around leisure-oriented topics to motivate participants to join the groups and discussions (e.g., music, sports, news, festivals, vacations). These groups are not primarily the focus of data collection, but were intended to give participants the possibility to exchange on less sensitive topics and to strengthen their fidelity to the network and the study.

Once the network was in use, we *sent out newsletters* to inform participants about new results of the study on the website and to announce the creation of new groups. We thereby wanted to remind participants of the network and the study and hoped to motivate them to log in by asking specific questions. Finally, we organised *raffles* (e.g., tickets for the movie theatre) to further motivate our participants to use the network.

With respect to *our role as researchers* on the network, all of the members of the research team had a user account with their first name and the mention "research team" in parentheses (e.g., Mouna (research team)). As such, we were readily identifiable by the participants as members of the research team. We updated our profile and sometimes posted comments in groups to stimulate the discussion. We could participate in discussions, but did not want to explicitly moderate the discussions between participants.

3.3   Some Results Regarding the Use of the Network

This section presents some preliminary results of the use of the network. The results are based on participants recruited from two institutions: The "Centre for Professional Formation and Orientation" (CPFO) and the "Municipality of Lausanne" (MOL). The CPFO is a centre for young adults who have difficulties finding an apprenticeship place or who do not know yet what type of apprenticeship they would like to do. Participants from this institution are thus particularly vulnerable regarding their professional trajectory. The MOL, in contrast, was chosen to get a comparison group of apprentices, as well as young employees, who are well integrated into the labour market. We were thus able to recruit participants at different stages of their professional development.

3.3.1 Participants and Procedure

Participants from the CPFO were either pre-apprentices or apprentices, and those from the MOL either apprentices or young employees aged 16–30. These four groups of participants differed with regard to their professional situation. The employees from the MOL were in stable employment with little job insecurity. In contrast to the employees, the apprentices from the MOL may not be employed by the MOL afterwards, but their apprenticeship at this institution is likely to give them good prospects for their job search after the apprenticeship. The apprentices from the CPFO were unable to find an apprenticeship within a company and were thus less integrated in the job market than their counterparts from the MOL. Finally, the pre-apprentices from the CPFO had usually not yet chosen their specific professional track yet or had trouble finding an apprenticeship. These four groups thus differ with respect to their present professional situation, but also in their prospects for finding a stable employment in the future.

At the CPFO, members of the research team personally presented the study with a short description of its goals and the different methods of participation to the pre-apprentices and apprentices during one of their courses. The website and network was also briefly shown to participants, along with some of its functions. All of the pre-apprentices and apprentices who attended the presentation completed the questionnaire, but the rate of course absenteeism was high (51.7 % for pre-apprentices, 31.9 % for apprentices).

At the MOL, participants were contacted with a letter describing the study and indicating the website of the study for further information, as well as a questionnaire with a return envelope. 28.9 % of the apprentices and 28.7 % of the employees completed the questionnaire. Table 1 indicates the socio-demographic characteristics of the sample of people who completed the first questionnaire.

3.3.2 Measures

The questionnaire included questions on regulation strategies and different types of vulnerability, as well as activities of young adults. Only the measures used in this chapter will be presented here.

Table 1 Means, standard deviations and percentages of socio-demographic variables of the sample that completed the first questionnaire

	CPFO		MOL		
	Pre-apprentices	Apprentices	Apprentices	Employees	Total
Age: M (SD)	16.68 (0.85)	19.35 (1.83)	19.07 (2.91)	26.42 (2.34)	22.24 (4.61)
Men: %	62.1	60.8	63.6	47.4	55.1
Swiss: %	43.9	53.2	78.2	89.0	72.7
N	58	79	55	173	365

Discrimination was assessed with one item, which was adapted from the European Social Survey: "Are you member of a group, which you believe is treated less well than other groups in Switzerland?" Answer options were *yes* (1) or *no* (0).

Financial worries were assessed with two items from the LIVES Daily Stress Inventory (Morselli et al. 2014). Participants reported to what degree they were worried about not having enough money to cover their living expenses (e.g., paying rent and bills) or needing financial aid (e.g., unemployment benefits, social aid). The items had to be rated on a scale from 1 (*it does not worry me at all*) to 4 (*it worries me a lot*).

Relational worries were assessed with two items from the LIVES Daily Stress Inventory (Morselli et al. 2014). Participants indicated to what extent they were worried about being alone or of having conflicts with family members on the same 4-point-scale as before.

Self-esteem was assessed with five items from the Rosenberg (1965) Self-Esteem scale, which had to be rated on a 6-point scale of 1 (*not at all*) to 6 (*absolutely*). One example item was "On the whole, I am satisfied with myself".

Lack of control was assessed with one item from the Perceived Stress Scale (Cohen et al. 1983), which had to be rated on a 6-point scale of 1 (*not at all*) to 6 (*absolutely*): "I feel that I am unable to control the important things in my life".

Internet use and computer access. In addition to these psychological questions, participants were asked about their use of internet and computer resources. They were asked what they did on the Internet and could select multiple answers: (1) read and write emails, (2) participate on an online social network, and (3) surf on websites. Additionally, they were asked how often they use the Internet on the following 5-point scale: 0 (*never or almost never*), 1 (*several times per month*), 2 (*several times per week*), 3 (*everyday*), and 4 (*several times per day*). Finally, they were asked whether they possessed or had easy access to a computer and/or a smartphone.

3.3.3 Who Has an Online Account?

In a first questionnaire, we asked all participants to indicate their name and contact details (i.e., postal and email address) to be able to contact them again. Additionally, we asked them to provide a username for the online social network. Of the 365 participants completing the questionnaire, 280 participants (76.7 %) indicated a valid email address so that we were able to create an account for each of them. In order to determine who is more or less likely to provide a valid email address, we ran a logistic regression analysis including socio-demographic variables in a first step and computer and internet use in a second step. In a final step we included the different types of vulnerability discussed in the introduction.

As our study focuses on vulnerability, it is important to know whether our methodology is adapted to our participants or if – on the contrary – the most vulnerable participants decide not to participate in the social network. We ran these analyses with the entire sample (*N* = 365 participants).

Table 2 Means, standard deviations and percentages of computer use and vulnerabilities of the whole sample ($N = 365$)

	CPFO		MOL		
	Pre-apprentices	Apprentices	Apprentices	Employees	Total
Access to					
Computer (%)	93.1	87.2	96.4	98.3	94.8
Smartphone (%)	41.4	50.0	76.4	75.6	64.7
Internet use					
Emails (%)	57.9	57.7	87.3	91.3	78.2
Social network (%)	80.7	80.8	89.1	75.6	79.6
Surfing (%)	73.7	76.9	90.7	94.8	87.0
Frequency (0–4)	2.85 (1.06)	2.96 (0.97)	3.41 (0.78)	3.47 (0.69)	3.25 (0.87)
Vulnerability					
External					
Discrimination (%)	26.8	11.3	18.2	30.8	24.3
Financial worries (1–4)	2.24 (0.88)	2.45 (0.79)	2.34 (0.82)	2.14 (0.81)	2.25 (0.82)
Internal					
Relational worries (1–4)	2.11 (0.98)	2.08 (0.93)	2.35 (0.89)	2.15 (0.90)	2.16 (0.92)
Self-esteem (1–6)	4.63 (0.99)	4.75 (0.93)	4.43 (0.79)	4.57 (0.71)	4.60 (0.82)
Lack of control (1–6)	2.61 (1.42)	2.63 (1.47)	2.27 (1.25)	2.30 (1.29)	2.41 (1.35)

Table 2 presents the means and standard deviations and percentages of computer and Internet use, as well as of the different vulnerability types. Table 3 shows the results of the logistic regression analysis on the indication of a valid email address.

The large majority of the participants owns a computer or has easy access to one, with employees from the MOL being more likely to have one than apprentices from the CPFO ($X^2(3) = 13.88, p = 0.003$). Participants from the MOL were more likely to own a smartphone than participants in the CPFO ($X^2 (3) = 33.40, p < 0.001$).

Regarding Internet use, the participants from the MOL read their emails and surfed on the Internet more than participants from the CPFO ($X^2 (3) = 52.90$, $p < 0.001$ and $X^2 (3) = 25.75, p < 0.001$). They also spent more time on the Internet (several times a day) than participants from CPFO (once a day, $F(3,359) = 12.30$, $p < 0.001$). Apprentices in the CPFO were less likely to report having experienced discrimination than employees from the MOL ($X^2 (3) = 11.83, p = 0.008$). This finding is surprising to the extent that the percentage of Non-Swiss is much higher in the CPFO than in the MOL. It therefore suggests that discrimination may be related to different groups within the different samples: Although most employees from the MOL are Swiss, they may be discriminated against based on gender, class, political orientation, and so on. There are no significant differences in the remaining vulnerabilities between the participants. All groups have relatively low levels of financial and relational (i.e., interpersonal) worries, as well as lack of control, while self-esteem is relatively high.

Table 3 Logistic regression analysis on the indication of a valid email address (unstandardized coefficients, standard errors and odds ratios) ($N = 365$)

DV: indication of valid email address	B	S.E.	Odds ratio	Sig.
Socio-demographic				
Age	0.12	0.073	1.12	0.112
Gender: Men	0.11	0.315	1.12	0.720
Nationality: Swiss	0.05	0.364	1.05	0.885
Group status				0.038
Group: Pre-apprentices CPFO	1.34	0.518	3.84	0.009
Group: Apprentices MOL	0.89	0.534	2.45	0.094
Group: Employees MOL	−0.45	0.655	0.64	0.490
Access to				
Computer	0.69	0.683	1.99	0.313
Smartphone	0.36	0.333	1.44	0.279
Internet use				
Emails	0.81	0.361	2.25	0.025
Social network	−0.16	0.380	0.85	0.674
Surfing	0.86	0.432	2.36	0.047
Frequency	0.22	0.192	1.25	0.251
Vulnerability				
External				
Discrimination	0.51	0.417	1.67	0.222
Financial worries	−0.35	0.204	0.70	0.083
Internal				
Relational worries	0.51	0.198	1.67	0.010
Self-esteem	−0.42	0.227	0.66	0.068
Lack of control	−0.02	0.129	0.98	0.876

Reference group for group status are apprentices from CPFO

Pre-apprentices from the CPFO (74.1 %) and apprentices from the MOL (85.5 %) were more likely to indicate a valid email address than apprentices from the CPFO (58.2 %). People who write emails and surf the Internet regularly were more likely to indicate an email address (81.7 % and 80.3 % respectively) than those who do not (60.8 % and 57.4 % respectively). Surprisingly, participating in an online social network had no impact on indicating a valid email address: Online social network users were neither more nor less likely to indicate an address (78.2 %) than others (73.0 %). Of the different types of vulnerability, financial worries were associated with lower likelihood of providing a valid email address, while relational worries predicted the indication of an email address positively. Additionally, people with high self-esteem were less likely to indicate a valid email address. These results suggest that people with internal vulnerabilities rather than material ones were especially interested in joining the online social network. Age, gender, and nationality did not have significant effects.

Table 4 Sample sizes and percentages of participants logging in and/or doing something on the network

	CPFO				MOL					
	Pre-apprentices		Apprentices		Apprentices		Employees		Total	
	N	%	N	%	N	%	N	%	N	%
Account	43	74.1	46	58.2	47	85.5	144	83.2	280	76.7
Log in: no	42	97.7	39	84.8	32	68.1	103	71.5	216	77.1
Log in: yes	1	2.3	7	15.2	15	31.9	41	28.5	64	22.9
Activity: no	0	0.0	1	14.3	11	73.3	34	82.9	46	71.9
Activity: yes	1	100.0	6	85.7	4	26.7	7	17.1	18	28.1

3.3.4 Who Uses the Online Account?

As mentioned above, an account was created for the 280 participants who provided a valid email address. We now turn to see who has been going online and/or been active on the network. Table 4 shows the sample size and percentages of participants logging in to the network and/or doing something on it.

The results show a dire picture of participation: Only about a quarter of the participants actually logged in at least once into the network. This percentage was low for pre-apprentices (2.3 %) and apprentices from the CPFO (15.2 %), while reaching almost a third for the participants from the MOL. This first step of actually logging into the network once is thus clearly a barrier for most participants.

The loss of participants at this stage may be due to two causes: (1) participants receive the username and are not interested to log into the network or (2) participants do not receive the username because the email address is not correct or they do not read their emails regularly.

Although we cannot determine the cause of the loss, the second explanation is supported by some indices. As we saw before, participants from the CPFO are much less likely than participants from the MOL to even log in even once, and they are also much less likely to regularly read their emails as indicated in Table 2. Additionally, when we sent an email to the winners of the first raffle, not all of the winners contacted us to collect their tickets, indicating that they may not have read the email in the first place (we asked them to verify their postal address so that we could send the tickets).

Interestingly, while the participants from the CPFO were much less likely to actually log in than participants from the MOL, once they did log in, almost all of them did something on the network. The opposite was true for participants from the MOL who were more likely to have a look around without doing anything. To investigate who is more likely to actually go online (independently of doing something or not), we ran a logistic regression analysis on those who had logged in at least once (as opposed to those who never logged in) including the same predictors as before. The only significant predictor was group status: Apprentices from the MOL ($O.R. = 12.13$, $p = 0.024$) and employees from the MOL ($O.R. = 8.25$, $p = 0.084$) were more likely to go online than those from the CPFO. None of the vulnerability types predicted more or less use of the network.

3.4 Difficulties

These findings show without ambiguity that participants are very reluctant to log in to the network to begin with, and when they do so, that it is highly likely that they will leave without leaving any trace. For the first log-in to the network, for example, more than two-thirds of the participants are lost. The difficulty of this participant loss is that we cannot determine whether people do not receive the log-in details and therefore do not log in, or whether they do receive them, but are not motivated to log in. Of those who do log in, only a small percentage of participants actively does something (those from the CPFO were somewhat more active than those from the MOL). These findings underscore the necessity to motivate participants actively and interactively, at least in the beginning, to join and to be active on the network. We tried to do this with raffles for network participants and asking questions for specific topic groups, but these measures can only be effective if participants actually read their emails.

Most of the activity on the network happens in areas less oriented towards research: Participants mostly updated their profile with a picture and their favourite music or sports, but without any self-description or discussion that could have been used for research purposes. Some joined groups without posting something and none actually joined the research-related groups at all. The fact that most activity happened in non-research-related domains like uploading pictures and joining "fun" groups does not, however, mean that the network cannot be used for research purposes. Participants may want to get used to the network and meet fellow users doing fun activities before posting personal comments on topics, which may be more sensitive (e.g., worries, projects).

Finally, the creation and maintenance of the network requires a considerable amount of *time* as well as *technical skill and knowledge*. Although the CMS in general, and Wordpress and Buddypress specifically, are developed for non-experts, users still need to invest time and effort to make such a network work. The utility of all the features and plug-ins, as well as their compatibility with each other, need to be tested and re-tested. Before going online, we did a pilot study with around 50 colleagues to see if the network and all the functions would work as they should. Now that the network is online, we still need to update the software and its plug-ins regularly to ensure the effective functioning of the website. Time is also needed for the regular update of the network and website. The calendar of regional events needs to be updated every few weeks and we try to create new groups around current topics to keep participants interested.

4 Conclusion and Future Directions

There can only be one conclusion with respect to the use of newly created social networks for research purposes, and it is rather disappointing: It is exceedingly difficult to attract participants to log in and then to use the network, not to mention to bring them to contribute to the network on a regular basis and to interact with others in a scientifically exploitable way. With hindsight, it may well be that as researchers we were overly optimistic not to say blinded by the scientific possibilities of a network and at the same time not sensitive enough to real-life constraints of young adults. Or more simply, the expectations of researchers were fundamentally incompatible with the everyday motivations of participants. We have the impression we did everything we could in order to set up an attractive and functional network only to observe that it did not make much of a difference. This outcome just seems to show that successful implementations of "high-tech" solutions to study social science problems require a tremendous amount of preparation, organisation and communication, and thus funding.

But not everything is lost. There are several possibilities that could make the network more attractive to young adults. First, with the necessary funding, it would be possible to financially compensate active participation in the network according to clear guidelines, thereby potentially creating a self-sustaining dynamic within the network.

Second, the network could be opened to the public at large so that the participants of our study could also communicate with their friends or other persons who do not participate in the study. This would make the network even more similar to the usual social networks with the advantage, however, that we would maintain data privacy. Opening up the network could also lead to a transformation of the website into a network on life transitions in general where individuals could share their experiences and life events. Websites, which follow a similar procedure are www.experienceproject.com and www.microaggressions.com for instance, which are regularly visited by people all over the world to "talk" about their everyday experiences.

Third, we might focus the network on topics that are most relevant to our participants. For instance, we could focus on topics like finding an apprenticeship position for pre-apprentices, thus creating a platform that has also practical instead of only scientific goals. Such a network would maybe also send a message to participants that the research team is sensitive to issues of concern for participants. We are presently evaluating these different options aimed at reinventing the network. The future will show whether these changes result in a different user behaviour among young participants, thus making it possible to address our original research questions.

References

Brandtstädter, J. (2009). Goal pursuit and goal adjustment: Self-regulation and intentional self-development in changing developmental contexts. *Advances in Life Course Research, 14*, 52–62.

Cohen, S., Kamarck, T., & Mermelstein, R. (1983). A global measure of perceived stress. *Journal of Health and Social Behavior, 24*, 385–39.

Eccles, J. S. (1994). Understanding women's educational and occupational choices. *Psychology of Women Quarterly, 18*, 585–609.

Eccles, J. S., & Wigfield, A. (2002). Motivational beliefs, values, and goals. *Annual Review of Psychology, 53*, 109–132.

Ellison, N. B., Steinfield, C., & Lampe, C. (2007). The benefits of Facebook "friends:" Social capital and college students' use of online social network sites. *Journal of Computer-Mediated Communication, 12*, 1143–1168.

Fleeson, W., & Cantor, N. (1995). Goal relevance and the affective experience of daily life: Ruling out situational explanations. *Motivation and Emotion, 19*, 25–57.

Heckhausen, J. (1999). *Developmental regulation in adulthood. Age-normative and sociostructural constraints as adaptative challenges.* Cambridge: Cambridge University Press.

Heckhausen, J., & Schulz, R. (1995). A life-span theory of control. *Psychological Review, 102*, 284–304.

Joinson, A. N. (2008). *Looking at, looking up or keeping up with people? Motives and use of facebook.* Florence: Online Social Networks.

Kiesler, S., Siegel, J., & McGuire, T. W. (1984). Social psychological aspects of computer-mediated communication. *American Psychologist, 39*, 1123–1134.

Köbler, F., Riedl, C., Vetter, C., Leimeister, J. M., Krcmar, H. (2010). *Social connectedness on facebook–an explorative study on status message usage.* Proceedings of 16th Americas Conference on Information Systems. Lima.

Morselli, D., et al. (2014). *LIVES Daily Stress Inventory.* Manuscript in preparation.

Nurmi, J.-E. (1993). Adolescent development in an age-graded context: The role of personal beliefs, goals and strategies in the tackling of developmental tasks and standards. *International Journal of Behavioral Development, 16*, 169–189.

Outten, H. R., Schmitt, M. T., Garcia, D. M., & Branscombe, N. R. (2009). Coping options: Missing links between minority group identification and psychological well-being. *Applied Psychology: An International Review, 58*, 146–170.

Pascoe, E. A., & Smart Richman, L. (2009). Perceived discrimination and health: A meta-analytic review. *Psychological Bulletin, 135*, 531–554.

Pimentel, E. E. (1996). Effects of adolescent achievement and family goals on the early adult transition. In J. T. Mortimer & M. D. Finch (Eds.), *Adolescents work and family: An intergenerational developmental analyses* (pp. 191–220). Thousands Oaks: Sage.

Postmes, T., Spears, R., & Lea, M. (1998). Breaching or building social boundaries? SIDE-effects of computer-mediated communication. *Communication Research, 25*, 689–715.

Postmes, T., Spears, R., & Lea, M. (2006). The formation of group norms in computer-mediated communication. *Human Communication Research, 26*, 341–371.

Putnam, R. D. (2000). *Bowling alone: The collapse and revival of American community.* New York: Simon & Schuster.

Reicher, S. D., Spears, R., & Postmes, T. (1995). A social identity model of deindividuation phenomena. *European Review of Social Psychology, 6*, 161–198.

Rosenberg, M. (1965). *Society and the adolescent self-image.* Princeton: Princeton University Press.

Salmela-Aro, K. (2009). Personal goals and well-being during critical life transitions: The four C's-Channelling, choice, co-agency and compensation. *Advances in Life Course Research, 14*, 63–73.

Socialbakers. (2012). *Switzerland facebook statistics*. Retrieved from: http://www.socialbakers. com/facebook-statistics/switzerland

Staerklé, C. (2009). Policy attitudes, ideological values and social representations. *Social and Personality Psychology Compass, 3*, 1096–1112.

Steinfield, C., Ellison, N. B., & Lampe, C. (2008). Social capital, self-esteem, and use of online social network sites: A longitudinal analysis. *Journal of Applied Developmental Psychology, 29*, 434–445.

Tajfel, H. (1978). *The social psychology of minorities*. London: Minority Rights Group.

Thomas, D. L., & Diener, E. (1990). Memory accuracy in the recall of emotions. *Journal of Personality and Social Psychology, 59*, 291–297.

Turner, J. C., Hogg, M. A., Oakes, P. J., Reicher, S. D., & Wetherell, M. S. (1987). *Rediscovering the social group: A self-categorization theory*. Oxford: Blackwell.

Turner, J. C., Oakes, P. J., Haslam, S. A., & McGarty, C. (1994). Self and collective: Cognition and social context. *Personality and Social Psychology Bulletin, 20*, 454–454.

Valenzuela, S., Park, N., & Kee, K. F. (2009). Is there social capital in a social network site? Facebook use and college students' life satisfaction, trust, and participation. *Journal of Computer-Mediated Communication, 14*, 875–901.

Valkenburg, P. M., & Peter, J. (2007). Preadolescents' and adolescents' online communication and their closeness to friends. *Developmental Psychology, 43*, 267–277.

Valkenburg, P. M., Schouten, A. P., & Peter, J. (2005). Adolescents' identity experiments on the internet. *New Media and Society, 7*, 383–402.

Attrition in the Swiss Household Panel: Are Vulnerable Groups more Affected than Others?

Martina Rothenbühler and Marieke Voorpostel

1 Introduction

One of the major difficulties of longitudinal surveys is panel attrition, the loss of panel members from one wave to the next. Attrition can lead to selective samples and make the interpretation of estimates problematic. The central concern in the analysis of attrition is therefore selection bias, that is, a distortion of the estimation results due to non-random patterns of attrition. Attrition may be especially problematic for vulnerable populations that are more difficult to survey, as they are more likely to drop out of panel surveys.

A common distinction is made between attrition that is completely at random, attrition that is selective on variables observed in the data and attrition that is selective on variables unobserved in the data. If the attrition is random, then the erosion of the sample does not lead to biased estimates. However, in most cases the attrition is non-random (Alderman et al. 2001). If attrition introduces a bias in the estimates of interest, selective attrition on observable variables is more amenable to statistical solutions than attrition on unobserved variables. Weighting strategies can help to reduce or even completely repair the effects of attrition on estimations. Using information from prior waves to model appropriate weights can contribute to reducing the amount of unexplained variation in the data due to attrition, but selective attrition on unobservable variables remains a problem.

M. Rothenbühler (✉)
Clinical Trials Unit, University of Bern, Bern, Switzerland

Swiss Centre of Expertise in the Social Sciences FORS, Lausanne, Switzerland
e-mail: martina.rothenbuehler@ctu.unibe.ch

M. Voorpostel
Swiss Centre of Expertise in the Social Sciences FORS, Lausanne, Switzerland

© The Author(s) 2016
M. Oris et al. (eds.), *Surveying Human Vulnerabilities across the Life Course*,
Life Course Research and Social Policies 3, DOI 10.1007/978-3-319-24157-9_10

We investigate the problem of attrition using the Swiss Household Panel (SHP). The SHP is a longitudinal survey with annual repetition and its main objective is the analysis of socio-economic change within households, in particular the dynamics of living conditions of the population in Switzerland.

In this contribution, we present two kinds of attrition analysis: first we show in Sect. 4 how variables can be affected by attrition by comparing means and frequencies of the answers given in the first wave by all respondents (all longitudinal sample members) with the longitudinal sample members still participating at a later wave. We also assess to what extent the use of weights correct for any bias. Second, we show which sociodemographic characteristics are most related to attrition patterns. This second part focuses on the relation between indicators of latent vulnerability and panel attrition and is addressed in Sect. 5. Using a discrete-time competing risk model, we analyse the impact of these variables on the dropout probability. Before turning to the analytical part, we describe in Sect. 2 the relation between being at risk of vulnerability and several demographic characteristics by using different theoretical approaches and point out how in turn these characteristics are related to attrition by presenting results from other studies. In Sect. 3 we give a short overview of the data used for our analyses. The last part of this contribution, Sect. 6 concludes the chapter by discussing the potential and limits of both analysing and countering selective attrition.

2   Attrition in Relation to Vulnerability

Nonresponse and panel attrition may be especially a problem for vulnerable populations. In this study we define people as vulnerable or at risk of being vulnerable if they possess traits that position them in low levels within the socioeconomic stratification. Several characteristics related to participation in surveys are associated with vulnerability, such as having a lower level of education, foreign nationality, being unemployed, in poor health, or being divorced (Loosveldt and Carton 2001; Kleiner et al. 2012; Stoop 2005; Watson and Wooden 2009). These characteristics indicate latent vulnerability; they tend to go together with a deficit in resources, creating a risky environment.

There are several reasons why vulnerable groups are in general more likely to drop out of surveys.

First, some vulnerable groups may be more difficult to locate or to contact, especially if they are more likely to move. For example, negative life events such as divorce usually involve the move of at least one of the partners, increasing the risk of losing track of the respondent. Unemployed and inactive people, older people, and people with children are more likely to be found at home, and these groups tend to include more women (Stoop 2005; Watson and Wooden 2009).

After locating and contacting sample members, they still have to be willing to cooperate. In making their decision sample members take the costs and benefits associated with participating into account (Dillman et al. 2002). Vulnerable groups may expect higher costs and lower benefits for several reasons. First, expected benefits may be lower or the costs higher if past experiences in a previous wave have been unpleasant, thereby decreasing the likelihood of participation (Loosveldt and Carton 2001). Respondents from vulnerable groups, such as those who experience a combination of factors such as unemployment, poverty and health problems, may experience talking about their negative situations as unpleasant, making the interview situation uncomfortable.

Another reason is that certain vulnerable groups may lack the skills needed to successfully complete the survey and make it a pleasant experience. Loosveldt and Carton (2001) provide evidence that participation in the second wave of a panel study is related to the respondent's ability to perform the task; an ability that is found to be lower for less educated respondents (Loosveldt 1997). Also language proficiency is an important skill necessary to successfully participate in an interview, which poses problems when interviewing certain minority groups (Kleiner et al. 2012).

Finally, benefits of participation are expected to be lower for groups who are less socially integrated, which is related to vulnerability as well. Studies have shown social integration and isolation to be correlated with the likelihood of responding to surveys (Stoop 2005; Watson and Wooden 2009). For the SHP, this correlation has been established in earlier studies as well (Lipps 2007; Voorpostel 2010). People who score high on social integration are more likely to participate in surveys for several reasons. One reason is that they tend to be guided by the norms of the dominant culture, in which participation in a survey may be seen as a "civic duty" (Dillman et al. 2002; Johnson et al. 2002). Second, less social integration is related to more cynicism about established institutions, an attitude which expected to influence response rates to surveys as well Stoop (2005). Third, individuals who score higher on social integration are more likely to find the topics that are usually covered in surveys relevant or important. One potentially useful indicator of social involvement is political interest. Research has shown that politically interested people are more cooperative irrespective of the survey topic (Stoop 2005). Possibly a wide variety of topics covered in most surveys are of interest to members' level of interest, however, is also judged on experiences made in previous waves. Generally speaking, more interest in the topic will lead to a higher probability of responding Groves et al. (2000, 2004).

Many of the usual background characteristics in nonresponse analyses can be linked to these processes behind non contact and noncooperation. For instance, employed people and people with a higher socio-economic status are often harder to contact, as they are less often found at home, but they are more willing to cooperate than people from a lower socio-economic stratum or unemployed people, as employed people and people with a higher socio-economic status might have better skills, experience lower opportunity costs and be more interested in the survey. Also, holding a paid job can be perceived as a way of participating in society, whereas unemployed people face more social isolation (Gallie and Paugam 2004). Older people, on the other hand, are easier to contact, because they are more likely to be at home, but they tend to be more reluctant to cooperate. Some groups are harder to contact and more reluctant to cooperate, such as men, singles, ethnic minorities, younger persons, and big city dwellers (Stoop 2005).

In Sect. 5 we examine the importance of several factors related to attrition and latent vulnerability, most importantly age, education, income, working status, civil status, nationality, health and political interest. In addition we also include gender, the presence of children in the household and whether the respondent is a home owner or a tenant. It should be noted that our indicators of latent vulnerability are not absolute proof of vulnerability, but only provide an indication of being potentially at risk for vulnerability.

3 Data

The analyses in this chapter are based on the Swiss Household Panel (SHP). Currently, the SHP consists of three samples. The first sample SHP_I started in 1999, when 5074 households were interviewed for the first time. In 2004 a refresher sample was added with 2538 additional households (SHP_II). The third sample (SHP_III) started in 2013. The interviews are done both at the household and the individual level using the computer assisted telephone interviewing (CATI) method. Every household member aged at least 14 is eligible to answer to the individual questionnaire.

In 2012, that is the 14th wave of SHP_I and the 9th wave of SHP_II, the combined panel SHP_I and SHP_II contained 4390 households. The SHP_I counted 2923 households who answered to the household questionnaire. This corresponds to 58 % of the number of household interviews conducted in the first wave in 1999. The second panel, SHP_II, had 1467 valid household questionnaires in 2012. This is also equivalent to 58 % of the number of household interviews conducted in 2004. In terms of personal interviews, there were 7446 individuals who answered the questionnaire, 5032 of them belonging to the SHP_I and 2414 to the SHP_II.

At the individual level we differentiate between the overall number of individual interviews and the fully longitudinal ones. The former include original sample members (OSM), that is individuals that were already present in the first wave, as well as their cohabitants, individuals who joined the household after the first wave and were thus not part of the sample as it was drawn. The fully longitudinal individual interviews refer to OSM who answered at each consecutive wave.

As can be seen in Table 1 the overall number of individual interviews in the SHP_I diminished until 2005. A number of changes[1] in the rules of follow-up in

---

[1] Since 2006, participants receive an unconditional incentive. If all household members participate, the household receives another, this time conditional, incentive. The incentives contribute to motivate the people to maintain cooperation throughout the duration of the panel. Together with the unconditional incentive, participants also receive some information about the survey in general and some results from the previous wave.

Table 1 Number of valid individual and household interviews in SHP_I and SHP_II for the years 1999–2012

Year	SHP_I			SHP_II		
	Individual interviews	Household interviews	Fully longitudinal individual interviews	Individual interviews	Household interviews	Fully longitudinal individual interviews
1999	7799	5074	7799			
2000	7073	4425	6335			
2001	6601	4139	5429			
2002	5700	3582	4480			
2003	5220	3227	3888			
2004	4413	2837	3076	3654	2538	3654
2005	3888	2457	2622	2649	1799	2395
2006	4091	2537	2399	2568	1684	1930
2007	4630	2817	2209	2350	1494	1601
2008	4494	2718	2060	2410	1546	1400
2009	4800	2930	1952	2309	1476	1289
2010	5057	2985	1876	2489	1557	1220
2011	5103	2977	1811	2481	1520	1155
2012	5032	2923	1739	2414	1467	1102

2006 and 2008 had a positive impact on the participation rate. Since 2006, the number of individual interviews has increased more or less steadily until 2011 and decreased slightly in 2012. On the other hand, the number of fully individual longitudinal interviews decreases steadily after the first wave. In 2012, 22 % of the OSM of the SHP_I had answered the individual questionnaire every year since 1999, compared with 30 % of the SHP_II.

The first part of the analysis, the comparison of means and frequencies (see Sect. 4) as well as the multivariate analysis of the characteristics of individuals in Sect. 5 is performed using only the data of the SHP_I. Furthermore, we only include the observations of OSM. Despite having an influence on the sample size, this restriction makes sure that we do not confound the effects of attrition with evolution, that is time and period effects, by allocating the same starting point to all the subjects included in the analysis.

4 Differences in Means and Frequencies due to Attrition

To analyse the effect of attrition we examine whether means and frequencies of a series of variables change if the sample composition changes due to dropout of panel members. One can assume that if attrition would be at random, means and distributions of variables would not change following attrition.

For each wave, we can define a new sample that is composed of individuals who participated both at the first wave and at the wave in question. Because of dropout this sample is smaller than the original one in the first wave. We then compare the answers given in the first wave using each of these samples on one side and the control sample, which is the sample of the longitudinal sample members of the first wave, on the other side. This means that we analyse the data of the first wave, but use different samples: the sample composed by all longitudinal sample members of the first wave on one hand and a subsample of longitudinal respondents in any later wave on the other hand. Differences in the statistics between these two samples indicate that dropout from the SHP is not random.

In order to identify the variables affected by attrition, we examine all variables that were included in the latest wave and in any of the previous waves. We consider attrition from the SHP_I.[2] We compare the means and frequencies calculated with the value of the first year of the variable ££ in (99, ...,12) on the sub-populations of longitudinal respondents still present in the latest wave as follows:

$$sL^{R££} = sL^{££}$$

$$sL^{R\$\$} = sL^{££} \cap sL^{\$\$}$$

$$\cdots$$

$$sL^{R12} = sL^{££} \cap sL^{12} \tag{1}$$

where $sL^{££}$ represent the longitudinal respondents (OSM) in 1999 and $sL^{\$\$}$ are the longitudinal respondents in year 20$\$\$$. Basically, we test to see if samples that still respond in a later year are representative of the same individuals that responded in the first year. The tests run through the SHP data of the wave 14 (year 2012).

The effect of attrition is analysed both on weighted and unweighted means and frequencies. The idea behind this approach is that the weight should correct for attrition e.g. that there should be no difference in means and frequencies when using different subsamples. The weights of the SHP represent a mixture of design weights and adjustment for nonresponse. The latter consists of several sociodemographic variables such as sex, age, civil status and nationality. As initial nonresponse to the first wave is also considered in the weighting scheme, the choice of the variables used for the adjustment to nonresponse is limited to information available in the sample frame.

As shown in Table 2, there are in total 1108 variables that appear in at least one wave of the SHP_I. Out of these, there are 306 variables that cannot be tested, either because they are proxy variables,[3] variables with the same response in all waves,

---

[2]The analysis is done for the first panel SHP_I that started in 1999. The analysis for the combined panel SHP_I and SHP_II was done in the same way and produced comparable results (not presented).

[3]Proxy-variables involve reports on other household members.

Table 2 Effect of attrition of means and frequencies for the SHP_I

Difference without weight	Difference with weight	Occurrences out of the 1108 variables (percent out of the 802 variables tested in parentheses)
–	–	306
No	No	644 (80.3 %)
No	Yes	9 (1.1 %)
Yes	No	85 (10.6 %)
Yes	Yes	64 (8 %)

variables with too few observations,[4] variables of which the modality is too high[5] or because it does not make sense to compare the variable.[6]

In the 14th wave of the SHP_I there are 644 variables out of the 802 tested variables that are not affected by attrition. This means that in 80.3 % of the variables there is no difference in means or frequencies when the sample of the first wave is compared to any subsequent longitudinal sample. The variables considered do not appear to be biased after attrition. The mean or the frequencies of 85 of the tested variables are different, but the difference disappears once the weights are used. These variables are therefore touched by attrition but the weighting corrects the phenomenon. In 64 cases we observe a difference without the weight and the difference persists even with weighting. The variable is therefore affected by attrition without the possibility of correction by weighting. With nine variables the estimates are biased only if the weights are applied. In these cases the weights clearly fail to correct for selective attrition.

The variables having been identified as being biased by attrition (in particular variables related to leisure and politics) need to be studied with care by the researchers who use them in their analyses. These results do not mean that these variables are unusable. However, they show that the phenomenon of attrition can certainly not be ignored. Most of the variables that are affected by attrition concern information on leisure activities, political and social participation, professional integration and health, which is in line with previous studies on attrition. One variable affected by attrition is, for example, political interest. Because politically uninterested individuals tend to drop out, the means of the political interest in the original sample SHP_I in 1999 and in a subsample consisting of individuals still present in 2004 or onwards differ even when using the weights that should correct for attrition. Other variables that have been affected by attrition are satisfaction with health, associational membership and working status.

---

[4] For categorical variables, at least one category needs to have 30 observations. Numeric variables are not tested if the total number of observations is less than 30.

[5] This is for categorical variables with more than 100 distinct responses, such as the isco job classification.

[6] This is the case for identification variables, dates or weights.

5 Participation Patterns and Sociodemographic Characteristics of Nonrespondents in the SHP

We now turn to the different causes for dropout and examine the characteristics of the individuals who participate in the SHP and those who drop out. We first give a short overview of the methods used to do this analysis (Sect. 5.1). We then describe the dropout rates according to the different reasons for nonresponse (Sect. 5.2). In Sect. 5.3 we describe the characteristics of the individuals for each participation pattern. The fifth part of this section is dedicated to the joint analysis of various characteristics in relation to dropping out of the SHP. We include the following characteristics: gender, age, education, working status, civil status, children in the household, Swiss nationality and legal status, income,[7] home ownership, political interest and satisfaction with health status. We analyse the effect of these variables on several causes of nonresponse.

5.1 Methodological Note

Participation in the SHP can be considered as exposure to the risk of dropping out. This risk arises each year when the interviewers call to realise an interview. Furthermore, there are different kinds of risks: people can drop out because they refuse to participate, because of missing contact information or because illness or frailty prevents them from answering to the questions. We differentiate seven causes for dropping out:

1. Not eligible
2. Left the household
3. Problems related to health and/or age
4. Family-related problems
5. Refusal
6. Non contact
7. Other reason

We grouped the individuals who are not eligible anymore because of death, emigration or institutionalisation into one group. The second group considers individuals who left the household either temporarily or permanently. There is no other information about the reason for nonresponse available for these panel members. A third group comprises the individuals who cannot participate due to health or age problems, whereas the fourth group includes individuals who state family-related problems such as the death of a family member or taking care of other household members as reasons for not participating. The fifth group contains

---

[7]To measure the effect of income we use the natural logarithm of the personal gross income.

the individuals who refuse to participate without any specific reason, either at the individual or the household level. Individuals who could not be contacted anymore due to missing contact information are included in the sixth group. The last group considers various causes for nonresponse with too few observations to be analysed separately, such as language problems or technical difficulties.

We provide a description of the variables of interest both separately for each participation pattern and by reporting the overall distribution. Continuous variables are presented as means and standard deviations (sd) if they are distributed normally, otherwise as medians and interquartile ranges (IQR). The corresponding statistical association with the participation pattern is evaluated using analysis of variance or the Kruskal-Wallis-test, respectively. Categorical variables are described by counts and percentages and are compared using the χ^2 test, Fisher's exact test or multinomial logistic regression where appropriate. All hypotheses are two sided and a p-value less than 0.05 is deemed statistically significant. We performed all the analyses using the statistical packages STATA version 13.1 and R version 3.1.0.

In our case, participation is equal to survival whereas the different reasons for nonresponse are treated as competing failures. In order to investigate the dropout patterns according to these different causes of failure, we use Kaplan-Meier estimates. The Kaplan-Meier procedure enables us to examine the distribution of the length of participation by estimating conditional probabilities for each cause of failure at each point in time (at each wave in our case) and by using these probabilities to estimate the corresponding survival rates (Kaplan and Meier 1958). Applying a survival model enables us to take into account that the probability of dropping out in any subsequent wave depends on the probability of having participated in all the previous waves. The probability of survival until the end of a specific interval (wave) corresponds to the product of the probabilities of not dropping out at one of the previous waves: the discrete time hazard function is the probability of an event occurring during interval t, conditional on the fact that the event did not occur before t (Mills 2011). We can therefore calculate a probability of not responding for each wave, given that there was no nonresponse up to this given wave.

In presence of competing events, the different dropout rates can also be understood as a cumulative incidence function. Cumulative incidence corresponds to the expected proportion of panel members experiencing a specific event in the presence of other risks (Beyersmann and Schumacher 2008; Gooley et al. 1999). Let us suppose that we observe an event of interest such as family-related problems which lead to nonresponse. This event has competing risks, events whose occurrence preclude or alter its own probability to happen.

As we interview the individuals once a year, there is only once in a year the possibility to participate or to nonrespond. We therefore have a limited number of occurrences and the duration data is intrinsically discrete. Because of the nature of this underlying transition process, we use a discrete time model and control for the intra-individual clustering of the data. As we are not only interested in general nonresponse, but also in the reasons leading to dropout, we will apply a competing risk discrete time model. Competing risk models make it possible to distinguish between different kinds of events and are thus applied in situations with more than one cause of failure (Allison 1982; Prentice et al. 1978; Putter et al. 2007). This is especially useful if there is reason to believe that the effect of the explanatory variables differs among the various types of competing failures.

A major aspect in favour of applying survival analysis to model attrition is that discrete time models make it possible to include time-varying covariates in the analysis. Applying a standard method could introduce bias and lead to a loss of information (Allison 1982). If we would use fixed values or a standard method, it would be difficult to decide which value to consider. Should we consider the last available value? This would mean that we would compare values of different years. Should we rather consider the value of the variable when the spell started, that is at the first wave of participation? This would mean that we do not take into account the evolution, like changing education, age or marital status, and thus ignore much information. By applying a survival model, we can overcome this problem, as we use for each transition the information of the previous wave, that is the most current information available independent of the participation status.

It should be noted that in all our analyses we only consider participation until the first dropout and ignore therefore the influence of the changes in the follow-up rules mentioned in Sect. 3. Those respondents who drop out temporarily and come back at a later wave are disregarded in this analysis after the first time they fail to respond. Because of these restrictions the analysis tends to overestimate attrition, as it cannot distinguish between permanent attrition or temporary nonresponse.

5.2   Dropout Patterns According to Causes for Nonresponse

If we consider the overall survival curve, we can see in Fig. 1 that the participation rate diminishes over the analysis period. The survival curve portrays that the dropout or first nonresponse rate is highest after the first wave of participation. The survival curve becomes flatter as the duration of the panel increases. This is illustrated by the fact that the vertical distance at each time point, that is the change in cumulative probability, becomes lower as the analysis time increases.

If we turn to the different reasons for dropping out, we can observe in Fig. 2 that the survival rates differ slightly according to the reasons for nonresponse. A vertical gap between two curves indicates that one group has a greater proportion of panel members surviving. The lower curves illustrate that the dropout rate among those participants is higher.

We can see in Fig. 2 that the dropout rate due to ineligibility was highest for this group at the start of the analysis period, but became the lowest compared to the other failure causes as time passes. The survival rate of the participants who state that the reason for their nonresponse are health problems is, compared to the other causes, mostly higher. We can also observe that non contact becomes a less important reason for dropping out: while its curve was steeper during the first five transitions, it became flatter afterwards. This change might be explained by analysis

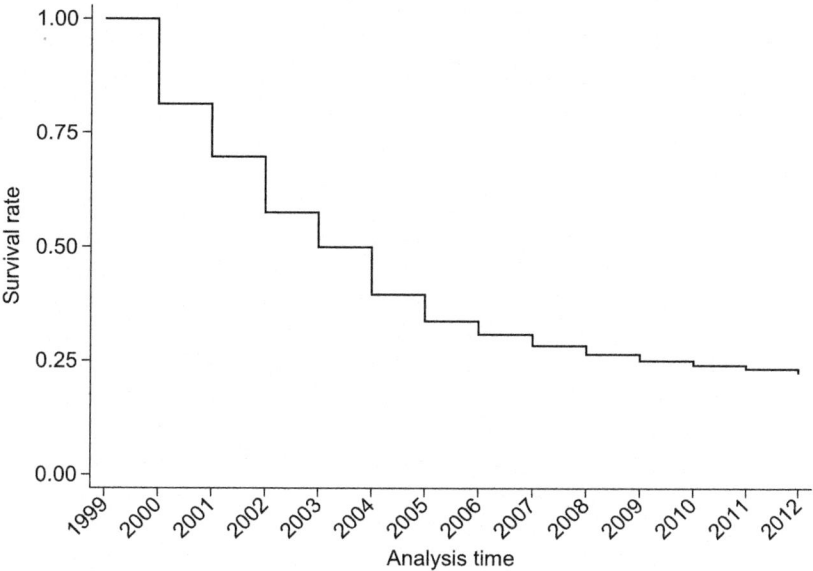

Fig. 1 Overall Kaplan-Meier survival estimates

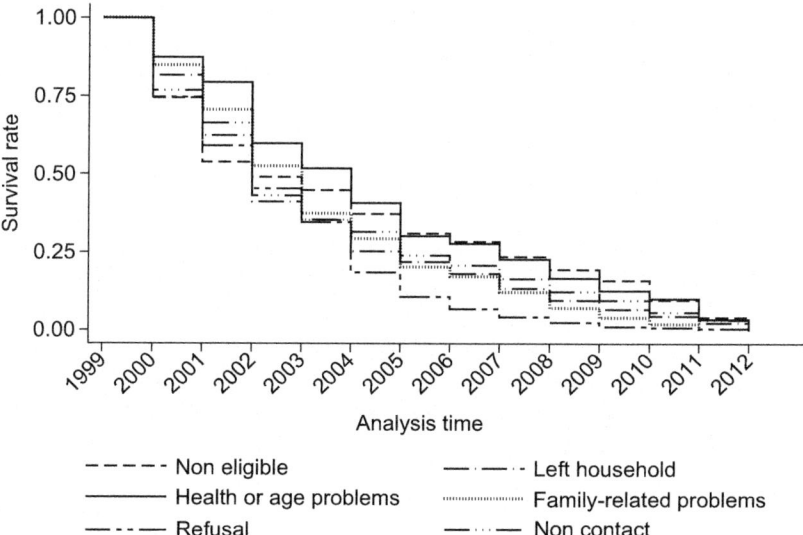

Fig. 2 Kaplan-Meier survival estimates according to failure cause

time: hard to reach individuals tend to drop out early. Once the panel members have participated during a few consecutive waves, their nonresponse is not because of a missing contact but rather because of other reasons like health problems, refusal or family-related difficulties. At the same time we can also suppose that it became easier to trace individuals due to the internet. Another explanation for the lower dropout rates due to missing contact information is that the interviewers put more effort in finding panel members after the change of the follow-up rules in 2006 and 2008 mentioned in Sect. 3. Figure 2 also suggests that refusal conversion and the use of unconditional incentives, two other measures enhanced in 2006 to counter attrition, had a positive impact on the participation rate, as the failure rate due to this cause becomes less important after 2006.

The cumulative incidence plot (Fig. 3) illustrates the dropout rates according to the different events. As in Fig. 2, we can see that refusal at individual or household level was the most cited reason for nonresponse, followed by non contact. It is also visible that both curves become flatter as time of analysis increases, which is partly due to a general lower dropout rate, but also due to competing risks that become more important such as health or age problems.

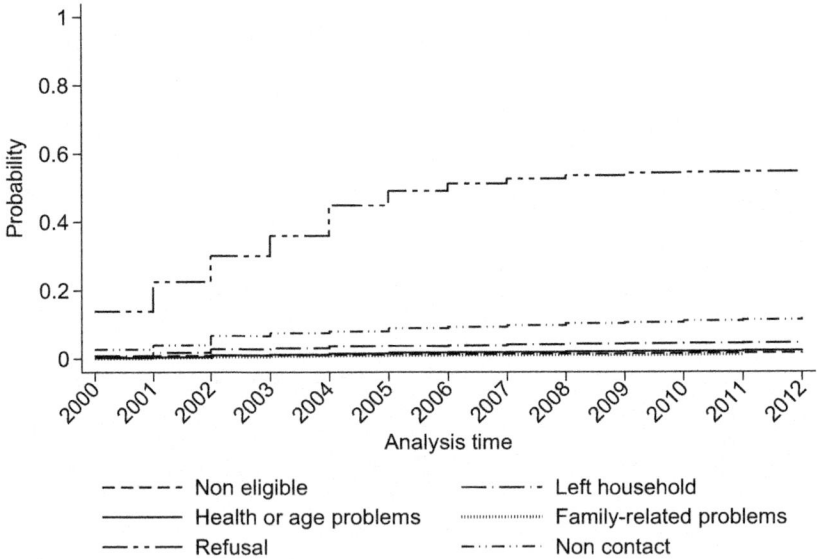

Fig. 3 Cumulative incidence of the different reasons for attrition

5.3 Description of the Characteristics of Nonrespondents Within the SHP

Before we turn to the competing risk model, we first provide a description of the variables of interest in relation to the different participation patterns. In total, we use the data of 7788 individuals. More than half of the panel members (55 %) refused at least once to participate during the observed period. The mean duration of participation among the nonrespondents varies from 2.7 ± 1.9 years for the individuals who dropped out because of different reasons than the ones specified here to 5.4 ± 3.5 years for the panel members who stopped participating because of health- or age-related problems.

Table 3 contains several variables related to vulnerability: level of education, income, working status, legal status and satisfaction with health. In addition to these variables we also included some general demographic variables (gender, age, civil status, children in the household, home ownership) and political interest as it is known to be a determinant of attrition and nonresponse (Groves et al. 2000, 2004). Moreover, political interest can be seen as a measure of social involvement, which in turn can be related to vulnerability. The association between the participation pattern and the variables in Table 3 is statistically significant in all cases, which is a first indication that causes of nonresponse differ according to both demographic characteristics and those related to vulnerability.

The overall participation rate is higher among women than men. However, nearly 70 % of the participants who state having family-related difficulties that prevent them from participating are women. The proportion of women is also higher among the participants having health problems or who do not participate anymore due to their age. The median age of the respondents is 57 (IQR $= 48 - 68$), whereas it is 25 (IQR $= 21 - 39$) among the individuals who left the household temporarily or permanently. This distribution is not surprising, as young adults tend to have a high geographic mobility due to educational reasons or in order to establish their own household. We can also see that the median age is highest among the group with health- or age-related problems (75, IQR $= 65 - 82$), followed by the ineligible sample members (62, IQR $= 41 - 77$). This last group includes deceased persons.

The groups also differ according to the education of their members. The lowest proportion of individuals having completed the obligatory school without any further education can be found among the individuals who have never dropped out until 2012 (11.7 %). At the same time the participants that are still involved have the highest proportion (37 %) of individuals with a tertiary education. The lowest proportion (16 %) of group members with a tertiary education can be found among the individuals who dropped out because of health and age problems. This group also has the largest share of individuals with a low level of education (35 %).

The median income, as measured by the personal gross income, is highest among the individuals who never dropped out (64,550; IQR $= 32,600 - 100,800$) and lowest among the individuals having health- or age-related problems that prevent them from participating (30,000; IQR $= 19,900 - 59,200$). The median income

Table 3 Description of the characteristics according to each participation pattern

Variable	Participation	Ineligible	Left household	Health- or age-related problems	Family-related problems	Refusal	Non contact	Other
Pattern: n (%)	1739 (22.3)	145 (1.9)	377 (4.8)	199 (2.6)	99 (1.3)	4283 (55.0)	918 (11.8)	28 (0.4)
Duration (years): mean (sd)	14.0 (0.0)	4.9 (4.0)	4.2 (3.2)	5.4 (3.5)	4.4 (2.9)	3.6 (2.4)	4.4 (3.5)	2.7 (1.9)
Men: n (%)	694 (39.9)	80 (55.2)	193 (51.2)	77 (38.7)	30 (30.3)	1887 (44.1)	433 (47.2)	15 (53.6)
Age (years): median (IQR)	57 (48–68)	62 (41–77)	25 (21–39)	75 (65–82)	46 (35–57)	45 (33–57)	38 (30–50)	26 (20–53)
Education: n (%)								
Primary level	204 (11.7)	36 (24.8)	83 (22.0)	69 (34.7)	16 (16.2)	1033 (24.1)	162 (17.7)	7 (25.00)
Secondary level	884 (50.8)	70 (48.3)	210 (55.7)	98 (49.3)	64 (64.7)	2331 (54.4)	507 (55.2)	16 (57.1)
Tertiary level	651 (37.4)	39 (26.9)	84 (22.3)	32 (16.1)	19 (19.2)	919 (21.5)	249 (27.1)	5 (17.9)
Income (thousands): median (IQR)	65 (33–101)	42 (20–70)	39 (14–63)	30 (20–59)	35 (18–64)	48 (19–79)	56 (31–80)	47 (24–75)
Home ownership: n (%)	1078 (62.0)	80 (55.2)	196 (52.3)	94 (47.2)	47 (47.5)	2234 (52.3)	251 (27.4)	10 (35.7)
Working status: n (%)								
Active occupied	1089 (62.6)	62 (42.8)	286 (75.9)	33 (16.6)	68 (68.7)	2892 (67.5)	698 (76.0)	23 (82.1)
Unemployed	12 (0.7)	2 (1.4)	10 (2.7)	2 (1.0)	2 (2.0)	67 (1.6)	29 (3.2)	0 (0.0)
Not in labour force	638 (36.7)	81 (55.9)	81 (21.5)	164 (82.4)	29 (29.3)	1324 (30.9)	191 (20.8)	5 (17.9)
Legal status/nationality: n (%)								
Swiss	1481 (85.2)	119 (82.1)	292 (78.3)	178 (89.5)	86 (86.9)	3387 (79.8)	661 (73.6)	19 (70.4)
Naturalised	186 (10.7)	8 (5.5)	41 (11.0)	14 (7.0)	8 (8.1)	363 (8.6)	100 (11.1)	4 (14.8)
Permit C	72 (4.1)	16 (11.0)	32 (8.6)	6 (3.0)	3 (3.0)	413 (9.7)	107 (11.9)	4 (14.8)
Permit B or other	0 (0.0)	2 (1.4)	8 (2.1)	1 (0.5)	2 (2.0)	79 (1.9)	30 (3.3)	0 (0.0)
Civil status: n (%)								
Single	206 (11.9)	32 (22.1)	253 (67.1)	21 (10.6)	16 (16.2)	1105 (25.8)	364 (39.7)	17 (60.7)
Married	1178 (67.7)	83 (57.2)	103 (27.3)	96 (48.2)	66 (66.7)	2629 (61.4)	348 (37.9)	9 (32.1)
Not married anymore	355 (20.4)	30 (20.7)	21 (5.6)	82 (41.2)	17 (17.2)	549 (12.8)	206 (22.4)	2 (7.1)
With children	689 (39.6)	35 (24.1)	268 (71.3)	24 (12.1)	53 (54.1)	2390 (55.8)	398 (43.5)	17 (60.7)
Political interest: mean (sd)	6.3 (2.5)	5.4 (2.9)	5.3 (2.8)	5.5 (2.8)	4.7 (2.9)	5.1 (2.9)	5.1 (2.9)	4.6 (3.6)
Satisfaction with health: mean (sd)	7.7 (1.6)	6.4 (2.7)	8.1 (1.6)	7.0 (2.2)	8.1 (1.6)	8.0 (1.8)	7.8 (2.0)	8.4 (2.0)

of the individuals who could not be contacted anymore was also relatively high (56,090; IQR = 31,380 − 80,340). Nearly three quarters of the individuals who could not be contacted anymore (73 %) lived in a rented home, whereas over 60 % of the individuals who never stopped participating live in a house or in a flat they own. This is an indicator that home ownership has a positive impact on the possibility to contact individuals, as they seem to be less mobile geographically, and thus, on the participation rate.

Most of the individuals who refused to participate without indicating any specific reason (68 %), who refused to participate because of family-related problems (69 %) or who could not be contacted anymore (76 %) were active in the labour market. Four out of five individuals who refused to answer because of health- or age-related problems were not in the labour force (anymore) whereas only one fifth of the individuals who could not be contacted anymore or who left the household temporarily or permanently were either unemployed or actively occupied.

The largest share (89 %) of Swiss without a second nationality can be found among the individuals having health- or age-related problems preventing them from participating at the survey, where as the lowest proportion is among the panel members who could not be contacted anymore. This group also contains the biggest proportion of individuals who became naturalised (11 %) and those who have a residence permit C (12 %).[8]

The civil status is another characteristic that differs among the participation patterns. Sixty-seven percent of the individuals who left the household that was selected for the SHP_I are single, whereas only 27 % among them are married. The lowest proportion of singles can be found among the individuals who do not participate anymore due to old age- or health-related problems (11 %). They also have the biggest proportion of individuals who are not married anymore (41 %), that is who are either divorced, separated or widowed. The group containing the individuals who never stopped participating has the largest share of married people (68 %) and nearly 40 % of them have at least one child living in the same household. Most of the individuals who left the household temporarily or permanently (71 %) lived in a household with at least one child before they moved out. It is very probable that the individuals of this group of nonrespondents are one of these children. Over half of the individuals who do not participate anymore because of family-related difficulties or who refused to participate without any specific reason live together with one or more child.

The findings suggest that the effect of the number of children in a household is not as straightforward as one might think. On one side, having children might be associated with being at home and therefore being accessible to answer to the questionnaire. On the other side, having children can prevent participation because of a tighter schedule or worries related to the children.

---

[8]Residence permit C is a long-term permit, whereas residence permit B is a short-term permit. This second category also includes other arrangements (for example asylum seekers or people with no permit).

On a scale between 0 and 10, the sample members who still participate have the highest political interest (6.3 ± 2.5) whereas those having family-related problems have the lowest (4.7 ± 2.9). Also on a scale going from 0 to 10, satisfaction with health was highest among individuals who had left the household (8.1 ± 1.6), while it was lowest for panel members who were no longer eligible (6.4 ± 2.7) and individuals who stated age- or health-related problems (7 ± 2.2).

5.4 Analysis of the Characteristics of Nonrespondents Within the SHP

As introduced in Sect. 2 and demonstrated in the previous parts, attrition is in general not random in longitudinal surveys. People with certain characteristics tend to drop out more often. Beside describing the participation rate of individuals according to unique variables, we can analyse the attrition using different characteristics at the same time. We do this using the same variables as in Table 3. Applying the discrete time competing risk model described in Sect. 5.1, we can see in Table 4[9] that panel attrition diminished with duration even when controlling for the other factors. Compared to individuals who drop out after the first wave, the probability of dropping out becomes lower with each transition (from one wave to the next).

If we turn to the individual characteristics, we can see that in general men drop out more often than women. The relative risk of dropping out because of ineligibility relative to non-stop participation increases by 2.50 (95 % CI: 1.45–4.31) for men compared to women. The relative risk of men having health-related problems preventing participation (1.61; 95 % CI: 1.04–2.50) or refusing to participate (1.13; 95 % CI: 1.03–1.24) is also higher compared to women.

The effect of age in all groups is not linear. We can see that age has the shape of an inverted "U", that is that the participation rate is higher as the age of an individual increases, but diminishes after a specific age. Correspondingly, getting older first has a negative impact on the probability of being among the nonrespondents, but later, when the maximum is reached, has a positive impact on the probability of dropping out. For the group of individuals who had left the household, this change in effect happened shortly after turning 55.[10] Until the age of 55, each additional year lowers

---

[9]Only results that are significant at least at the 5 %-level and where the variable has strictly positive counts are displayed in Table 4.

[10]This example illustrates the inter-operation of the influence of age for the group who left the household:

$$y = \beta_0 + \beta_1 * x + \beta_2 * x^2$$

$$\frac{\partial y}{\partial x} = \beta_1 + \beta_2 * 2 * x = 0$$

$$x = -\beta_1/(2 * \beta_2) = 0.2669914/(2 * 0.0023951) = 55.287874$$

Table 4 Competing risk discrete time model for various causes of dropout from the SHP

Variable	Non eligible	Left household	Health- or age- related problems	Family- related problems	Refusal	Non contact	Other
Duration of participation	0.92*		0.91**	0.90**	0.83**	0.97*	0.70**
	(0.03)		(0.02)	(0.03)	(0.01)	(0.01)	(0.07)
Men (ref: women)	2.50*		1.61***		1.13***		
	(0.69)		(0.36)		(0.06)		
Age (centralised)	0.89*	0.77**			0.97*	0.92**	0.81***
	(0.04)	(0.02)			(0.01)	(0.02)	(0.07)
Age squared (centralised)	1.00**	1.00**	1.00**		1.00*	1.00***	1.00***
	(0.00)	(0.00)	(0.00)		(0.00)	(0.00)	(0.00)
Education (ref: primary school)							
Secondary level		1.53***					
		(0.32)					
Tertiary level			0.51***		0.76**		
			(0.17)		(0.06)		
Income (ln)		1.30*		0.72*		1.16***	
		(0.11)		(0.09)		(0.07)	
Home owner-ship (ref: tenant)					1.11***	0.53**	
					(0.05)	(0.06)	
Working status (ref: active occupied)							
Unemployed					1.54***		
					(0.29)		
Not in labour force			1.82***				
			(0.55)				
Legal status/nationality (ref: Swiss (only))							
Swiss and other					1.24*	1.36***	
					(0.10)	(0.20)	
Permit C					1.31**	1.54*	
					(0.10)	(0.23)	
Permit B or other					1.75*	2.36*	
					(0.32)	(0.68)	
Civil status (ref: single)							
Married		0.43**		3.08***	0.85***	0.63**	
		(0.09)		(1.40)	(0.06)	(0.08)	
Not married anymore		0.21**			0.78*	1.55*	
		(0.08)			(0.07)	(0.22)	
Children (ref: none)		1.87*			1.23**		
		(0.38)			(0.07)		
Political interest			0.91*	0.90***	0.95**	0.96***	
			(0.03)	(0.05)	(0.01)	(0.02)	
Satisfaction with health	0.66**		0.84**			0.92**	
	(0.04)		(0.04)			(0.02)	

$n = 7027$; * $p < 0.01$; ** $p < 0.001$; *** $p < 0.05$

the relative risk of dropping out because of leaving the household temporarily or permanently. Afterwards, getting older has a positive effect on the relative risk of dropping out because of having left the household. For the individuals who drop out because of ineligibility, the maximum of the negative age effect is reached at 38. After 38, each additional year increases the relative risk to becoming ineligible compared to the non-stop participants. For the group who refused to participate, the maximum is reached at 44, for the individuals who dropped out because of other reasons at 50 and for those who could not be contacted anymore at age 78.

The participation rate is also influenced by education. Depending on the cause of nonresponse, the influence is positive or negative. On one side, a higher educational level has a positive impact on the probability of leaving the household (1.53; 95 % CI: 1.02–2.30). On the other side, compared to individuals whose highest education is primary school, tertiary education is associated with a lower relative risk to drop out due to age- or health-related problems (0.51; 95 % CI: 0.27–0.99) or refusal (0.76; 95 % CI: 0.66–0.89).

If we consider the effect of a higher income, we can also observe different patterns according to the failure cause. The relative risk for individuals who dropped out because of family-related problems relative to the constant participants decreases by 0.70 (95 % CI: 0.57–0.91) for each unit change of income.[11] In this case, a higher income has a negative effect on the probability of dropping out. On the other hand, a higher income increases the probability of leaving the household temporarily or permanently (1.30; 95 % CI: 1.11–1.53) or of having missing contact information (1.16; 95 % CI: 1.03–1.32).

One aspect that is linked to income is home ownership. Besides acting as an indicator for income and wealth, home ownership also influences geographical mobility, in the sense that these individuals move less and can thus be contacted more easily. This is visible in our data: the relative risk for individuals who cannot be contacted anymore relative to the constant participants is lowered by home ownership (0.53; 95 % CI: 0.43–0.65). However, compared to tenants, individuals who own a house or a flat tend to refuse more often without specifying the reason (1.11; 95 % CI: 1.01–1.22).

Working status is another aspect that influences participation in the SHP positively, in the sense that unemployment affects the probability of refusing to participate without specific reason or for not responding for another reason. Compared to individuals who are employed, individuals who are unemployed have a lower participation rate (1.50; 95 % CI: 1.07–2.24). Compared to the individuals who are active on the labour market, not being in the labour force increases the relative risk of being in the group having health- or age-related problems relative to the participants (1.82; 95 % CI: 1.01–3.31).

---

[11]Because income is not distributed normally, we use the natural logarithm of it in this analysis.

The legal status or nationality is another characteristic of nonrespondents. Individuals who received the Swiss nationality or have for some other reason two nationalities tend to drop out more often due to refusal (1.24; 95 % CI: 1.06–1.44) or non contact (1.35; 95 % CI: 1.01–1.82) than those having only the Swiss nationality or who have it since birth. In general, a long- or short-term permit leads to higher dropout rates. Furthermore, the relative risk to drop out is higher for those having a short-term permit than for individuals with a long-term permit.

Another characteristic related to dropout is marital status. Compared to individuals that have never been married, the dropout rate of married individuals or of those that are no longer married (widowed, divorced or separated) is in general lower, except for the individuals who drop out because of family-related problems. Here, being married increases the relative risk for this group relative to the respondents by the factor 3.10 (95 % CI: 1.27–7.48) compared to the singles. Being no longer married also increases the relative risk of being among the individuals who cannot be contacted anymore (1.55; 95 % CI: 1.18–2.05). Living in a household with children influences the dropout rate positively when the reason for not responding is moving out of the household (1.87; 95 % CI: 1.25–2.79) or refusing without any specific reason (1.23; 95 % CI: 1.10–1.38).

Political interest, which is associated with social integration, is another aspect that influences loyalty to the survey. On a scale going from zero (not interested at all) to ten (very interested), each additional point leads to a lower dropout rate, except when nonresponse is due to ineligibility or because of moving out, where it has no statistically significant influence. Politically interested individuals seem to be more motivated to participate in the survey. The same applies to health satisfaction. On a scale going from zero (very unsatisfied) to ten (very satisfied), each additional point diminishes the probability of dropping out of the panel due to ineligibility (0.66; 95 % CI: 0.59–0.74), age- or health-related problems (0.84; 95 % CI: 0.77–0.91) and missing contact information (0.92; 95 % CI: 0.87–0.96). Individuals who are satisfied with their health status tend to participate more often in the survey.

6 Conclusion

We have shown that attrition in the Swiss Household Panel is not completely at random, but that individuals with certain characteristics tend to drop out more often, as is usually the case in panel surveys (Groves 2006; Watson and Wooden 2009). Many of these characteristics can be associated with the concept of "vulnerability". Individuals with a migration background, who are unemployed, who are socially less integrated or whose health status is poor drop out more frequently. Moreover, a lower income is also associated with higher dropout rates when the reason for not responding is family-related problems and a higher educational level tends to have a positive impact on participation, except if the reason for dropping out is leaving the household. This means that in general population surveys such as the SHP vulnerable groups tend to be underrepresented. Whereas a survey such as the SHP allows for a comparison of vulnerable groups with other groups in society, researchers should be aware that such datasets underestimate the degree of vulnerability in the general population. Weights allow to adjust to a certain extent for unit nonresponse, but, as has been shown in Sect. 4, for a number of variables, the correction is not sufficient.

Furthermore, one has to be cautious with the results related to the bias in estimates resulting from dropout, as the variables are compared from their first year of appearance and not imperatively in the first year of interviewing the sample. So it is possible that there is left handed bias already introduced in the sample when the question is asked the first time, in the sense that the estimates are already biased due to selective attrition. That is to say that a selective attrition may have occurred before the variable was introduced. This is undetectable by this method. These calculations are done on the entire sample of longitudinal respondents. There are no comparisons on the sub-populations (by sex, age class, nationality, etc.). Such comparisons could reveal differences which are not observed at the aggregated level. The inverse is also possible.

A difficulty related to the analysis of attrition is that the underlying patterns are complex. Our results contribute to the existing studies on attrition by specifically analysing different causes for nonresponse. This has revealed that the relationship between variables and dropout is often complex. For example, married individuals are less likely to drop out than other groups, except when family-related issues prevent their continued participation. Similarly for home ownership, compared to tenants home owners are less likely to drop out because they cannot be contacted, but they are more likely to refuse participation. When introducing group-specific measures to counter attrition one should, therefore, bear in mind that a single intervention might have an impact on a specific reason for nonresponse, but might not affect all the causes.

Another difficulty related to this kind of attrition analysis is that the imminent factors leading to irregular participation or complete dropout might often be unob-served, because there is no data for the wave in question: because individuals drop out, we don't know their most current situation, but only the one from the previous year, when they last answered the questionnaire. If someone gets ill between two waves and cannot participate anymore because of this illness, it is not possible to consider this in the statistical model, because the last available observations of this individual would not reflect the illness. In our data, this individual might still state that the satisfaction with health is high, because the data refer to the situation in the previous year. Therefore it is likely that we tend to underestimate the influence of the explanatory variables. Although efforts are made to collect information about why a household or an individual does not want to participate anymore, the data is incomplete and cannot, therefore, be incorporated into the model. Also related to the variables that were used here is that when doing this kind of analysis, we suppose that attrition is based on variables that can be observed in the dataset. However, attrition is also likely to be partly due to variables that are not included in the questionnaire. If this is the case, models estimating the factors influencing attrition fall short. Moreover, the available weights, whose construction is based on the variables available in the dataset, would run the risk of not fully correcting the bias introduced by attrition. Although this can be a problem, our analysis has shown that for over 90 % of the variables estimates are unbiased or the bias is corrected by applying the weights.

References

Alderman, H., Behrman, J., Watkins, S., Kohler, H.-P., & Maluccio, J. A. (2001). Attrition in longitudinal household survey data. *Demographic Research, 5*, 79–124.

Allison, P. D. (1982). Discrete-time methods for the analysis of event histories. *Sociological Methodology, 13*, 61–98.

Beyersmann, J., & Schumacher, M. (2008). Time-dependent covariates in the proportional subdistribution hazards model for competing risks. *Biostatistics, 9*(4), 765–776.

Dillman, D. A., Eltinge, J. L., Groves, R. M., & Little, R. J. (2002). Survey nonresponse in design, data collection, and analysis. In R. M. Groves, D. A. Dillman, J. L. Eltinge, & R. J. Little (Eds.), *Survey nonresponse*. New York: Wiley.

Gallie, D., & Paugam, S. (2004). Unemployment, poverty and social isolation: An assessment of the current state of social exclusion theory. In D. Gallie (Ed.), *Resisting marginalization: Unemployment experience and social policy in the European Union*. Oxford, UK: Oxford University Press.

Gooley, T. A., Leisenring, W., Crowley, J., & Storer, B. E. (1999). Estimation of failure probabilities in the presence of competing risks. *Statistics in Medicine, 18*(6), 695–706.

Groves, R. M. (2006). Nonresponse rates and nonresponse bias in household surveys. *Public Opinion Quarterly, 70*(5), 646–675.

Groves, R. M., Singer, E., & Corning, A. (2000). Leverage-saliency theory of survey participation: Description and illustration. *Public Opinion Quarterly, 64*(3), 299–308.

Groves, R. M., Presser, S., & Dipko, S. (2004). The role of topic interest in survey participation decisions. *Public Opinion Quarterly, 68*(1), 2–31.

Johnson, T. P., O'Rourke, D., Burris, J., & Owens, L. (2002). Culture and survey nonresponse. In R. M. Groves, D. A. Dillman, J. L. Eltinge, & R. J. Little (Eds.), *Survey nonresponse*. New York: Wiley.

Kaplan, E. L., & Meier, P. (1958). Nonparametric estimation from incomplete observations. *Journal of the American Statistical Association, 53*(282), 457–481.

Kleiner, B., Lipps, O., & Ferrez, E. (2012). Satisficing and language proficiency. *FORS working paper series* (Paper 2012-1). Lausanne: FORS.

Lipps, O. (2007). Attrition in the Swiss Household Panel. *Methoden – Daten – Analysen, 1*(1), 45–68.

Loosveldt, G. (1997). Interaction characteristics of the difficult-to-interview respondent. *International Journal of Public Opinion Research, 9*(4), 386–394.

Loosveldt, G., & Carton, A. (2001). An empirical test of a limited model for panel refusals. *International Journal of Public Opinion Research, 13*(2), 173–185.

Mills, M. (2011). *Introducing survival and event history analysis.* London: SAGE Publications Ltd.

Prentice, R. L., Kalbfleisch, J. D., Peterson, A. V., Jr., Flournoy, N., Farewell, V. T., & Breslow, N. E. (1978). The analysis of failure times in the presence of competing risks. *Biometrics, 34*(4), 541–554.

Putter, H., Fiocco, M., & Geskus, R. B. (2007). Tutorial in biostatistics: Competing risks and multi-state models. *Statistics in Medicine, 26*(11), 2389–2430.

Stoop, I. A. L. (2005). *The hunt for the last respondent: Nonresponse in sample surveys.* The Hague: SCP.

Voorpostel, M. (2010). Attrition in the Swiss Household Panel by demographic characteristics and levels of social involvement. *Swiss Journal of Sociology, 36*(2), 359–377.

Watson, N., & Wooden, M. (2009). Identifying factors affecting longitudinal survey response. In P. Lynn (Ed.), *Methodology of longitudinal surveys* (pp. 157–182). London: Wiley.

CPSIA information can be obtained
at www.ICGtesting.com
Printed in the USA
LVOW04*1623030516
486513LV00008B/54/P